Twinning and Twins

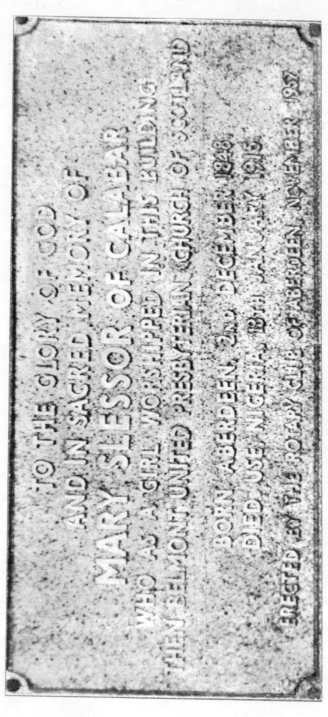

TO THE GLORY OF GOD
AND IN SACRED MEMORY OF
MARY SLESSOR OF CALABAR
WHO AS A GIRL WORSHIPPED IN THIS BUILDING
THEN BELMONT UNITED PRESBYTERIAN CHURCH OF SCOTLAND

BORN ABERDEEN 2ND DECEMBER 1848
DIED USE NIGERIA 13TH JANUARY 1915

ERECTED BY THE ROTARY CLUB OF ABERDEEN NOVEMBER 1957

An early Aberdeen contributor to the care of twins.

Twinning and Twins

Edited by

Ian MacGillivray and Doris M. Campbell
*Department of Obstetrics and Gynaecology**

and

Barbara Thompson
*MRC Medical Sociology Unit**

**University of Aberdeen, Aberdeen, UK*

A Wiley Medical Publication

JOHN WILEY & SONS
Chichester · New York · Brisbane · Toronto · Singapore

RG 567

Library of Congress Cataloging-in-Publication Data:

Twinning and twins/edited by Ian MacGillivray, Doris M. Campbell, and
   Barbara Thompson.
      p.   cm.—(A Wiley medical publication)
   ISBN 0 471 92033 9
   1. Pregnancy, Multiple.   2. Birth, Multiple.   3. Twins,
I. MacGillivray, Ian.   II. Campbell, Doris M.   III. Thompson, Barbara.
IV. Series.
RG567.T85 1988
618.2′5—dc19   88-14385
                                                         CIP

British Library Cataloguing in Publication Data:

Twinning and twins.
   1. Newborn babies., Twins. Medical aspects
I. MacGillivray, Ian   II. Campbell, Doris M.   III. Thompson, Barbara.
618.92′01
ISBN 0 471 92033 9

Typeset by Acorn Bookwork, Salisbury, Wiltshire
Printed in Great Britain by
St Edmundsbury Press Ltd, Bury St Edmunds, Suffolk

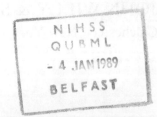

Contents

List of Contributors

ELIZABETH M. BRYAN, MD, MRCP, DCH
Honorary Consultant Paediatrician, Queen Charlotte's Maternity and Hammersmith Hospitals, London, UK; Consultant to the Twins and Multiple Births Associaton.

JOHN BURN, B. Med Sci, MBBS, MRCP
Consultant Clinical Geneticist, Royal Victoria Hospital, Newcastle-upon-Tyne, UK.

DORIS M. CAMPBELL, MD, MRCOG
Senior Lecturer, Obstetrics and Gynaecology and Reproductive Physiology, University of Aberdeen, Aberdeen, UK.

GERALD CORNEY, MD, DRCOG, DCH
Medical Geneticist, Medical Research Council Human Biochemical Genetics Unit, The Galton Laboratory, University College, London, UK.

CYNTHIA FRASER, MA, DIP Ed
Psychologist, Medical Research Council Medical Sociology Unit, University of Aberdeen, Aberdeen, UK.

JULIAN LITTLE, PhD, MA
Lecturer, Department of Community Medicine and Epidemiology, University of Nottingham, Nottingham, UK.

IAN MACGILLIVRAY, MD, FRCP, FRCOG
Emeritus Professor, Department of Obstetrics and Gynaecology, University of Aberdeen, Aberdeen, UK.

PERCY P. S. NYLANDER, MD, FRCP (Ed) FRCOG,
Professor of Obstetrics and Gynaecology, University College Hospital, Ibadan, Nigeria.

MIKE SAMPHIER, BSc (Soc.),
Sociologist, Medical Research Council Medical Sociology Unit, University of Glasgow, Glasgow, UK.

BARBARA THOMPSON, OBE, PhD, BA
Social Scientist, Medical Research Council Medical Sociology Unit, Honorary Research Fellow, Department of Obstetrics and Gynaecology, University of Aberdeen, Aberdeen, UK.

Acknowledgements

Many people have contributed in many different ways to this book and we are grateful to them all, but especially to our obstetric colleagues and those who have given specific help.

John Burn and Gerald Corney wish to thank Mrs Linda Burn and Mrs Debbie Seedburgh for assistance with data and the preparation of Chapter 2.

Julian Little wishes to thank Mrs Anne Davies-Mulloy and Mrs Janet Mawby for help with the Library Search and Mrs Sheila Kelsey for secretarial assistance. He also acknowledges access to data and help received from Dr S. K. Cole (Scottish Home and Health Department); Dr R. C. Graham (Tayside Health Board); Professor R. C. Nevin (Queens University, Belfast); Dr J. G. Paterson (Grampian Health Board) and Dr A. L. Walby (Department of Health and Social Security, Northern Ireland) as well as Dr W. H. James (London) for helpful comment and advice.

Julian Little and Elizabeth M. Bryan are grateful for help and comments received from Professor R. Derom (Akademisch Ziekenhuis, Ghent); Professor J. M. Elwood (University of Nottingham); Professor C. Rodeck (Queen Charlotte's Maternity Hospital, London); Dr K. Shiota (Kyoto University) and Dr M. Snow (MRC Mammalian Development Unit).

Cynthia Fraser acknowledges the preliminary work on 'The Reading Survey' twin data undertaken by Dr Fiona Wilson.

We are grateful to Mr John Lemon (Computing Centre, Aberdeen University) for some analyses of data and to Mrs Irene Morrison who through many vicissitudes has so cheerfully borne the brunt of the typing and secretarial responsibilities.

Above all we are indebted to the mothers of twins and to twins themselves for their co-operation and collaboration without which this book would not have been produced.

Ian MacGillivray
Doris M. Campbell
Barbara Thompson

Twinning and Twins
Edited by I. MacGillivray, D. M. Campbell and B. Thompson
© 1988 John Wiley & Sons Ltd

Chapter 1

Introduction

IAN MACGILLIVRAY

*Department of Obstetrics and Gynaecology, University of Aberdeen,
Aberdeen, UK*

Twins have figured prominently in history and mythology from ancient times, possibly because of their rarity. Rome is said to have been founded by Romulus and Remus, the twins who were suckled by a she-wolf, after the cradle in which they had been condemned to be drowned became stranded. Castor and Pollux became famous in Greek mythology as guardians of the wind and the waves and are immortalised in the heavenly constellation, Gemini. Twins have often figured in literature and Shakespeare, who was himself the father of twins, developed the theme of twins in 'Twelfth Night' and 'The Comedy of Errors'.

Many customs and beliefs grew up around twins throughout the world. In some places twin births were abhorred while in others they were welcomed. In some communities both twins would be killed, while in others only one of the twins would be killed, or alternatively adopted by another family. In some societies twins were thought to result from the mother having had intercourse with a god or another man as well as her husband, and many cruel customs developed because such behaviour was likened to that of the lower animals who were multiple-bearing.

It is curious that in one area of Nigeria both the mother and her twins might be killed, whereas in another area close by, the twins might be greatly revered (Corney, 1975a). For example, in the small area west of Lagos, the Popo people welcomed twins, but in the rest of Yorubaland there was a marked aversion to them. Elsewhere in Africa, as recently as 1910, Matabele parents were tried for ritual twin murders, and about ten years later Basuto parents were also tried for the same crime (Harris, 1922). Abhorrence of twins has been reported from Japan, from Australia, and from the Pacific Islands, and also amongst eskimos (Corney, 1975a).

In Europe similar beliefs and customs were found. In mediaeval Europe the mother was thought to have been unfaithful to her husband because twins implied two fathers (Giles, 1908). In Wales twins were associated with good luck and fertile influences. In contrast, in both England and Scotland it was believed that infertility would follow a twin birth and that twins themselves would be childless. A twin birth was said to be ensured by drinking a tumblerful of water from the well of St Mungo in Scotland. However, this was overcome by Scots women who took only half a glass of water from the well (Corney, 1975a)!

This book was initiated from Aberdeen, Scotland, where interest in twin births was recorded over a century ago. James Matthews Duncan, a graduate of Aberdeen University, wrote in 1865 'The rarity of plural births in women and increased danger to mother and offspring in these circumstances renders such an event in a certain limited sense a disease or abnormality' (Duncan, 1865).

At about the same time Mary Mitchell Slessor, who had been born in 1848 in a suburb of Aberdeen, was a weaver in the textile mills in Dundee to where her family had moved in 1859. At the age of 11 Mary went to work for half the day in the mills; for the other half of the day she went to school. She was a very devout Christian and became a Sunday School teacher. She was able to obtain books from the library of the Sunday School and she laid a book on the loom and glanced at it in her free moments (Livingstone, 1918). Early in 1874 with the news of the death of Dr David Livingstone, Mary, who had become very interested in foreign missions, was stimulated to action. Her mother had wished her son, John, to become a missionary, but his health had failed and he died. Mary decided to take his place in the mission field, and so she sailed on August 5th, 1876 to Calabar on the west coast of Africa, to become a missionary of the Scottish Missionary Society. At that time large areas of what is now Nigeria had not been explored by the white man. Against tremendous odds, Mary Slessor established her mission and refuge for orphans and abandoned children. Many of the children were twins who had been abandoned because of the taboos which existed at that time in West Africa. Mary Slessor's work amongst the children, particularly twins, gained international recognition.

The chances of survival of twins were known to be much less than those of singletons, and the woman with a twin pregnancy was also known to be at greater risk. The risks to the babies were not only of death, but of handicap. At that time provisions for medical care during pregnancy, particularly in places like Africa, were very poor. Indeed, it was not until the beginning of this century that antenatal care was introduced. A pioneer of antenatal care was Dr Ballantyne of Edinburgh, and one of the things which he suggested would be beneficial for fetal growth was rest for the pregnant woman (Ballantyne, 1902). This is a subject which is still hotly debated. However, the avoidance of strenuous manual work, particularly in the later months, would seem to be desirable for any pregnant woman.

It was in association with rest that the next recorded interest in twin pregnancies in Aberdeen was made. Russell (1952), under the influence of

Dugald Baird, then Regius Professor of Midwifery and Gynaecology in the University of Aberdeen, showed that women with twin pregnancies being delivered in a private nursing home and, therefore, presumably of the more affluent upper social classes, did better than women who were delivered in hospital. The perinatal mortality rate was halved and the average twin birthweight was 5 lb 8 oz. in the private patients compared with 4 lb 13 oz. in the hospital delivered women. He suggested that these differences might be due to the upper social class privately delivered women having more rest and 'a better' diet in pregnancy. He, therefore, recommended that women with twin pregnancies should be admitted to hospital at 30 weeks gestation, so that they could have 'a better diet' and more rest. Although no clinical trial was carried out to support this recommendation, it became common practice in Great Britain to admit all women with multiple pregnancies into hospital for rest.

It was clear, however, from the pioneer work of Dugald Baird on the social aspects of obstetrics that there were many factors other than rest and diet which could account for the differences in the reproductive performance of upper and lower social class women, and that the outcomes of their pregnancies were to a large extent determined prior to the conception. In a later study in Aberdeen, Anderson (1956) looked in detail at stillbirths and neonatal mortality in twin pregnancies and concluded that there was no social class difference. This finding is somewhat surprising in view of the differences in the outcome of singleton pregnancies between the social classes, but may be accounted for by twin pregnancies being less likely to occur in thin and small women (Anderson, 1956; Campbell *et al.*, 1974). Such women are likely to be of lower social class.

The great stimulus to twin research in Aberdeen was due to Percy Nylander from Nigeria who came as a medical student to Aberdeen University. After graduation in 1958 he stayed on to undertake specialist training in obstetrics and gynaecology. He was responsible for initiating the liaison with Dr Gerald Corney of The Galton Laboratory, University College, London, and arranging for the determination of zygosity from cord blood samples and placental specimens. This arrangement was continued after Percy Nylander left Aberdeen until 1985 when it was arranged that blood specimens would be sent to the local blood transfusion service for the necessary typing to give an accurate determination of zygosity. On his return to Ibadan, Nigeria where he later became Professor and Head of Department of Obstetrics and Gynaecology, Nylander established twin pregnancy research in Nigeria while continuing his association with the Aberdeen work.

An increasing worldwide interest in twinning and twins was manifest in the formation of the International Society for Twin Studies in 1975. A subsection which meets regularly at a Workshop on Multiple Pregnancies is particularly flourishing. The controversies raised at these meetings highlight the complexities of the subject—particularly where apparently contradictory results are presented. Some of the problems raised are about the fall in twinning rates in many parts of the world, differential changes in monozygotic and dizygotic (or like and unlike sex), twinning and the possible influence of contraception and of abortion policy and practices. On the other hand is the new phenomenon of multiple births associated with treatment for infertility including in vitro fertilisation. The representativeness of samples, method of zygosity determination, differences in classifications and analytical method are always issues. Lively debates about the management and outcome of twin pregnancies can be guaranteed.

The present book aims to review the current state of knowledge, including the physiology, obstetric implications, management and outcome of twin pregnancies, augmented by new or updated analyses of data from Aberdeen population-based studies.

Aberdeen Populations

The populations referred to in several chapters of this book are as follows.

Twins

1. All twin maternities to women resident in Aberdeen City District for the years 1951 to 1983 inclusive.
2. All twin maternities to women resident in Aberdeen City District for the years 1969 to 1983 and for whom zygosity of the twins was determined in collaboration with The Galton Laboratory, University College, London.
3. All twin maternities for north-east Scotland (Grampian Region) for 1969 to 1983 for whom zygosity was determined as for 2. This population is labelled the 'Galton Series'.

Singletons

Data on singleton pregnancies for comparison with 1 and 2 above have been extracted for the appropriate years from the Aberdeen Maternity and Neonatal Data Bank (Samphier and Thompson, 1981). This Data Bank, started in 1949, contains details of all obstetric and fertility related gynaecological events to women resident in Aberdeen City District; it is now computerised and continuously updated.

All data presented refer to total populations from geographically defined areas. This is particularly important for epidemiological purposes as hospital-based data are usually biased.

Many studies have been carried out in Aberdeen relating to twin pregnancies, particularly with respect to the epidemiology, and to the physical responses and complications of twin pregnancies. Although there is a very considerable interest in comparative studies using twins as models, apart from the comparison of the reproductive performance of twin sisters (see Chapter 13) this has not been an aspect of the work in Aberdeen.

It has been possible to determine the physiological responses to twin pregnancies in considerable detail, partly because of the tremendous co-operation and willingness of mothers expecting twins to participate in research studies. With the co-operation of all the obstetricians it has been the practice in Aberdeen in recent years for all the women with multiple pregnancies to attend a research antenatal clinic. Thus, it has been possible to make many observations on the women as outpatients and also to recruit them for studies involving stays in the metabolic unit, particularly for assessment of nutritional needs.

All of the twin babies were seen by a neonatologist shortly after birth, and if they were of low birthweight or had any major abnormality or problem they were followed up for at least a year. No complete follow-up study, however, was made comparing the development of the twins with singletons for the total population, but for a subgroup of twins, subsequent physical and mental development was assessed (see Chapter 12).

In this review of the literature and presentation of new data, the various authors have identified some of the pitfalls to be avoided in interpreting findings on twinning, clarified some issues and answered certain questions, although in some cases confirmation from other studies may be desirable. However, many problems remain unanswered and further research is indicated which has important implications for the understanding of twinning as well as for clinical practice. Such research is increasingly being facilitated by the development of new scientific techniques, e.g. for zygotic or genetic determination and by advancements in computing.

Twinning and Twins
Edited by I. MacGillivray, D. M. Campbell and B. Thompson
© 1988 John Wiley & Sons Ltd

CHAPTER 2

Zygosity determination and the types of twinning

JOHN BURN
Royal Victoria Hospital, Newcastle-upon-Tyne, UK
and
GERALD CORNEY
Medical Research Council Human Biochemical Genetics Unit, The Galton Laboratory, University College, London, UK

The determination of whether twins are dizygotic or monozygotic is often regarded as a complex problem requiring extensive and expensive laboratory facilities. In fact, the differentiation can be simple and the complexity applies, particularly in the newborn, only to a minority of pairs.

With the very rare exception of twins discordant for sex chromosome anomalies—heterokaryotypic twins—(Dallapiccola *et al.*, 1985) all pairs discordant for sex are dizygotic. One-third of all twin pairs in populations of Western European origin are of unlike sex (Corney *et al.*, 1983; Nylander, 1970d) and thus can definitely be said to have originated from the fertilisation of separate ova.

In the same populations, about one-fifth of all twin pairs share a single placenta, i.e. are monochorionic (Corney, 1975b). With one convincing documented exception (Bieber *et al.*, 1981), all monochorionic twin pairs can be regarded as monozygotic (Corney and Robson, 1975). Dichorionicity is not helpful in assessing zygosity.

Thus, if placentation is identified reliably, the zygosity of half of all twin pairs can be determined at birth from these simple observations. In later childhood physical appearance can be used. While monozygotic twins are never completely identical in appearance, they can be sufficiently alike to be indistinguishable to all but their close relatives. Twin pairs found to be 'as alike as two peas in a pod' can be regarded as almost certain to be derived from a single zygote. Similarly, twins found to differ in eye and hair colour may be regarded as dizygotic.

This combination of sex, placentation and physical similarity can assign zygosity with reasonable accuracy to most twin pairs. Whether resort to the laboratory investigation of blood groups and other polymorphisms is made will depend on circumstance. For very large twin populations, testing of blood samples is likely to be both impractical and uneconomic. In such circumstances, questionnaires may be used. Alternatively, for pairs suspected of being monozygotic (MZ), but discordant for some anomaly, or in the case of a pair of twins between which organ transplantation is contemplated for example, as much precision as possible is desirable and as many methods as are conveniently available will then be used.

If such twins are found to differ in one or more genetically determined markers such as blood groups, then in the absence of a recent transfusion, the twins may be taken to be dizygotic (DZ). If, however, they are alike in sex and all markers tested then their probability of dizygosity needs to be calculated.

Sex

Twins of unlike sex are, for practical purposes, dizygotic. The proportion of pairs of unlike sex will vary between different countries and racial groups as the proportion of DZ pairs is not the same all over the world (Bulmer, 1970; Nylander, 1983). In Europe and North America the proportion of unlike-sex pairs amongst white populations is about 30% but in Japan it is only about 18% (Imaizumi and Inouye, 1979). In south-western Nigeria, Nylander found 46% of twins to be dizygotic, though a recent study (Marinho et al., 1986) has revealed a marked decline in DZ twinning in this population, perhaps related to dietary changes.

Before laboratory methods became available and when the relationship between zygosity and placentation was not clear, sex was the only available information for determination of zygosity. Assuming that the sex of each zygote would be determined independently, the French mathematician Bertillon (1874) reasoned that the number of DZ pairs would equal twice the number of pairs of unlike sex. The remainder of pairs in a sample would presumably be MZ. Some thirty years later Weinberg (1902) re-stated this idea and the calculation has come to be known as Weinberg's method. The small excess of males at birth is not usually thought to affect the validity of this theory (Bulmer, 1970). This method has stood the test of time and is still in use. It should, however, only be used for relatively large groups. It is not suitable for small samples of twins or those in which the proportions of like- and unlike-sexed pairs might deviate from those expected for that population. For example, among deliveries in a referral maternity hospital there may be selection in favour of pairs of like sex (Nylander, 1975b; 1983).

Comparison between the results from the Weinberg method and those obtained by laboratory testing for determination of zygosity has revealed an interesting discrepancy and James (1979) has suggested that this might indicate a flaw in Weinberg's method. He studied data from various twin surveys in which blood typing was carried out on *all* pairs, i.e. both of like and unlike sex. By excluding sex as a marker he was, therefore, able to obtain samples of DZ pairs ascertained by blood typing only. He found that there was a significant excess of DZ pairs of like sex, i.e. in these samples there were not, as is assumed in Weinberg's method, equal numbers of DZ pairs of like and unlike sex. James postulates that this could be accounted for by the fact that the sex of the zygote might be determined by the timing of conception in relation to the menstrual cycle. This topic will be discussed further later in this chapter.

Placentation

There are two types of twin placentation according to the number of chorionic membranes, *dichorionic* or *monochorionic*.

It was originally supposed that dichorionic placentation (two placentae be they separate or partially or closely fused) meant that the twins had arisen from two zygotes. Conversely it was thought that monochorionic placentation was consistent with monozygosity. With very rare exceptions the latter statement has subsequently been shown to be correct, but the belief that dichorionic placentation means dizygosity has been known to be untrue for most of this century. Even so the belief still holds in some quarters and many twin pairs think that they are DZ because the mother was told at their delivery that there were two placentae (Lykken, 1978; King *et al.*, 1980). The inaccuracy of placental observation as a sole indicator of zygosity was demonstrated by the discrepancy between the proportions of DZ and MZ twins shown by this method and by the twin pair sex-distribution calculation described above. There was found to be a smaller proportion of MZ pairs from placental observation. The reason for this discrepancy suggested by Danforth (1916), was that some dichorionic pairs must be MZ. This hypothesis was later confirmed by twin studies using physical similarity as a method of zygosity determination. Waardenburg (1926) published a detailed account of his own twin daughters (Figure 2.1) who were 'identical' but had separate placentae. Further confirmation has come from newborn twin studies which have compared the type of placentation with the results of testing the many blood types which have subsequently become available (Corney and Robson, 1975). Some of these are summarised in Table 2.1. It seems that some 3–18% of dichorionic twin pairs have similar blood types and thus are likely to be MZ (Tables 2.2 and 2.3).

The same prospective studies of newborn twins, their placentation and blood types, have also shown that monochorionic pairs were consistently alike in sex and all blood markers tested (Tables 2.1 and 2.3) and thus are highly likely to be MZ. Reports to the contrary over the years in the literature

Table 2.1. Placentation and zygosity of twin pairs in various populations. Note: the figures from some surveys have been adjusted. Reproduced by permission of W. B. Saunders & Company Ltd from Corney (1975b). For details see Corney (1975b)

Country	Reference	Ethnic group	Dichorionic		Monochorionic		Total
			MZ	DZ	MZ	DZ	
England	Edwards, Cameron and Wingham (1967)[a]	Caucasian	47	429	116	0	592
	Corney, Robson and Strong (1972)[b]	Caucasian	28	377	123	0	528
USA	Potter (1963)[a]	Caucasian	38	188	67	0	293
	Fujikura and Froehlich (1971)[b] {	Caucasian	16	124	55	0	195
		Negro	26	124	54	0	204
Nigeria	Nylander and Corney (1977)[c] {	Hausa	4	51	7	0	62
		Others	8	56	12	0	76
		Yoruba (northern Nigeria)	0	63	3	0	66
	Nylander (1970c)[c]	Yoruba (Ibadan)	45	1316	75	0	1436

[a] Corrected for inefficiency of markers from original data according to method explained in Corney (1975b).
[b] Markers sufficiently efficient to require no further correction.
[c] Corrected for inefficiency of markers in the original papers.

Table 2.2. Dichorionic placentation and zygosity in various populations. Note: the figures from some surveys have been adjusted. Reproduced by permission of W. B. Saunders and Company Ltd from Corney (1975b). For details see Corney (1975b)

Country	Reference	Ethnic group	Total no. of pairs	Percentage of MZ twins who are dichorionic	Percentage of dichorionic twins who are MZ
England	Edwards, Cameron and Wingham (1967)[a]	Caucasian	592	28.8	9.9
	Corney, Robson and Strong (1972)[b]	Caucasian	528	18.5	6.9
USA	Potter (1963)[a]	Caucasian	293	36.2	16.8
	Fujikura and Froehlich (1971)[b] {	Caucasian	195	22.5	11.4
		Negro	204	32.5	17.3
Nigeria	Nylander (1970c)[c]	Yoruba	1436	37.5	3.3

[a,b,c] See footnotes to Table 2.1.

Table 2.3. Results for sex, placentation and zygosity from the Aberdeen survey of twins delivered during the period 1968–1982. Criteria for monozygosity were either monochorionic placentation or probability of dizygosity of 0.02 or less

			Twin pairs
Sex		Unlike	230 (28.3%)
		Like	582
Placentation		Dichorionic	578 (80.4%)
		Monochorionic	141
Zygosity		DZ	452 (64.9%)
		MZ	244
Zygosity and Placentation	DZ	⎰ dichorionic	415
		⎱ monochorionic	0
	MZ	⎰ dichorionic	94 (40.0%)
		⎱ monochorionic	141

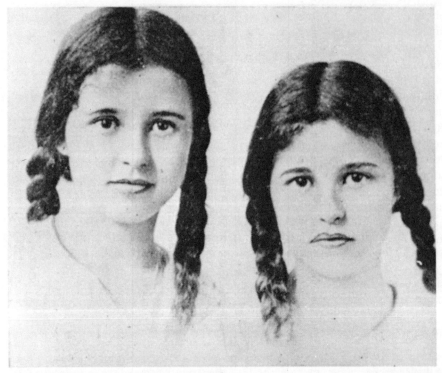

Figure 2.1. The twin daughters of the geneticist and ophthalmologist Waardenburg, pictured at 11 years in the 1920s. They were monozygotic on physical traits, but had separate placentae. From Gedda, L. *Twins in History and Science* (1961) Courtesy of Charles C. Thomas, Publishers, Springfield, Illinois.

probably represent inaccurate observation of the placental membranes. An illustration of this is the case reported from Nigeria in which twins of unlike sex were initially thought to have a monochorionic placenta, but closer examination (including histology) showed that this was a dichorionic placenta from which the intervening membranes had disappeared; the twins were subsequently found to be chimeras (Nylander and Osunkoya, 1970; Corney, 1975b; Tippett, 1983). A rare exception to the rule that monochorionic placentation invariably indicates monozygosity has been reported (Bieber *et al.*, 1981). In this case the placentation was monochorionic but the twins were of unlike sex—XY and XXX (acardiac). Further studies showed that although they were monovular they were not MZ as two spermatozoa had been involved in the conception. It was concluded that this was a case of polar body twinning.

With this unique exception, present evidence indicates that if the placentation is *reliably* identified at delivery, it can be assumed that twins with monochorionic placentation are MZ. In fact this represents the strongest item of evidence for monozygosity available. Conversely, with pairs of dichorionic twins of like sex, very little information with regard to zygosity can be obtained from the placentation. In European populations the DZ : MZ ratio among like-sexed dichorionic twins is 3 : 1.

About 20% of twin pairs have monochorionic placentation in Europe and North America (Table 2.4). As already stated, in these countries about 30% of all pairs are of unlike sex and thus blood studies will be needed to differentiate the remaining 50%. This, of course, assumes reliable identification of the type of placentation. Unfortunately despite a 'plea to the obstetrician' by Benirschke (1961a) placental information in maternity hospital notes is often not adequate for zygosity determination. The method in use in Aberdeen—a simple sketch diagram in the delivery notes, has much to commend it and this can, of course, be supplemented by a short verbal description. This method is probably preferable to histological examination; the pathologist can only report on material sent to the laboratory and this may have been incorrectly taken. Determination of the composition of the dividing membranes is best accomplished by preparing a full thickness jelly-roll-like tissue sample for histological section (Johnson and Driscoll, 1986). During the Aberdeen twin survey samples were routinely taken for histological examination for a period. However, when the histological reports were compared with information from observation of the placental membranes and blood typing there were various discrepancies. The histological method was therefore abandoned.

One approach to the confirmation of monochorionicity is the injection of a contrast liquid into a clamped cord to determine whether this crosses to the other cord. In the delivery suite milk is a suitable choice (Strong and Corney, 1967) though it is important to avoid excessive pressure and to remember that without preparation, with dextran for example, small vessels may become

Table 2.4. Placentation of twin pairs in various populations (Adapted from Corney, 1975b)

Country and reference	Ethnic group	Dichorionic	Monochorionic		Total
			Diamniotic	Monoamniotic	
Japan					
Yoshida and Soma (1984)	Japanese	68 (38.2%)	103 (57.9%)	7 (3.9%)	178
England					
Cameron (1968)[a]	Caucasian	534 (79.9%)	134 (20.1%)		668
Corney, Robson and Strong (1972)	Caucasian	405 (76.7%)	115 (21.8%)	8 (1.5%)	528
USA					
Benirschke (1961a)	Caucasian	173 (69.2%)	74 (29.6%)	3 (1.2%)	250
Potter (1963)	Caucasian	431 (78.6%)	116 (21.2%)	1 (0.2%)	548
Fujikura and Froehlich (1971)	Caucasian	169 (75.6%)	52 (23.2%)	3 (1.3%)	224
	Negro	177 (76.6%)	47 (20.4%)	7 (3.0%)	231
Nigeria					
	Hausa	130 (87.8%)	18 (12.2%)	0	148
	Others (northern Nigeria)	140 (87.5%)	20 (12.5%)	0	160
Nylander and Corney (1977)	Yoruba (northern Nigeria)	146 (93.6%)	10 (6.4%)	0	156
Nylander (1970c)	Yoruba (Ibadan)	1361 (94.8%)	73 (5.1%)	2 (0.1%)	1436

[a]Figures estimated from percentage data in original publication.

occluded (Robertson and Neer, 1983). This latter paper investigated 139 fused placentae of which 124 gave satisfactory results. In the monochorionic group 55 of the 56 showed positive transplacental circulation whereas 67 of 68 dichorionic placentae did not. The one dichorionic case which did have a vascular communication illustrates the rare but recognised possibility of error in assigning zygosity using this approach (Cameron, 1968).

Twin Transfusion Syndrome

An imbalance in blood flow between the twins can produce the enigmatic disorder known as the twin transfusion syndrome. This condition is of interest in zygosity determination since its presence can be taken as proof of mono-zygosity while, paradoxically, its effect is to produce sometimes a quite striking dissimilarity of the 'identical' twin pair.

The clinical presentation of a polycythaemic–anaemic twin pair was first described by Herlitz in 1941, and has been recorded frequently since (for reviews see Benirschke and Driscoll, 1967; Strong and Corney, 1967; MacGil-livray et al., 1975; Tan et al., 1979; Bryan, 1983). The placentation of such pairs is usually monochorionic and the assumption is that there has been an imbalance in the flow of blood through the various vascular communications which are known to occur almost invariably in this form of twin placentation. The presence of such anastomoses has been known for many centuries and the classic morbid anatomical work of Schatz and others on such placentae about a hundred years ago has yet to be surpassed (Strong and Corney, 1967). The *pathophysiology* of the fetofetal transfusion syndrome is not understood, despite the numerous theories in the literature, though there is some compa-rative supporting evidence now available (Dudley and D'Alton, 1986).

When it has been possible to examine the placenta of such a clinically diagnosed twin pair, placental vascular anastomoses have usually been seen and sometimes shown, by various means, to be patent. It seems not unreason-able to assume, therefore, that there is an association between the apparent haematological differences between the twin babies and their conjoined placental circulations. However there is substantial variability within such a conjoined (or 'third' as it has sometimes been called) circulation. This includes variation in quality (artery–artery, vein–vein and artery–vein or vein–artery) and in quantity, including the dimensions and patency of the vessels (Arts and Lohman, 1971). To say the least, therefore, the problem is a very complicated one and almost certainly will not have a single solution. Quite reasonably, the anastomotic culprits are thought to be the artery–vein channels, but detailed supporting evidence for this assumption is awaited and the other communications may have some role to play in the severity, or in the appearance or absence, of the clinical syndrome in monochorionic pairs.

There is considerable variation in severity; the striking appearance of red and white twin babies represents only the tip of a harlequin iceberg. If haemoglobin estimations are carried out on a series of twins at birth, it can be seen that there is a subclinical discrepancy between the haematological results of many pairs. To determine an estimate of prevalence, diagnostic criteria are, of course, required. Rausen *et al.* (1965) suggested that these might include a haemoglobin difference between the twins of 5 g/100 ml as they had not found a difference greater than this amongst dichorionic pairs. Using this and a variety of other criteria, they suggested that up to 15% of monochorionic pairs might have the syndrome. More recent studies have found the incidence to be of a similar order (Dudley and D'Alton, 1986).

There must also be additional variables. In some cases, in the so-called 'chronic' form, there is evidence, including, for example, birthweight differences between the twins, that the interfetal transfusion must have been in progress for some months and pathological findings indicating this have been demonstrated in the twins and in their placenta (Naeye, 1965; Aherne *et al.*, 1968; Klebe and Ingomar, 1972; Tan *et al.*, 1979), the latter sometimes having a striking appearance on the maternal surface. These observations about the relatively long duration of intrauterine shunt of blood if such be the case have more recently been supported by ultrasound findings during pregnancy, showing for example, polyhydramnios and oligohydramnios and discrepancy in fetal size (Wittmann *et al.*, 1981; Brennan *et al.*, 1982; Schneider *et al.*, 1985). The use of Doppler ultrasound and the consequent study of umbilical artery wave-forms is another method of intrauterine diagnosis of this syndrome (Giles *et al.*, 1985). A full assessment of the significance of the findings using this technique has yet, however, to be made (D'Alton and Dudley, 1986).

The so-called 'acute' cases which display no evidence of long-term effects, are presumably associated with events during labour and delivery, but might also, for example, be due to fetomaternal haemorrhage (Strong and Corney, 1967; Bryan, 1983).

The syndrome has been reported, though rarely, in dichorionic pairs (Corney, 1975b). It is known that, as in twins with blood group chimerism (Gilgenkrantz *et al.*, 1981; Tippett, 1983), such pairs uncommonly have placental vascular communications (Robertson and Neer, 1983).

In the extreme form the clinical effects can be serious and the anaemic–polycythaemic twins might both need treatment (Galea *et al.*, 1982; Bryan, 1983). The disorder can be lethal to one or both twins and indeed any assessment of the frequency of the condition should allow for those pairs who die in utero. One twin might survive, but it is clear that this infant is also subsequently at risk, and should be kept under observation (Szymonowicz *et al.*, 1986; Dudley and D'Alton, 1986; Johnson and Driscoll, 1986).

It is not clear why this dramatic intrauterine event should happen only to some twin pairs; many variables are presumed to be involved (Benirschke,

1984). Some believe, with little supporting evidence, that the superficial artery–artery and vein–vein anastomoses compensate for exchanges in the deep arteriovenous channels and that the syndrome presents when the superficial anastomoses are small or few in number. Kloosterman (1963) suggested that some of these anastomotic vessels are too small to allow for a substantial exchange of blood during the pregnancy and that intrapair differences in plasma proteins might play a part in causation. Surprisingly little attention has been paid to biochemical (as opposed to haematological) parameters. This aspect merits further study as many of the features, particularly birthweight and individual organ size, suggest intrauterine malnutrition, though why this should be is not at all clear. Studies of IgG (Bryan and Slavin, 1974; Bryan, 1976; Bryan et al., 1976; Bryan, 1977) suggest that there might be some defect of maternofetal transfer in the placenta of the donor, which is interesting as morbid anatomical placental studies have shown that there are, in some cases, chorionic changes which might be expected to affect transfer of substances from the mother to that fetus (Aherne et al., 1968).

Erythroblastosis was mentioned in Herlitz's original report (1941). Many of the features of the syndrome are similar to those found in haemolytic disease of the newborn due to blood group incompatibility, though such has never been demonstrated in any reported pairs. Why should there be this erythroblastotic response and why, for example, should nucleated red cells be found mainly in the placental territory of the donor twin (Corney and Aherne, 1965; Aherne et al., 1968)?

Twenty years ago the alternative name for this phenomenon was 'parabiotic syndrome' (Naeye, 1963; Rosenquist, 1963) because of the analogy with a similar syndrome in experimental rats. The salient features of 'runt disease' found in rats due to an immunological response are, however, not found in human twins (Naeye, 1963). One possibility is that, if the elusive 'third type' of twins with monochorionic placentation (Bieber et al., 1981) are commoner than has been supposed and are capable of sustained normal development, then one could have genetically non-identical twins with placental anastomoses. In theory an immunological response could then produce some of the features of the syndrome. In practice lack of immune competence, particularly in early pregnancy, makes such an effect unlikely. The pioneering work of Naeye (1963, 1965) in this area deserves to be pursued (Johnson and Driscoll, 1986).

Comparison of Blood Group and Serum Polymorphisms

The identification of many blood group, serum protein and enzyme polymorphisms, particularly in the past thirty years, has provided a more precise objective test for zygosity determination. A polymorphism is a common population variant. If, for example, the father of twins has the ABO blood group AB and the mother is group O their offspring may be group A or group

B. If the twins are monozygotic they will both be either A or B whereas dizygotic twins could differ. To be precise, there would be a half chance of DZ twins being different for this blood group system. On the other hand, there would be a half chance of DZ twins being the same. If the twins are alike in a whole range of polymorphic markers the probability that they are dizygotic (pDZ) becomes very small. How small depends on whether the parents have been tested to discover the number of informative systems. If both parents have the Duffy type aa then all offspring will be the same regardless of twin zygosity so the Duffy group provides no information.

If the parental genotypes are *not* known, the likelihood of DZ twins being different depends on the population gene frequency. If, for example, a hypothetical locus has two alleles Q and q in the population, individuals can be QQ, Qq or qq. If the gene frequency of q is only 1/100, however, the great majority of the population will be QQ, to be precise $99/100 \times 99/100$ or $9880/10\,000$, so most parents are QQ. If the twins are QQ the marker is not particularly informative. If, on the other hand, both twins are qq the marker is informative. Since qq individuals are rare $(1/10\,000)$ the parents of these twins are both likely to be Qq. If both parents are Qq there is a 1 in 4 chance of having produced a qq zygote which went on to form monozygotic twins and $\frac{1}{4} \times \frac{1}{4}$ or $\frac{1}{16}$ chance of two such zygotes to form dizygotic twins. Therefore for this marker the ratio of probability MZ : DZ would be 4 : 1. To be accurate the calculation should be worked out using different parental genotypes and the relative probabilities combined in proportion to the incidence of the different mating types in the population. One or both of the parents could be qq which would reduce the value of the system as a discriminant, but only if such parents are relatively common in the population.

If the parental types are known much of the complexity is avoided, but not all. This is because some systems have silent alleles, in particular the ABO and P blood groups (not fully expressed in the newborn). In the first example above the parents are AB × OO. However, if the parents are both group A1 a calculation is necessary if both twins are also group A1, because the parents may be A10, A1A2 or A1A1, all of which give a group A1 phenotype. Whenever a parent is group A or group B a calculation is necessary to take account of the possible genotypes in the population. Even for those acquainted with such calculations, the process is tedious. Fortunately, tables are available which provide relative probabilities for the blood group and other systems in common use (Race and Sanger, 1975; Corney and Robson, 1975). The methods used to combine information from the study of different markers make use of Bayesian calculation (based on Bayes' theorem). These calculations, presented in tabular form seem incomprehensible to the casual observer, yet the principle is not complex. For example, using two of the above markers, an Aberdonian twin pair present who are both female, both

Table 2.5a. A simplified calculation of the probability of dizygosity using 'standard' format for Bayesian analysis

	MZ	DZ
Prior probability	$0.35 = \frac{7}{20}$	$0.65 = \frac{13}{20}$
Conditional probabilities		
Like sex	1	$\frac{1}{2}$
Parents AB × 0, twins both B	$\frac{1}{2}$	$\frac{1}{4}$
Parents Qq, twins qq	$\frac{1}{4}$	$\frac{1}{16}$
Joint probability	$\frac{1}{8} \times \frac{7}{20}$	$\frac{1}{128} \times \frac{13}{20}$

i.e. ratio of probabilities MZ : DZ is $\frac{1}{8} \times \frac{7}{20} : \frac{1}{128} \times \frac{13}{20}$

Simplify by multiplying both sides by 128 and by 20

Ratio becomes   112 : 13

and the probability of dizygosity is $\frac{13}{125}$ or 10.4%

Table 2.5b. The same calculation reconstructed to allow the relative probability of dizygosity to be expressed for each variable. Most published tabulations use this format

	MZ	DZ
Prior	1	$\frac{0.65}{0.35} = \frac{13}{7}$
Like sex	1	$\frac{1}{2}$
Blood group B	1	$\frac{1}{2}$
Type qq	1	$\frac{1}{4}$
Joint	1	$\frac{1}{16} \times \frac{13}{7}$
Probability DZ =	$\dfrac{\frac{13}{112}}{1 + \frac{13}{112}}$	
=	$\dfrac{13}{112 + 13}$	
=	10.4%	

ABO type B and are qq at our hypothetical locus. The prior probability of them being MZ is 0.35 (35%) and DZ 0.65. We know the father is ABO type AB and mother is O, and the q allele is rare so we assume both parents are Qq. We now have three pieces of information which tip the balance in favour of the twins being MZ. To combine these 'conditional' probabilities with the prior probability requires six questions; if the twins are MZ, what is the

chance of being the same sex?—100% or a probability of 1. If the twins are
DZ the chance of being like sex is 0.5. The same approach is taken with the
two markers; if the twins are MZ, the chance of these parents having type B
children is 0.5 and if they are DZ the chance is 0.25. The chance of qq twins is
a quarter for the MZ side and a sixteenth for the DZ option, i.e. each Qq
parent has a half chance of passing on the q allele to each child hence the
quarter chance for qq MZ twins since these are, in effect one child. DZ twins
are separate conceptions and so the chance of both being qq is a quarter
multiplied by a quarter. Table 2.5a shows how these figures are combined by
simple multiplication to give the joint probability of MZ and DZ options.
These awkward fractions represent ratios and can be simplified as shown to
the ratio 112 : 13. There are thus 13 chances out of a total of 125 that these
twins are DZ, or 10.4%. A further glance at the table will show that each line
represents a ratio which can be simplified by dividing by the figure in the MZ
column (Table 2.5b) making the figure on the right the relative probability of
DZ status for each piece of information. It will be noted that despite being
alike in the two systems tested these twin girls still have a greater than 10%
chance of being DZ. The twins in Figure 2.2 were alike in all blood groups

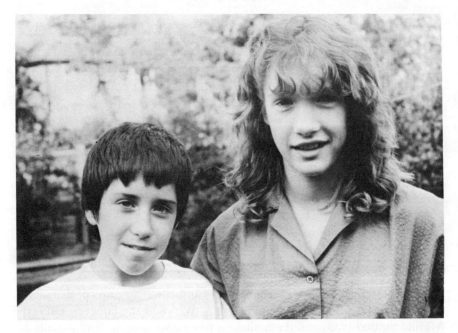

Figure 2.2. Twin sisters adjudged probably monozygotic on the basis of concordance
for a range of blood group markers. Subsequent demonstration of differences in serum
markers between the girls confirmed what physical examination made obvious, that
they were dizygotic.

and were adjudged probably MZ. The truth, obvious on examination, was revealed in the laboratory by differences in the serum polymorphisms. The need for such Bayesian calculations is likely to diminish in the near future with the development of genetic fingerprinting techniques. The approach uses gene probes which identify repetitive sequences in the DNA. These are extremely variable between individuals so that the likelihood of DZ twins having the same pattern is very small (Jeffreys *et al.*, 1985; Hill and Jeffreys, 1985). Once widely available, this approach will become the method of choice. Additional advantages are that it can be used on placental material and will thus be helpful with stillborn babies and that tissue samples from the baby and/or placental samples can be frozen and tested at a later date.

Biological Exceptions

In addition to the various methodological problems in zygosity determination, true exceptions to the rules may occur. In the case of DZ twinning the rare events superfetation and superfecundation are of interest, but do not present diagnostic problems since they enhance the differences between the twin pair; superfetation may be defined as the implantation of a fertilised ovum in a uterus containing a pregnancy of at least 1 month duration. This would require a failure of luteal suppression of the second ovulation and while it is theoretically possible, existing evidence, based on birthweight disparities in occasional twin pairs, is not convincing (Corney and Robson, 1975). Superfecundation, on the other hand, does occur rarely. For example, Majsky and Kout (1982) have shown on the basis of tissue typing that a twin pair had different fathers, making them genetically less alike than normal sibs.

Heterokaryotypic twins have differing chromosome complements as has already been mentioned. There have been several examples of MZ twins where one is a normal male while the other has Turner's syndrome (45X) and is thus a phenotypic female (Edwards *et al.*, 1966). The presumed polar body twins described by Bíeber *et al.* (1981) included one with the karotype 69XXX and, therefore, may be included in this category.

Burn *et al.* (1986) reported a pair of twin girls who were monozygotic on the basis of physical similarity, placentation and a full range of blood group, tissue type and serum polymorphisms and yet were discordant for Duchenne muscular dystrophy. Discordance was such that one was an accomplished gymnast whilst the other had the full features of a disease normally confined to males. Investigation of the X inactivation pattern using mouse human hybrids provided evidence in support of the theory that the affected girl was using exclusively the maternal X whilst in the case of her twin, only the paternal X was active. This was attributed to chance asymmetry in the X inactivation process in the cells of the inner cell mass at the blastocyst stage.

This was the third such MZ twin pair to be reported in the literature, yet severe manifestation in singleton female carriers is very rare; a reasonable deduction was that the difference in X inactivation had precipitated the developmental separation of the zygote into a twin pair. This 'clonal separation' theory could also explain the development of twins discordant for Turner's syndrome, a mosaic zygote having divided because the two cell masses failed to recognise each other.

Causes and Prevalence of MZ Twinning

The interest in such rare cases is enhanced by the need to explore further the causes of MZ twinning. While much is known of the factors which influence DZ twinning (Bulmer 1970; Nylander 1975c; 1983; Elwood 1985), very little light has been shed on the reasons for developmental separation within a single zygote. The concept of developmental separation is important as it emphasises the issue of timing. The fact that the early zygote is confined within a rigid zona pellucida makes the common perception of some form of 'celestial meat cleaver' splitting apart the blastomeres at the two cell stage biologically improbable. The sharing of a placenta by the majority of monozygotic pairs makes it more likely that in most cases separation begins at the blastocyst stage at about 4 days (Benirschke and Kim, 1973; Boklage, 1981) with physical division following some time later. The latter author develops this concept with the suggestion that dichorionic, monochorionic, monoamniotic and conjoined twins represent points on a time continuum extending over the first 2 weeks of gestation. The proportions in each category in published series quoted by Boklage comply reasonably well with the concept of a random separation through this time span with the proportions on each day obeying a Gaussian distribution. This idea is in keeping with the observation that the birth prevalence of MZ twinning is remarkably constant in all human populations at about 3.5/1000 deliveries in contrast to the marked global variations in DZ twinning (Bulmer, 1970; Nylander, 1983; Elwood, 1985). It is, however, possible that the incidence of MZ twinning does vary in time and place but that early gestational loss conceals this variation. The development of ultrasound has revealed that 'the disappearing twin' may be a common phenomenon though there are a number of technical artefacts which may be mistaken for multiple gestation sacs.

The idea of MZ separation being decided according to a basic physical law of particle decay is appealing. This would not preclude other influences contributing to a background level. Reports of geographical and temporal clusters of conjoined twins (Harrison and Rossiter, 1985; Viljoen *et al.*, 1983), for example, might be looked on as rare teratogenic exceptions made more easy to identify by the low prevalence of conjoined twins. Conversely, exaggerated first trimester loss could prevent such clusters from seeing the light of day. Even allowing for this possibility, the remarkable constancy of MZ twinning in human populations argues against major environmental factors open to fluctuation in time and place.

Genetic factors must be considered; though rare, families have been described where MZ twinning appears to behave as an autosomal dominant trait with incomplete penetrance (Harvey *et al.*, 1977; Segreti *et al.*, 1978; Shapiro *et al.*, 1978). It remains possible, of course, that occasional two generation families are mere coincidences. What cannot be dismissed as observer bias, however, is the remarkable reproductive behaviour of the armadillo.

When it was first suggested that the armadillo produced invariably monozygotic litters, the claim was dismissed as being biologically implausible (Newman and Patterson, 1909). Nevertheless, subsequent investigation has confirmed that this is the case. *Dasypus novemcinctus*, or the nine-banded armadillo, normally produces monozygotic quadruplets and the mulita (*Dasypus hybridus*) produces seven to fifteen monozygotic offspring (Benirschke, 1981). The unique nature of this phenomenon among vertebrates suggests that a rare genetic change has become established in this species which affects the interaction of blastomeres in such a way as to precipitate their developmental separation. Setting aside the interesting question of the possible evolutionary effects of such a change, the important question in the obstetric context is how this effect is achieved.

A change in early cell surface receptors mediated through the nuclear genome is a possibility. An alternative is the effect of cytoplasmic factors.

Clonal separation on the basis of 'unequal X inactivation' could also provide an explanation for the marked excess of female pairs known to be present among conjoined twins (Milham, 1966) and the less marked female excess in other monochorionic twins (James, 1980b), since it would provide a mechanism for late twinning exclusive to females. A similar effect could be related to preferential loss of male twins. A male excess is evident among spontaneous abortuses (Byrne and Warburton, 1987) though the difference is unlikely to account for the markedly low sex ratio in the 'late twinning' groups.

An experiment using the mouse human hybrid approach on fibroblasts from a pair of female conjoined twins has provided some support. Four independent hybrids from the left hand twin were equally divided with two using the maternal X and two the paternal. The right hand twin, however, appeared to have non-random X inactivation with all six informative hybrids showing the same X to be active (Holt, 1987). If these results are borne out by further studies, it may be that the 'unequal inactivation' theory will need to be slightly modified to suggest that one group of cells would need to be using one X chromosome almost exclusively to precipitate developmental separation— it takes two to make a marriage but only one (cell cluster) to make a divorce!

A critical issue is the timing of X inactivation. Recent studies have shown this to occur on a tissue specific basis triggered by the commencement of differentiation (Gartler and Riggs, 1983). It may thus precede developmental separation in the inner cell mass. Precipitation of dichorionic twinning by this means is very unlikely since recent evidence suggests that in the trophectoderm of mammals, including man, there is preferential inactivation of the paternal X (Harrison and Warburton, 1986) presumed to be due to persistence of the damage to methylation associated with sperm formation.

Ovum Cytoplasm and Twinning—Developmental Clock?

Bomsel-Helmreich and Papiernik-Berkhauer reported in 1976 an important experiment; they showed that by delaying ovulation in the rabbit, where it is coitus dependent, for 60 hours after the induction of follicular maturation using pregnant mare serum gonadotrophin, they were able to generate six pairs of MZ twins among 387 blastocysts. MZ twinning is otherwise rare in the rabbit.

Harlap (1979) in a study of orthodox Jewish couples, whose religion requires intercourse to take place 7 days after the last day of the menstrual period, found a significant variation in sex ratio. Coitus just prior to ovulation produced an excess of males as did late coitus whereas coitus at ovulation produced more females. In a subsequent study this author (Harlap *et al.*, 1985) reported a marked excess of twins in late conceptions, though the large proportion of unlike-sex pairs made it likely that the majority of these were DZ. This may have been an indirect effect, since longer menstrual periods are more common in older mothers, making an adherence to the 7 day rule more difficult. DZ twinning is associated with increased maternal age, probably as a result of greater parity. These authors did not rule out an association with MZ twinning particularly if aberrant twinning occurred with delayed fertilisation such that mitotic division of the ovum permitted access by two sperm of different sex. It is perhaps more likely, however, that this event would result in a chimera (Tippett, 1983) rather than viable twins, Shahar and Morton (1986) have provided a mathematical model based on centromere mapping which will allow the possibility of dispermic twins to be explored further. Edwards *et al.* (1986) reviewed twinning in pregnancies following in vitro fertilisation. In addition to the predictable excess of DZ twins in view of replacement of multiple zygotes, they found nine MZ pairs among over 600 reported births. Even allowing for under-reporting of singletons, this represented a significant excess for which no obvious precipitant could be found.

How can these observations be tied to the excess MZ twinning in delayed ovulation? One attractive possibility would be that the timing of all these early events relates not only to the time of fertilisation but also to the timing of follicular maturation. The possibility that 'overripeness' of the egg might be deleterious has been the subject of debate for many years (Witschi, 1952). If a 'clock' started when the ovum was prepared for its final launch and this 'clock' decided, via the ovum cytoplasm, the commencement of embryonic development, a delay in fertilisation would result in the cell mass being too small and immature to respond appropriately. A 'clock' set at 10 days with a cell mass equivalent to only, say, 4 days would result in more than one area being capable of the initiation of development and thus would produce more than one blastocyst. A less striking disparity would mean 'premature' development in the inner cell mass of the blastocyst leading to the formation of two 'bodies' but a single placenta. This challenge to the usual assumption of the relationship between cell mass and stage of development would fit well with the 'unequal X inactivation' theory if this too was dependent on the 'ovum clock' since the greater the delay in the commencement of cell division, the fewer cells would be involved and so the greater would be the capacity for clumping of cells according to X chromosome type. The induction of monozygotic twinning in mice with the antimetabolite vincristine (Kaufman and O'Shea, 1978) may result from a similar reduction in cell number.

In summary, the determination of zygosity has been examined from the practical viewpoint and some of the underlying theories of cause discussed in relation to the types of twinning. The march of obstetric progress brings with it multiple implantations of zygotes fertilised outside the womb, frozen embryos capable of being born months or years after their 'twins' and the prospect of induced MZ twinning as a means of preimplantation prenatal diagnosis. There seems little doubt that interest in the biology of twinning is set to increase.

Twinning and Twins
Edited by I. MacGillivray, D. M. Campbell and B. Thompson
© 1988 John Wiley & Sons Ltd

CHAPTER 3

Aetiology of twinning

DORIS M. CAMPBELL

Department of Obstetrics and Gynaecology, University of Aberdeen, Aberdeen, UK

The types of twinning and placentation have been discussed in the previous chapter. This one concentrates on factors that promote either monozygotic twinning or dizygotic twinning in human multiple pregnancies. The study of the process of human twinning has been helped by observations from a number of animals in which twinning occurs much more commonly and evidence from the animal kingdom may help clarify the reasons for monozygotic and dizygotic twins.

Monozygotic Twinning and Placentation

The armadillo is one of the few known species where the embryo regularly splits into several monozygotic offspring (Bulmer, 1970). It has been established that the placentae of such animals are monochorionic with apparently no vascular communication, but some of these identical animals differ in genotype. This is of interest because in humans the frequency of certain abnormalities is greater in monozygotic twins (see Chapter 11).

It may be significant that implantation of the ovum is delayed in the armadillo, as Stockard (1921) theorised that monozygotic twinning could be regarded as a congenital abnormality caused by developmental arrest. He based this theory on his work with frog and fish eggs, but later work with armadillos supports the concept. He suggested that developmental arrest was due to lack of oxygen caused by failure of implantation. However, in other mammals there is delayed implantation, e.g. roe deer, badger (Bulmer, 1970), but no association with monozygotic twinning. Apart from an increased frequency of congenital malformations in monozygotic twins in humans (see Chapter 11) in keeping with Stockard's theory, there is now some other evidence that developmental delay may be true also for humans as monozygotic twins have been reported following in vitro fertilisation (see below). Increased congenital anomalies, however, may be due to differences in placentation.

Vascular communication in a dichorionic placenta is common in cattle and other animals (Benirschke, 1970), but the effect produced by the common circulation in dichorionic placentation is very different from the common circulation of monochorionic placentation. Also there are major differences between animal species (Corney, 1975b). Such a communication with dichorionic placentation allows exchange of blood elements known as chimerism, and the individual twin is termed a chimera. In cattle when there are unlike-sexed twins, this usually results in a sterile female member known as a freemartin. Such a phenomenon does not occur in marmoset monkeys (Benirschke, 1970), although there is regular and extensive blood exchange between the twins starting early in fetal life.

Although chimerism is said not to occur in man, Nylander and Osunkoya (1970) described the placenta of a pair of unlike-sex twins. This placenta was originally thought to be monochorionic, but subsequent histological examination suggested that it was a dichorionic placenta in which the two layers of chorion had fused and virtually disappeared leaving only traces of two chorions at the base of the septum. Although the twins were normal on clinical examination and the genitalia showed no abnormalities, subsequent chromosomal studies (Corney, 1975b) showed a mixture of male and female karyotypes in each twin. Other investigations on lymphocyte cultures from the children provided strong evidence that blood interchange had taken place between these twins with dichorionic placentation. Such a phenomenon would appear to be very rare in humans in contrast to animals.

Dizygotic Twinning

Dizygotic twinning results from simultaneous fertilisation and development of two ova released from the ovaries. Changes in dizygotic twinning rates can, therefore, be caused by change either in the frequency of double ovulation, or in the proportion of times both ova are fertilised, or in embryo mortality usually ending in a singleton birth (Bulmer, 1970). Superfecundation, dizygotic twinning resulting from fertilisation at different times from different acts of coitus in a single menstrual cycle, has only been recorded in an isolated case (Gedda, 1961). James (1984) has reported a higher frequency of intercourse in couples who have dizygotic twins compared with those who have singleton births, but as the difference is not large he considered that superfecundation was likely to be a rare event.

Superfetation may also be considered in respect of the implantation of a second fertilised ovum in a uterus already containing a pregnancy of at least one month's duration, but has not yet been proven in humans. Although there are reports of possible occurrence of this phenomenon in the literature (Meyer, 1919; Studdeford, 1936; Scrimgeour and Baker, 1974; Bulmer, 1970) they are based on gross discrepancies in birthweight between the twins which are quite common in monochorionic monozygotic twins.

Hormone Levels

Injection of pituitary gonadotrophin leads to superovulation in many species including rabbits, rats, sheep and cattle (Bulmer, 1970) although the exact mechanism by which the pituitary gonadotrophins and ovarian hormones exercise control on the release of ova is not clear. In humans, one maturing follicle usually becomes dominant, inhibiting the development of others. If this inhibition fails, or if there is excess pituitary stimulation, or if other as yet unknown factors influence this process, two or more ova will be released, from which dizygotic twins can result.

Milham (1964) put forward his hypothesis that excess maternal pituitary gonadotrophins was related to dizygotic twinning rates. He commented that epidemiological findings were consistent with this hypothesis. First, dizygotic twinning rates increase with maternal age; second, multiparous women have a higher dizygotic twinning rate than primiparae; third, dizygotic twinning rates are higher in negroes than in whites, which in turn are higher than those of the Japanese; and fourth, that dizygotic twinning repeats itself within the same family (see Chapter 5). He commented that anatomical features of the pituitary gland were compatible with the epidemiological findings, i.e. the pituitary reaches a maximum weight in the fourth decade, its weight is greater in multiparae than primiparae and it is larger in negroes than in whites. He proposed four questions which it would be necessary to answer in order to confirm his hypothesis: (i) Pituitary gonadotrophin levels in women of child-bearing age should vary with age with an age distribution similar to that of dizygotic twinning rates. It has been now shown that the levels of these hormones in ovulating blood do increase with maternal age (Guyton, 1981). (ii) Pituitary gonadotrophin levels should increase with parity within a given maternal age. As yet there is no conclusive proof for this. (iii) Negro women should have higher levels of gonadotrophins than white women who in turn should have higher levels than Japanese women. (iv) Mothers of dizygotic twins should have higher gonadotrophin levels than mothers of singletons. Evidence is now available to answer these third and fourth questions.

Mean follicle stimulating hormone levels in serum reached a higher peak and were higher for 4 days before and after the peak in women who had twins compared to those who had had singletons (Nylander, 1973). Levels were higher still in women who had two sets of twins though the number of these was small.

Mean luteinising hormone levels were less clearly related to the twinning history. Only a small number of Nigerian women were studied and Nylander considered that further work was needed to compare mothers of twins and mothers of singletons after standardisation for maternal age, parity and social class.

Martin et al. (1984) measured several hormones, in six Australian mothers who had had two sets of dizygotic twins and whose menstrual cycles were regular. They found that follicle stimulating hormone and, to a lesser extent, luteinising hormone levels were significantly higher in the twin mothers than in a control group of six women with no history of twinning. Oestradiol levels were also noted to be higher in mothers of twins, particularly in the follicular phase. The two groups of women did not differ in age, height, weight, or parity. A recent study has reported lower serum gonadotrophin levels, both follicle stimulating hormone and luteinising hormone, in Japanese women who are known to have a low dizygotic twinning rate (Soma *et al.*, 1975).

It is difficult to compare directly the findings of these separate studies on gonadotrophin levels on account of the different timing of samples in the menstrual cycle and possible differences in results due to laboratory variation, although the methods used in Japan and Nigeria were similar. Soma *et al.* (1975) claimed both follicle stimulating hormone and luteinising hormone levels were lower than in American women (Yen *et al.*, 1970) whose levels were in turn lower than those of Nylander's Nigerian women. It is known that Nigerian dizygotic twinning rates are extremely high, whereas in Japan they are very low. Nylander (1979a) has proposed that yams, common in the diet of the Yoruba, might contain a constituent which affected the hypothalamic–pituitary–ovarian axis and thus, twinning in Nigeria. This theory has been further supported by the work of Peal (1965) who examined various East African crops, including yams, for steroidal compounds as hormone precursors. From such findings it is possible to speculate that high intake of such cereals in the diet might inhibit or augment pituitary function.

Ovulation Induction

In the treatment of infertile women, regimens for inducing ovulation have been introduced. There is no doubt that stimulation of the ovaries by human gonadotrophins leads to multiple follicles developing and rupturing. This was initially reported by Gemzell and Roos (1966) who noted that in 43 women treated with human pituitary follicle stimulating hormone and human chorionic gonadotrophin, the resulting pregnancies were 20 singleton, 14 twin and 9 triplets or higher multiple. These authors concluded that to avoid multiple births, the daily dose of human pituitary follicle stimulating hormone needed to be carefully adjusted, taking into consideration endogenous gonadotrophin production for individual women. There are now many regimens for 'superovulation' related to obtaining ova for in vitro fertilisation, some based on giving clomiphene prior to the use of human gonadotrophins. Hack *et al.* (1970) reported 78 pregnancies after ovulation induction: 47 were singleton, 23 twin, 5 triplet, 2 quadruplet, and 1 sextuplet births, giving a multiple birth rate of 39.7%. Interestingly enough these authors commented that the secondary sex ratio for single births was 0.88, while that for twin births was significantly lower at 0.43. Caspi *et al.* (1976) in a study of 110 women in whom ovulation was induced found a multiple pregnancy rate of 26.8% with again a predominance of female births. Dor and co-workers (1980) who had a high success rate following gonadotrophin therapy did not comment on the rate of twinning or multiple pregnancy. However, they noted that age was crucial, there being an improved cumulative pregnancy rate in women under age 35 compared with the older women.

Klopper (1976) after reviewing reports on induction of ovulation, concluded that there were many different regimens in practice, but none was ideal. Assuming that multiple pregnancies occur when many mature follicles rupture and that numerous follicles produce more oestrogens than one follicle, he suggested that multiple ovulation and multiple pregnancies could be avoided by giving human chorionic gonadotrophin (hCG) only to patients with oestrogen levels within the normal preovulatory range. From practical experience, however, it was often necessary to attain oestrogen levels in excess of normal cycle peak in order to achieve ovulation at all, and he thought that there was some factor missing in the system when ovulation was induced. In normal cycles there seemed to be a mechanism for inducing atresia in some of the follicles well short of ovulation, but this was lacking when ovulation was induced artificially. The missing factor controls follicles becoming atretic. Having ripened a large number of follicles by stimulating the ovary, attempts have been made to control the number ovulated by varying the dose of hCG, but there is no evidence to link hCG dosage and multiple pregnancies.

Wyshak (1978a) quantified the statistical effect of the use of 'ovulation inducing' drugs on multiple births. She found that between 10 and 15% of twin births followed the use of ovulation stimulants. A similar estimate has been reported more recently from Nottingham (Webster and Elwood, 1985).

In Vitro Fertilisation

The importance of in vitro fertilisation (IVF) in relation to changes in twinning rates has recently become an issue. Edwards and Steptoe (1983), referring to the experiences at Bourn Hall where stimulation of follicle growth is by clomiphene and human menopausal gonadotrophin as their 'superovulation' regimen for egg retrieval, have reported that the success rate of IVF increases with the number of embryos replaced following IVF. They proposed a theoretical model for the influence of maternal factors on the incidence of pregnancy and in particular, multiple pregnancy after replacing one or more embryos. They predicted that pregnancy rates would rise sharply when more than one embryo was replaced, up to 32.9% when three embryos are replaced. In practice their success fell well short of the predicted, but this they concluded was due to the inclusion of patients aged over 40 years. The results were particularly poor indicating that any model must take account of maternal age (Edwards, 1985). It is well known that multiple conceptions are higher than multiple births (syndrome of the vanishing twin, see Chapter 4). This can be illustrated from experience with IVF, where it is found that many singleton births occur although multiple pregnancies are noticed at ultrasonic scanning performed in early gestation. When either two or three embryos are replaced, more than 50% of pregnancies are noted to be multiple between 4.5 and 7 weeks (Edwards, 1985). The incidence of multiple implantation is far higher than that predicted by Edwards, usually binomial expansion. Other factors must interfere in aiding embryos to implant, such that once one embryo is implanted it helps another embryo to implant. The phenomenon termed 'helping' results in immediate multiple pregnancies being established at implantation. Further detail of the physiological evidence for 'helping' is required, namely the factors that lead to delayed implantation and those which help embryos to increase their chance of implantation. Edwards *et al.* (1984), after reviewing data from various centres practising IVF, concluded that in some centres the number of multiple pregnancies fitted their model very closely, whereas others obtained many more multiple births than expected. Some centres have to replace four or more embryos to obtain any pregnancies at all (Quigley and Wolf, 1984; Kerin *et al.*, 1983). Gronow *et al.* (1985) suggest that four or more embryos need to be transferred because their data indicate that embryos were of poorer quality or the endometrium was less receptive, or a combination of both these factors in cycles when IVF was less successful compared with those cycles giving better results. Their only predictive factor relating to outcome was the multiplicity of embryos transferred. They also commented that a predictor of embryo health was urgently required in order to enhance the rate of implantation.

Type of Twinning following Induced Ovulation and IVF

In both ovulation induction and IVF programmes twin pregnancies are usually dizygotic, resulting from double ovulation, fertilisation and implantation, or the replacement of two or more separate embryos in IVF. However, there are now several reports of the birth of identical, monozygotic twins following IVF (Edwards *et al.*, 1986). Some of these monozygotic twins were easily identified since only one embryo had been replaced. Others arose after multiple embryos had been transferred followed by the birth of triplets consisting of an identical monozygotic pair and a singleton. Edwards reported that at Bourn Hall after 320 births following IVF, no identical twins had been born. He thought that ovarian stimulation used in the IVF programme might promote embryo division or the enhanced survival of identical twins. Dor *et al.* (1980) have shown no increase in monozygotic twinning following ovulation stimulation. Derom *et al.* (1987) determined the zygosity, using genetic markers and chorion type from both naturally occurring triplets and triplets born after induction of ovulation. They showed that irrespective of the type of ovulation, naturally occurring or induced, the number of monozygotic pairs was higher than estimated from other published work of the known incidence of splitting of the single human zygote. They suggest, therefore, that with ovulation stimulation, whatever the method, the use of clomiphene and gonadotrophins may in some way lead to early division of the embryo, and thus MZ twins.

Edwards *et al.* (1986) speculate that malformation or weakness in the zona pellucida of the embryo in vitro might also predispose to twinning. Many blastocysts may fail to hatch fully from their zona pellucida and others remain half hatched. It is possible that two separate embryos could form if the inner cell mass divided during hatching as it does in animals. It is possible, too, that the drugs used as ovulation stimulants alter the human zona pellucida. Further studies of monozygotic pregnancies which result from IVF and, therefore, better understanding of the physiology of embryo transfer and implantation, might indicate other environmental factors, which may be implicated in monozygotic twinning.

In the Aberdeen series, multiple pregnancy following the induction of ovulation was 6.7%, but varied from 3.8 to 15.6% in different years (Table 3.1). Zygosity, accurately determined using genetic markers, and the sex of the infants are given in Table 3.2. One of the two sets of twins was definitely monozygotic, and the other was presumed to be monozygotic as the placenta was monochorionic and some (those tested) of the markers were identical; sixteen sets of twins were dizygotic and the remaining six sets were not tested. The sex ratio at birth was 1.00 which is slightly less than the population figure for Aberdeen, 1.06. James (1980d) reported that the human secondary sex ratio was low following ovulation induction.

James (1984) speculated that other factors might affect endogenous gonadotrophin levels resulting in double ovulation. These included psychological

Table 3.1. Multiple pregnancy rate by year, Aberdeen City District, in women who have had ovulation induced

	Twin/multiple	Singleton	Multiple rate (%)
1976	3[a]	74	3.9
1977	3	34	8.1
1978	3	36	7.7
1979	2	51	3.8
1980	2	26	7.1
1981	1	25	3.9
1982	7	38	15.6
1983	4	66	5.7
Total	25	350	6.6

[a]Including one set of quins.

Table 3.2. Distribution of zygosity and sex of infants of ovulation-induced twins (24 pairs)

Sex of infants	Monozygotic (2)	Dizygotic (16)	Not known (6)
Male/male	–	3	3
Female/female	2	1	3
Male /female	–	8	–
Female/male	–	4	–

factors, coital rates, and the length of fertile period. He considered that in a small number of cases, frequent coitus may give rise to DZ twinning, but it seemed more likely that in human beings as opposed to animals, the corpus luteum will usually inhibit fertilisation of a further ova. Harlap et al. (1985) studying orthodox Jews for whom both the day of ovulation and the earliest possible day of conception could be estimated, concluded that there was an excess of multiple births in late conceptions although rather surprisingly the excess was of unlike-sex twins.

Additionally, Wyshak (1981) from a self-administered questionnaire sent to mothers of twins, found an earlier age at menarche and a shorter menstrual cycle length than in a group of singleton mothers. This comparison group, however, was obtained from friends of a 'similar nature' to the twin mothers. Although there are flaws in this study, e.g. overall design and no attempt to correct for maternal age, the findings support the hypothesis of altered hypothalamic and pituitary function with respect to twinning as both age at menarche and cycle length are likely to be a reflection of this endocrine function.

Oral Contraception

Twinning rates have declined over the past twenty years in developed countries including Scotland, England, Wales, Hungary, Canada, Australia, Denmark (see Chapter 4). This has been mainly due to a fall in dizygotic twinning although more recently there has been a slight increase reported in the monozygotic twinning rates. MacGillivray (1981) examined the data for Scotland and concluded that the main explanation for the decrease in DZ twinning was a continuation of a decrease in maternal age and parity. He admitted, however, that there was a possibility that oral contraception introduced about 1964 which became very popular and widely used might have an adverse effect on hypothalamic–pituitary function and thereby on twinning. More recently, both James (1980c) and Emery (1986) have suggested that the slight increase in monozygotic twinning rates could be related to prior oral contraceptive use leading to delayed implantation of the fertilised ovum with early division to two embryos. Vessey et al. (1976)

reported that multiple pregnancy was less common following oral contraceptive use. In contrast to this Rothman (1977) reported that twinning was increased when conception occurred following the use of oral contraception. Bracken (1979) also reported an increased rate of twinning, but concluded that the rate of delivering twins doubled if conception occurred within 2 months of the cessation of oral contraceptive use, and particularly affected dizygotic twinning based on identification of unlike- and like-sex pairs. Neither Rothman (1977) nor Bracken (1979) studied a total population, zygosity was not properly determined, and details of use of oral contraception was obtained retrospectively, one using a questionnaire, and the other an interview some time after the birth of the twins.

Two other studies relating the types of twinning to oral contraceptive use have been reported from France (Hemon et al., 1981a) and from Australia (Macourt et al., 1982). The French study included 673 mothers of twins delivering at several different hospitals, compared with the mothers of preceding singleton births at each place. Thus, the twin and singleton control births were matched for the time and place of delivery. Hemon et al. (1981a) concluded that there was a decrease in dizygotic twinning rate after oral contraceptive use. In the Australian study Macourt et al. (1982) sent questionnaires to approximately 2000 mothers of twins and obtained a 50% response. They reported an alteration in the ratio of monozygotic to dizygotic twins which they attributed to an increase in monozygotic twins following the use of oral contraception. There are several problems associated with both the French and Australian studies. Data on the use of oral contraception were collected retrospectively. In the French study, the mothers of twins and the controls were interviewed in hospital soon after the birth, whereas the mothers of twins in Australia were filling in a questionnaire at home an unspecified time after the birth. Zygosity was not determined accurately in either study. The French study relied on the Weinberg formula which, as has been indicated elsewhere in this book (see Chapter 4) may give an inaccurate result, whereas the Australian study based zygosity on whether the mothers said like-sex twins looked alike. It is well known that maternal age and parity affect twinning, and the French study considered these as possible confounding variables, but they were ignored in the Australian study as was any secular change in the use of oral contraception. Neither study was based on a total population of twin pregnancies. Earlier work from Aberdeen suggested that dizygotic twinning was reduced after the use of oral contraception in multiparae only. This study highlighted, however, some of the problems of considering twins and adjacent singletons (control births) in the same hospital (Thompson et al., 1982). More recent work from Aberdeen (Campbell et al., 1987) showed no association between oral contraceptive use prior to pregnancy for either monozygotic or dizygotic twinning. In contrast to the other studies mentioned, the Aberdeen findings were based on total births in a geographically defined population with zygosity determined from blood samples and placentation, and with data on the use of oral contraception routinely collected prospectively. In this study, three mutually exclusive control groups of singletons were used to take account of age, parity and secular trend.

Conclusion:

Although there is a definite familial tendency to twinning (see Chapter 5) suggesting a genetic aetiology of predisposition to both dizygotic and monozygotic twinning, it can be concluded that the aetiology of twinning depends on modification of the genetic state by environmental factors. Such factors as psychological stress, nutrition or climate might modify hypothalamic–pituitary–ovarian function, leading to increased ovulation with many follicles being developed, ripened and ruptured, and also to modification to the uterine environment for implantation, either aiding or delaying implantation resulting in differences in twinning rates both monozygotic and dizygotic, as are now being reported (see Chapter 4).

Twinning and Twins
Edited by I. MacGillivray, D. M. Campbell and B. Thompson
© 1988 John Wiley & Sons Ltd

CHAPTER 4

Descriptive epidemiology

JULIAN LITTLE
Department of Community Medicine and Epidemiology, University of Nottingham, Nottingham, UK
and
BARBARA THOMPSON
Medical Research Council Medical Sociology Unit and Department of Obstetrics and Gynaecology, University of Aberdeen, Aberdeen, UK

Introduction

Until recently, it was generally accepted that twins occur in about one in 80 pregnancies, but the observation of James (1972) that dizygotic twinning rates had been declining dramatically, together with the evidence from ultrasound scanning that many twin pregnancies end in singleton deliveries, a phenomenon known as the 'vanishing twin' (Landy *et al.*, 1982) has prompted further studies. The aim of this chapter, therefore, is to review recent data on the descriptive epidemiology of multiple pregnancy: i.e. group or population based rather than based on comparisons between twin and singleton individuals. Some results of an analysis of data from north-east Scotland and Northern Ireland, described in the Appendix to Chapter 5, are included.

Prevalence of Twinning

(a) Abortions

As the estimation of the true incidence of twinning is hampered by the difficulty of studying early prenatal losses, it is at present possible only to consider prevalence at various later stages of development. Recent evidence suggests that twin pregnancy occurs more frequently than the number of twins observed at birth suggest. A summary of some published reports of twins amongst consecutive series of pregnancies ending in spontaneous abortion is presented in Table 4.1. Many other large series of spontaneous abortuses have been described but the focus has been on the frequencies and types of chromosomal anomalies: twins are not mentioned in most reports even though they are likely to have been present (Uchida *et al.*, 1983b). In the

studies summarised in Table 4.1 the number of twins identified is likely to be a
minimum. Earlier spontaneous abortions will have been missed and, as there
is some evidence of an association between MZ twinning and 'early malformation' (see Chapter 11), it is possible that a greater proportion of twin
conceptions than of singletons are aborted in early pregnancy. Many of the
products of conception sent to the laboratory arrive as empty ruptured sacs
or fragmented tissue. In the study of Uchida *et al.* (1983b), for example, only
eight specimens were recognisable as twins on anatomical examination. In the
absence of two discrete specimens, it is virtually impossible to detect MZ
twins and difficult to identify DZ twins of the same sex. Again, in the absence
of two discrete specimens, it can be difficult to identify twin pairs of unlike sex
as the 46, XX cells of the female members of these pairs may be attributed
mistakenly to maternal contamination if their chromosomal banding patterns
are similar to those of the mother. In view of these difficulties, therefore, the
finding of a consistently higher twinning rate observed in series of spontaneous abortions than in series of births is impressive.

At variance with these findings at first sight, however, is the report by
Tanimura and Tanaka (1977) of 78 twin pairs amongst 20 339 pregnancies
ending in induced abortion in Japan, a rate of 0.38%, which is low as
compared to the 0.64% of pregnancies at and over the 4th month of
pregnancy as recorded by national statistics. The authors suggest that this is
due to erroneous diagnosis of twin conceptuses as singletons because of
damage incurred during the procedure to effect pregnancy termination.
Another possible explanation for the low rate is selection bias—reporting of
induced abortions in Japan is known to be incomplete (Tietze, 1983) and the
material investigated by Tanimura and Tanaka (1977) was selected for the
presence of a complete embryo or fetus. On balance, therefore, this one
report on a series of induced abortions does not contradict the findings of the
studies of series of spontaneous abortions.

Recent data from ultrasound screening early in gestation suggests,
moreover, that the death of one twin in utero is not infrequent. For example,
among a series of 6990 pregnant women, multiple pregnancy was diagnosed
by ultrasound before 10 weeks in 28 patients (Levi, 1976). Only fourteen of
these patients were followed up, of whom ten subsequently delivered singletons. Levi is of the opinion that the twin echo pattern from which the
diagnosis was made was not an artefact in most of the cases. Conversely,
Ramzin *et al.* (1982) point out that it is not always easy to differentiate
between a second gestational sac and the early separation of embryonic
membranes. A summary of some reports on spontaneous abortion in multiple
pregnancy diagnosed by ultrasound is presented in Table 4.2. Accurate
assessment of the incidence of death of one of a twin pair in utero is difficult
because (1) it is not routine for women to undergo early first trimester
ultrasound examination; (2) there are a number of sources of false positive

Table 4.1. Summary of published reports on products of multiple pregnancy detected by pathological examination of material from spontaneous abortions

Study location	Study period	Study population	Examination technique	Modal gestational age	Number of pregnancies ending in spontaneous abortion investigated	Number of pregnancies from which identifiable fetus or sac recovered	Number of twin pregnancies diagnosed	Estimated prevalence of twin pregnancy amongst pregnancies ending in spontaneous abortion (%)	Prevalence of twin deliveries amongst pregnancies ending in birth (%)	Reference
UK (South-east England)	Sept. 1971 – April 1974	Consecutive series from 15 large hospitals	Dissection and standard karyotyping	12 weeks	2 607	1 803	36	2.0	1.0[a]	Creasy et al. (1976)
Japan	Not stated	Material selected for presence of complete embryo or fetus. 1) spontaneous abortions 2) ectopic pregnancies	Dissection	Not specified		441 / 216	7 / 4	1.6 } 1.9	0.6	Tanimura and Tanaka (1977)
Switzerland (Geneva)	Jan. 1971 – Nov. 1974	Consecutive series[b] from 1 maternity hospital	Dissection and standard karotyping	12 weeks	862	621	11	2.0[c]	0.9[a]	Kajii et al. (1980)
Canada (British Columbia)	11 years (no further details)	Consecutive series from 1 hospital plus opportunistic referrals	Dissection; karyotyping only in selected cases	Not specified; 25 sets of embryos, 26 sets of fetuses, 2 sets embryo/fetuses	2169	1886	53	2.8	0.9 (live births in a 5 year period)	Livingston and Poland (1980)
Canada (Hamilton)	Aug. 1977 – July 1981	Consecutive series from 3 obstetric units	Dissection and comparison of Q-band variants of conceptuses with maternal variants	Not specified		646	15[d]	2.3	1.0 (all births 1978/1980)	Uchida et al. (1983b)

[a]Calculated from data on live births 1972–1974 in UN *Demographic Yearbook* (1981).

[b]Study also included data from a selected series. These are excluded from this table.

[c]As 67 specimens 100 mm or more in crown–rump length were excluded, denominator is 554.

[d]Includes two sets of conjoined twins

Table 4.2. Summary of published reports on the spontaneous abortion of multiple pregnancies which had been detected by ultrasound scanning techniques (modified and expanded from Landy, 1982)

Reference	Number of pregancies investigated	Ovulation-stimulating therapy		Number of multiple pregnancies detected	Estimate of overall incidence of multiple pregnancy	Estimated range of gestational age	Number of multiple pregnancies detected within range	Number of detected multiple pregnancies which were followed up	Outcome		
		Yes	No						Number of multiple[a] abortions	Number of multiple[a] pregnancies from which delivery of singleton birth	Number of Multiple[a] pregnancies from which delivery of multiple birth
Hellman, Kobayashi and Cromb (1973)	140 with 'abnormalities of gestation'		131	13		First trimester	13	13	13	—	—
		9		9	9.9%		9	9	1	3	5
Kohorn and Kaufman (1974)	65	—		3	4.6%	First trimester	3	3	—	3	—
Levi (1976)	6 990	—		118	1.7%	10 weeks	28	14	—	10	4
						10–15 weeks	11	8	—	5	3
						15 weeks	79	79	—	1	78
Robinson and Caines (1977)		6	24	24		First Trimester	24	24	5	10	9
				6			6	6	1		5
Levi and Reimers (1978)	3 161	—		159	5.0%	4–9 weeks	47	32	—	26	6
						10–14 weeks	23	22	—	8	14
						14 weeks	89	89	—	—	89

Reference[a]			% twins	Gestation at diagnosis					10 + 3 elective abortions	
Finberg and Birnholz (1979)	(22)		14	—	First trimester	14	14	1	—	—
Kurjak and Latin (1979)	(20 000)		41	—	First trimester	41	41	13	28	20
Schneider, Bessis and Simonnet (1979)	Not stated	54	54	—	First trimester	54	54	—	34	17
Varma (1979)	1 500	24	30	2.0%	First trimester	30	30	8	7	15
Jeanty et al. (1981)	300		23	7.7%	First trimester	23	23	—	7	18 from twin pregnancies + 1 from quadruplet pregnancy
Ranzin, Stucki, Napflin et al. (1982)	17 500		150	0.8%	20 weeks	150	150	—	6	3 sets of twins + 1 set of triplets
									144	

[a]Twin, unless otherwise stated

diagnosis of multiple pregnancy by ultrasound prior to the 12th week of gestation (Landy *et al.*, 1982). Pooling of the data in Table 4.2 relating to first trimester pregnancies where no ovulation-stimulating therapy had been used shows that of the 278 multiple pregnancies detected, 14% ended in multiple abortion and 58% in a singleton birth, but these figures should be regarded with caution in view of the difficulties just mentioned. Clearly, further data are needed, but this newer form of investigation may in the longer term provide what has formerly been impossible, namely some assessment of the rate of twin conception, which it seems might be higher than is generally supposed.

Edwards (1986) has reviewed the outcome of pregnancies following in vitro fertilisation in one clinic. Of 148 twin pregnancies confirmed clinically, 26 (18%) ended in the delivery of a singleton; of 51 triplet pregnancies, eight (16%) ended in the delivery of twin babies only and one in the delivery of a singleton infant. These figures suggest lower rates of 'vanishing twins' than indicated by the ultrasound studies. The difference may be due, at least in part, to the operation of different selection biases in the two types of study, the in vitro fertilisation group having by definition a history of reproductive problems while the reasons for ultrasound scanning in early pregnancy in the studies listed in Table 4.2 are not specified.

(b) Births

Geographical variation in the prevalence of twinning at birth has been reviewed extensively by Bulmer (1970), Hytten and Leitch (1971) and Nylander (1975b; 1983). Most of the studies reviewed by these authors were carried out between the end of the Second World War and the 1960s. More recent data available from national statistics are collated in the United Nations *Demographic Yearbooks* for 1975 and 1981, but the material is difficult to interpret because of ambiguity of the distinction between twin maternities and twin births. For example, in the most recent *Yearbook*, the numbers entered under twin livebirths for Canada in the years 1973 and 1974 are 5766 and 2853 respectively. Further difficulties are that still births are excluded and it is not certain whether both members of a pair are excluded if only one is born dead. Also the figures are not adjusted for maternal age.

The studies of Europe, Japan and the USA were based on national statistics which are thought to have been complete. James (1972) and (1982a) reviewed time trends in data from Australia, Canada and New Zealand which are also likely to have been complete. Virtually all the other data available relating to twins from parts of America other than Canada or the USA, and from Africa, Asia and Oceania are derived either from national statistics based on birth registration which may be incomplete (UN *Demographic Yearbooks*, 1975; 1981 technical notes) or from hospital series. Data based on hospital series may lead to over-estimation or under-estimation of twinning rates (Nylander, 1983). Over-estimation will arise when emergency admissions are included because obstetric complications occur more frequently in twin than in singleton pregnancies or from preferential booking of women suspected to be carrying twins. Under-estimation will occur if (1) primigravidae, who have a relatively low twinning frequency, are booked preferentially or (2) only uncomplicated maternity cases are accepted, the difficult ones being referred to other hospitals with better facilities. Quite apart from these problems of recording, data on twinning in Africa, South America, Asia and Oceania (other than Australia and New Zealand) are scanty. In essence, generalisations about the epidemiology of twinning have been made from populations in North America, Europe, Japan and Nigeria and hospital series in (1) Africa—the British Cameroons, the Gambia, Natal and Zimbabwe, (2) Asia—India, Pakistan and Singapore. In Table 4.3, therefore, specific figures are given from the UN *Demographic Yearbooks*, however unsatisfactory, and from published ad hoc reports for selected countries in Africa, America, Asia and Oceania, and ranges of figures for Europe.

As noted in an earlier review (Nylander, 1983), analysis of the available data suggests that populations can be classified into three broad groupings on the basis of their crude (i.e. not adjusted for maternal age) twinning rates:

1. *Low prevalence*: notably Hawaii, Japan and Taiwan, with twinning rates between 2 and 7 per 1000.
2. *Intermediate prevalence*: most countries in Africa, America, Asia and Oceania from which data are available, and all of Europe, with twinning rates between 9 and 20 per 1000.
3. *High prevalence*: in parts of Africa, especially Nigeria, the Seychelles, the Transvaal and Zimbabwe; in parts of America into which there has been migration from West Africa, notably the Bahamas, the Dominican Republic, and Jamaica; in one hospital series in Asia—Lehore in India; with twinning rates in excess of 20 per 1000.

On a global scale, there appears to be a fifteen-fold variation in crude rates. Variation in twinning rates amongst and within populations in each of the three groups is now considered.

Low Prevalence Except for Japan and for migrant groups in Hawaii, there are few data from areas of low prevalence. Within Japan, twinning rates increase from a low level in the south and west to a high level in the north and east (Kamimura, 1976; Imaizumi and Inouye, 1979). Geographical correlations between twinning rates and, (1) the proportion of twin pairs born in the

Table 4.3. International variation in twinning rates[a]

Continent, country or area	Type of study[b]	Period of study	No. of twin maternities	Twin-ning rate	Reference
AFRICA					
Algeria		1963	2 181[c]	13.3	
Ghana, Korle Bu	H	1954–56	291	52.4	Hollingsworth and Duncan (1966)
Libyan Arab Jamahiriya		1972–75	5 260	12.3	
Mali	H	1968	761	21.8	Imperato (1971)
Nigeria, lowest rate	H	1976–79	352	23.7	Harrison and Rossiter (1985)
highest rate		1964–68	216	45.1	Nylander (1969)
Seychelles		1972–76	236	27.2	
South Africa[d]		1963	2 784	16.8	
Tunisia		1972–74	10 972	27.9	
Uganda, Mbale	H	1971–80	1 104	16.3	Zake (1984)
AMERICA, NORTH					
Antigua and Barbuda		1972–75	56	10.3	
Bahamas		1972–76	482	21.8	
Barbados		1960	80	11.1	
Canada		1972–76 and 1976–79	20 786[e]	9.0	
Costa Rica		1974	579	10.2	
Cuba		1973 and 75	5 871	14.1	
Dominican Republic		1972–76	28 626	32.5	
El Salvador		1972–76 and 1978–80	12 455[f]	9.6	
Greenland		1972–76	59	13.2	
Jamaica		1960	1 652	25.7	
Mexico		1972–78	89 945[g]	5.3	
Nicaragua		1967	520	6.7	
Panama		1972–75 and 1977–80	6 899	16.2	
Former Canal Zone		1974–78	21	7.4	
Puerto Rico		1972–80	10 275	15.9	
Trinidad and Tobago		1972–76	1 929	14.5	
USA		1972–75	116 464	9.2	
		1978–79	65 511	9.6	
AMERICA, SOUTH					
Brazil		1974–76	147 353	16.8	
Chile		1972–80	31 245	14.7	
Ecuador		1972–74 and 1976–77	22 109	18.7	
Venezuela		1963	3 439	9.7	
ASIA					
Burma	H	1972–73	462	11.7	Kyu et al. (1981)
Cambodia, Pnom-Penh	H	1957–60	242	15.2	Olivier et al.
		1964	90	10.6	(1965)
Cyprus		1972–77 and 1979–80	1 889	19.2	

Table 4.3. *Continued*

Continent, country or area	Type of study[b]	Period of study	No. of twin maternities	Twin-ning rate	Reference
Hong Kong		1972–77 and 1979–80	8 117	12.5	
India, sample of townships		1963–73	2 564	16.0	Goswami and Wagh (1975)
Ahmedabad	H	1965–75	1 026	14.7	Bildhaiya (1978)
Palgar Block					Junnarkar and
sample townships		1966–75	154	9.0	Nadkarni (1979)
Tamilnadu		1969–75	96	8.6	Rao *et al.* (1983)
South Delhi		1969–73	81	9.8	Ghosh and Ramanujacharyulu (1979)
Bombay	H	1983–84	149	8.4	Shah and Patel (1984)
Israel		1961–64	1 769	9.7	Modan *et al.* (1968)
Israel		1972–80	6 309[h]	9.8	
Japan		1972–74 and 1976–80	82 647[i]	5.6	
		1955–67	151 709	6.4 ⎱	Imaizumi and
		1974	12 392	5.8 ⎰	Inouye (1984)
Korea				9.7	Kang and Cho (1962)
Ryukyu Islands		1968	188	8.4	
Singapore		1972, 1973 and 1975–80	4 457	13.1	
Singapore	H	1960–70	3 276	8.1	Tan *et al.* (1971)
Singapore	H	1969–70	174	7.9	Foong (1971)
	H	1970–72	234	7.5	Dawood *et al.* (1975)
Taiwan, Cheng-Chung		1956–65	122	5.7 ⎱	Lin and Chen
whole country		1963–64	4 703	5.6 ⎰	(1968)
Taipei		1972–77	?	4.5	Cheng *et al.* (1986)
Turkey, Ankara	H	1965–	149	14.9	Say *et al.* (1967)
Vietnam, Saigon	H	1952–62	1 266	10.7	Olivier *et al.* (1965)
EUROPE[j]					
lowest: Spain		1951–53		9.1 ⎱	
highest: East Germany		1950–55		12.4 ⎰	Bulmer (1960a)
lowest: Bulgaria		1978	891	6.5 ⎱	UN *Demographic*
highest: Ireland		1977	800	11.6 ⎰	*Yearbook* (1981)
OCEANIA					
American Samoa		1972	18	16.7	
		1976	10	9.2	
Australia		1973–79	15 455[i]	9.5	
Fiji		1976–81	802	7.6	Pollard (1985)
Guam		1972–79	393	15.9	
New Guinea, selected communities in west		?–1946[k]	790	10.3	Groenewegen and van de Kaa (1967)

Table 4.3. *Continued*

Continent, country or area	Type of study[b]	Period of study	No. of twin maternities	Twin-ning rate	Reference
New Zealand		1972–79	4 406[l]	9.8	*New Zealand*
New Zealand Maoris			122	9.4	*Yearbook* (1982)
Pacific Islands		1973,4,6,8,9	344	18.2	
Papua New Guinea	H	1970–71	421	19.1	Archer (1973)
New Britain		1953–67	87	31.2 ⎫	Scragg and Walsh
New Ireland and Bougainville		1949–69	37	11.5 ⎭	(1970)
Philippines	H	1959–65	1 911	8.5	Bayani-Sioson *et al.* (1967)
Tonga		1975–78	64	17.9	Felszer (1979)
USSR					
Arctic region		1944–50		7.7	Kandror (1961)
Moscow		1956		11.9 ⎫	Lipovetskaya and
		1973		7.8 ⎭	Yampol'skaya (1975)

[a]Unless otherwise stated, data are from the United Nations *Demographic Yearbooks* (1975, 1981). Although these data are purported to relate to maternities, this is not always certain, as indicated in the notes below. Literature sources suggest that the rates in Japan and Australia are about half those indicated in the 1981 *Yearbook*, and hence the published figures have been taken as relating to babies (footnote [i]).

The figures obtained from the *Yearbooks* for some other countries appear sufficiently high for it to be surprising that no reports appear to have been published, and the figures may therefore relate to babies rather than maternities. The countries involved are the Seychelles, Tunisia, Brazil, Chile, Ecuador, Cyprus, Singapore, Guam and the Pacific Islands.

These data from the *Yearbooks* mostly relate to pregnancies ending in live birth, whereas the data for which other references are given relate to maternities with delivery of live or stillborn babies.

[b]H—hospital series, otherwise deliveries in a defined geographical area.

[c]Includes maternities ending in births other than of known twins or singletons.

[d]UN *Demographic Yearbook* 1975 provides breakdown by 'race'; the method of classification is uncertain and therefore the figures have been pooled.

[e-h,j]Figures appear to change from maternities (M) to individual babies (B), or vice versa:

Canada	B → M in 1974
El Salvador	M → B in 1980
Mexico	M → B in 1976
Israel	M → B in 1973; B → M in 1979; M → B in 1980
New Zealand	M → B in 1975

[g]According to the 1981 *Yearbook*, the data from Mexico relate to confinements ending in live births or fetal deaths for all years except 1976.

[i]Figures in 1981 *Yearbook* have been taken as referring to individual babies rather than to maternities.

[j]Excluding countries for which it is unclear whether figures relate to maternities or individual babies.

[k]All previous deliveries of women surveyed in 1945–1946 who were aged 15 or more.

[l]According to the 1981 *Yearbook*, the data from New Zealand relate to confinements ending in live births or fetal deaths in the period 1972–1974.

first 6 months of 1974 with multiple births among relatives (not defined) as assessed by self-administered questionnaire with a response rate of just 70%, and (2) age-specific fertility rates in 1960 (but not in 1975, the other year considered), have been reported (Inouye and Imaizumi, 1981). The proportion of mothers of twins who had been treated with ovulation-stimulating hormones in the 1974 sample is negatively correlated with the DZ twinning rate, but this is not statistically significant.

Intermediate Prevalence In Europe, the continent for which the data are most complete, variation in twinning rates is 1½-fold–2-fold.

Davenport (1930) suggested a positive correlation between twinning rates and latitude which, in the main, appears to be confirmed by data from Europe, Japan, and the USA. Bulmer (1960a) reported that the twinning rates increased from a low level in the south-west of Europe to a high level in the north-east, similar to the pattern observed in Japan. DZ twinning rates appear to increase with latitude in France in different time periods (Lazar *et al.*, 1978; Hemon *et al.*, 1979a), in England and Wales in the late 1940s and within the USA in 1964 (James, 1985). Variations between European countries during the late 1950s and early 1960s also fit this pattern (James, 1985). However, within Italy and Spain, DZ rates decrease with latitude (Bulmer, 1960a). There is no substantial variation in twinning rates amongst the provinces of Canada (Elwood, 1978), but in this instance analysis by province is a test of variation by longitude rather than by latitude.

Bulmer (1970) suggested that the geographical variations within Europe may, in part, be due to genetic factors. Population consanguinity levels increase from northern to southern Europe (McCullough and O'Rourke, 1986), i.e. are negatively correlated with DZ twinning rates. This is consistent with the finding that inbreeding has no effect on twinning rates (Morton and Schull, 1953). From a study of reproductive outcome consequent on mating between migrant groups in Hawaii, Morton *et al.* (1967) concluded that DZ twinning is a partially recessive maternal trait. Further evidence on the possible role of genetic factors in twinning, from family studies within populations is discussed in Chapter 5.

James (1985) argues that the genetic hypothesis is implausible in view of the correlations between twinning rates, mean birthweight and latitude observed in both Europe and the USA. It is highly unlikely that similar genetic clines would have become established in both continents. In the UK, birthweight varies substantially between the social classes (Butler and Bonham, 1963; Illsley and Samphier, 1985) and there is a high correlation in international data between birthweight and income (Boldman and Reed, 1977). James (1985) found no correlation between income and latitude within the USA and noted that incomes decline with increasing latitude in the UK. He concluded that there was no association between the general level of affluence and DZ

Table 4.4. Variation in twinning rates in Nigeria

Region and population	Main ethnic group	Period of study	No. of twin maternities	Twinning rate (per 1000 maternities)	Reference
WESTERN					
Igbo-Ora	Yoruba	1963–69	289	47.0 ⎫	Nylander (1978)
Ibadan: Adeoyo and UCH	Yoruba	1967–69	1 459	66.5 ⎬	Nylander (1971b)
Oke-Offa and UCH	Yoruba only	1967–69	580	54.2 ⎭	
Ilesha: Wesley Guild Hospital	Yoruba	1940–57	158	53.2	Knox and Morley (1960)
Wesley Guild Hospital	Yoruba	1960–68	822	76.1	Mulligan (1970)
MIDWESTERN					
Delivered in Ibadan	Edo, Urhobo and others	1967–69	35	33.4	Nylander (1971b)
EASTERN					
Delivered in Ibadan	Ibo and Ijaw	1967–69	11	41.7	Nylander (1971b)
Ama Achara: Methodist Hospital	Ibo	1958–60	117	55.7	Cox (1963)

Location	Hospital	Ethnic group	Years	Number	%	Reference
Anua:	St Luke's Hospital	Ibo and Ibibio	1956–60	35	33.4	Nylander (1967)
Calabar:	Maternity Hospital	Efik	1964	44	50.5	Waboso (1966)
Enugu:	Teaching Hospital	Ibo	1974–78	558	34.1	Azubuike (1982)
	Maternity Hospital		1974–75	166	31.3	
Oko:	Community Hospital	Ibo	1977–78	40	40.0	
Umuahia:	Queen Elizabeth Hospital	Ibo	1958–60	112	34.1	Cox (1963)
NORTHERN						
Delivered in Ibadan		Hausa, Fulani and others	1967–69	2	19.4	Nylander (1971b)
Kano: General Hospital		Hausa and Fulani	1965–66	174	30.2	Imam (1967)
Katsina: Maternity Hospital		Hausa	1974–78	228	39.7	Rehan and Tafida (1980)
Zaria, General Hospital		Hausa and Fulani	1968	44	27.9	Lister (1969)
Zaria, Ahmadu Bello University Hospital		Hausa and Fulani	1976–79	118	26.3	Harrison and Rossiter (1985)

twinning, which would be supported by the inconsistent findings regarding
social class (see Chapter 5). By contrast, twinning rates may be positively
correlated with per capita milk and potato consumption. Photoperiodicity is
another possible explanation, but the evidence of seasonality in DZ twinning,
which would be expected on the basis of this hypothesis, is inconclusive. Data
are required on levels of pituitary action in those latitudes where the photoperiodicity is most extreme (James, 1985).

Hemon *et al.* (1979a) found statistically significant, but moderate (maximum 0.49), positive correlations between birth rates and DZ twinning rates
in France. This was regarded as consistent with the hypothesis (Lazar, 1976;
Lazar *et al.*, 1978) that there is a higher probability that a fetus from a DZ than
from a MZ pair or a singleton pregnancy will be aborted spontaneously. The
authors suggest that the risk of abnormality in each member of a DZ twin pair
is independent and therefore a fetus in such a pregnancy is more likely to be
abnormal. In a later paper, however, the association between birth rates and
DZ twinning rates was regarded as consistent with the hypothesis first
advanced by Allen and Schachter (1970) that twin-prone mothers conceive
with greater ease than other women (Hemon *et al.*, 1981b) but this has not
been confirmed in an analytical study by Wyshak (1985). Zahalkova and
Zudova (1984) found a geographical correlation between twinning rates and
rates of recognised spontaneous abortion in Czechoslovakia.

High Prevalence   Nigeria is the only country for which there are consistent
reports of high twinning rates. Variations in twinning rates reported from
Nigeria are shown in Table 4.4. All of the data except from the study in
Igbo-Ora (Nylander, 1978) are from hospital series but the differences appear
to persist when only booked cases are considered and when rates are
standardised for maternal age and parity (Nylander, 1971a). Twinning rates
are highest amongst the Yoruba in the western part of the country and
amongst the ethnic groups in the eastern area. The next highest rate is for the
midwestern area, but there is only one report (Nylander, 1971b). Rates are
lowest among the various ethnic groups of northern Nigeria, most notably the
Hausa and Fulani. The rate reported by Rehan and Tafida (1980) appears to
be high. Although more than three-quarters of the mothers of twins in this
series were unbooked, the authors argue that the various referral factors
'cancel out' and refer to a small community-based study in which a similar
twinning rate was found. However, the MZ twinning rate as estimated by
Weinberg's rule (10.4 per 1000) is high and therefore suggestive of some
peculiarities of referral or recording. It is clear that twinning rates in Nigeria
do not correlate with latitude. Nylander (1978) suggests that the variation by
geographical area and ethnic origin is related to social class, which has a very
marked influence on twinning in Nigeria (see below).

Inferences about Zygosity Distribution

As described in Chapter 2, there are at least two types of twin, monozygotic (MZ) and dizygotic (DZ). Most investigations on the epidemiology of the two types of twinning have had to be based on series of twins where the only indication of zygosity is sex-pairing, from which estimates of zygosity distributions are made by Weinberg's difference rule. The keystone of the Weinberg rule is that DZ pairs should be equally likely to be of the same or of the opposite sex. The method is based on three assumptions:

1. The sex ratio is 1 : 1.
2. The sexes of DZ co-twins are determined independently and with the same probability in all parents.
3. Selective factors, taken to include prenatal loss and ascertainment at birth, are the same among unlike-sexed and like-sexed DZ twins.

Departure of the sex ratio from 1 : 1 in either direction reduces the expected proportion of pairs of opposite sex, and thus the estimated number of DZ pairs of the same sex, in turn leading to an over-estimation of the number of MZ pairs. In practice, such over-estimation is small and correction is inappropriate in view of other potential sources of error (Bulmer, 1970; Allen, 1981; Boklage, 1985).

If there were a negative association between the 'sex' of the two fertilising sperm, then the proportion of DZ pairs of the same sex would be over-estimated and the proportion of MZ pairs would be under-estimated. The converse would apply if there were a positive association between the 'sex' of the fertilising sperm. There is some evidence in favour of a positive association but none published supporting a negative association (Boklage, 1985). Sperm has been separated into fractions with different proportions of X and Y bearers (Roberts, 1972). If such separation occurs in the male or female genital tract, the sex of two embryos conceived at the same time would be correlated. Sex ratio appears to vary markedly with time between ovulation and insemination (Guerrero, 1970, 1974; Harlap, 1979; James, 1979).

Selection bias as regards sex distribution is particularly important in studies based on adults (Allen, 1981). It may be of importance in studies based on hospital populations of births if certain complications in twin pregnancy (e.g. intrauterine death, hydramnios and retained second twin) induce mothers expecting a particular type of twins (i.e. like or unlike sex) to seek admission to hospital (Nylander, 1983). More importantly, bias would arise as a result of differential prenatal loss of dizygotic twins of like and unlike sex. Boklage's (1985) reanalysis of the data of Myrianthopoulos (1970) suggests that the fetal mortality of like sex DZ twins resembles that of MZ twins much more than that of DZ twins from pairs of unlike sex.

It would appear that the combined effects of non-independence of the sex determination of DZ pairs and differential prenatal loss as between DZ pairs of like and unlike sex are complex. Overall, there appears to be an excess of DZ pairs of the same sex, due primarily to males (James, 1971). On the one hand, this is consistent with the observation that the primary sex ratio is less than 1 : 1 only when insemination is close to the estimated time of ovulation whereas the DZ twinning rate has been reported to increase with increasing interval between these two events (Harlap et al., 1985). On the other hand, the relationship between pregnancy loss and the interval between ovulation and insemination parallels that for the sex ratio (Guerrero and Rojas, 1975), and there is known to be excess prenatal mortality of males (Lindley and Migeon, 1979; Lowry, 1979; McMillen, 1979). An alternative explanation for the observed positive association between the sexes of members of DZ twin pairs is that the sexes of the fetuses may be related to maternal hormone levels at the time of conception (James, 1986a) and the times of formation of the two zygotes may be close (James, 1984). The net effect of an excess of DZ pairs of the same (male) sex would be a consistent over-estimation of the MZ twinning rate when Weinberg's rule was applied (Boklage, 1985). In terms of estimating the frequencies of twinning by zygosity, the effect is probably small in most populations. However, where the true DZ twinning rate is high, the extent to which MZ rates are over-estimated by Weinberg's rule may be substantial, and this effect is also important when analyses require the assumption that pairs of unlike sex are biologically representative of all DZ pairs.

In the rest of this chapter, unless otherwise stated, twinning rates by zygosity have been estimated by the Weinberg rule. Thus, we adhere to the conventional use of the terms 'dizygotic twinning' and 'monozygotic twinning' as relating to unlike-sex twinning and like-sex twinning respectively.

Monozygotic Twinning

It is generally accepted that most of the geographical variation is due to variation in DZ twinning rates, and that MZ twinning rates are remarkably constant at around 3.5 per 1000 maternities. MZ twinning rates as high as 10 or 11 per 1000 have been reported (Cox, 1963; Bulmer, 1970; Rehan and Tafida, 1980). However, such high rates have related to hospital series and are generally regarded as an artefact of selection bias consequent upon the higher rate of complications associated with like-sex than with unlike-sex twin pregnancy. Whilst Allen and Hrubec (1986) have been able to identify constant values within populations for the MZ rate and constant, or nearly constant, values for the DZ same sex : opposite sex ratio, the values of these constants differ between different populations. On the other hand, there appear to be few reported associations betwen MZ twinning rates and maternal or environmental factors (Elwood, 1985). A sharp rise in MZ twinning rates at maternal ages over 40 has been noted amongst USA blacks (Enders and Stern, 1948) and amongst African and Asian born migrants to Israel (Modan *et al.*, 1968) and in north-east Scotland (see Appendix to Chapter 5). Bulmer (1970) reported a small but consistent increase in the MZ twinning rate with maternal age in data from Denmark, England and Wales, France, Italy and the USA. The pattern has also been observed in Canada (Elwood, 1978), Hawaii (Morton *et al.*, 1967), Japan (Inouye and Imaizumi, 1981; Imaizumi and Inouye, 1984), Nigeria (Harrison and Rossiter, 1985) and Taiwan (Lin and Chen, 1968). James (1974) suggested that this association with maternal age could be an artefact produced by inclusion of like-sex DZ pairs as the proportion of DZ pairs which are of like sex may be greater than 0.5. Elwood's (1978) analysis took account of this possibility and the maternal age effect persisted. Maternal age effects were noted in two series in which zygosity was determined directly—Ibadan (Nylander, 1971b) and the National Collaborative Perinatal Project (NCPP) in the USA (Myrianthopoulos, 1970)—but not in a third in Aberdeen (Nylander, 1971a) (see Appendix to Chapter 5). Excesses at young maternal ages have been recorded in Hungary (Czeizel, 1974) and in India (Rao *et al.*, 1983). Variations in MZ rates with parity (Waterhouse, 1950; Morton *et al.*, 1967) (see Appendix to Chapter 5), and over time (Parisi and Caperna, 1981; James, 1983) have also been observed. In general, such variations are small and hence minor violations of the assumptions of the Weinberg rule may be important, making the variations difficult to interpret (Elwood, 1985).

Secular Trends

Evidence regarding the ubiquity of a decline in opposite sex twinning rates has been considered by James (1972 and 1982a) and Elwood (1985). Starting in the middle or late 1950s, opposite sex twinning rates declined substantially in Europe, Canada, Japan, Australia and New Zealand. As adequate data are not available, evidence of a decline in the USA is less certain (Allen, 1986); if one occurred, it seems to have been confined to white women aged more than 30 and black women aged more than 25 (James, 1982a; Elwood, 1985). The data from the USA also suggest an end to the decline in the 1970s. The decline appears to have ceased in Czechoslovakia, Denmark, Hungary, Norway, Sweden and Switzerland around the end of the 1960s, and in Canada and Great Britain in the mid 1970s, but to have continued in other countries into the 1970s (Elwood, 1985; James, 1986b).

Data from other countries and for further years are required in order to determine whether or not the stabilisation or slight increase in the cases of Canada, Czechoslovakia, Great Britain, Hungary and Switzerland is transient (Elwood, 1985). The pattern is complicated by the increased use of ovulation-stimulating preparations in the treatment of infertility. James (1986b) suggests that an additional factor may be increased legislative control of the environment.

Two recent studies, one in France and one in Nottinghamshire, England, showed at least 11% and up to 15% of twin births occurred after the use of ovulation-stimulating preparations as compared to 2% of singletons (Hemon *et al.*, 1981a; Webster and Elwood, 1985). The figures from a recent study in the USA were 4.3% and 3.4% respectively (Wyshak, 1985). In Japan in 1974, 4.5% of mothers of twin pairs of like sex and 9.2% of mothers of pairs of unlike sex had received ovulation-stimulating agents; no data were presented on mothers of singletons (Inouye and Imaizumi, 1981). It would be relevant to know the figures for the Eastern European countries mentioned and for Canada.

Data on series of twins studied over 40 years or more are summarised in Table 4.5. There were large peaks in twinning rates in Italy in 1919 and in the USA in 1946. There are also signs of a peak at the end of the Second World War in data from Canada, Denmark, Scotland and perhaps Hungary. Allen and Schachter (1970, 1971) showed that the peak in California followed exactly 9 months after the peak number of military discharges following the end of the Second World War. The peak in twin births occurred 2–3 months before the peak in all births, suggesting that women prone to bearing twins find it easier to conceive than other women rather than superfecundation. The 1919 peak in the USA is not associated with large-scale demobilisation and in some regions in Italy, the twinning rate peaked before the demobilisation following the First World War (Parisi, 1986). The low rate in the Netherlands in 1945 may be a chance fluctuation but might be linked with the famine (Bulmer, 1959b).

Rates declined in the inter-war years in Canada, Denmark, France, the Netherlands and Sweden, but not in Finland, Germany, Hungary, Italy or the USA. It would be interesting to relate these figures to indices of the state of the economies of these countries. Parisi (1986), for example, notes that twinning rates started to decline in northern Italy after the unification of the country whereas there was no decline in southern Italy until after the Second World War. He suggests that both declines are related to industrialisation, but as the nature of change in exposures associated with industrialisation differ between the two periods, he speculates that emotional factors provoking neuroendocrine responses, rather than specific environmental exposures, may be involved.

Bulmer (1959b) examined trends in twinning rates during the period 1936–1950 in five European countries. There was no change in the rate of decline of twinning rates in Denmark, north-west France or Sweden during this period, in all of which there is no evidence of under-nutrition during the Second World War. By contrast, DZ twinning rates fell sharply in 1941, and less markedly in 1942 in the rest of France, the Netherlands and Norway, all of whose populations suffered considerable under-nutrition. The rates in these countries returned to the pre-war levels in 1947. In the Netherlands alone, there was a further sharp fall in twinning rates in 1945, which may have been due to the 'famine winter' of 1944–1945. Time trends are consistent with this hypothesis, but geographical variations in twinning rates within the Netherlands are not (Eriksson *et al.*, 1986). Bulmer suggests three possible explanations for the link between low twinning rates and under-nutrition:

1. Decrease in gonadotrophin secretion by the pituitary; this is known to follow prolonged underfeeding in other mammals.
2. Decline in male fertility.
3. Increase in prenatal mortality; as estimated MZ twinning rates did not change over the 15 year period, the increased prenatal mortality would have to be confined to the period before MZ splitting occurs.

In contrast to this work, some authors are of the opinion that the twinning rate increases in times of food shortage. Cristalli (1924) noted an increase in the number of multiple births in Naples during and after the First World War and suggested that food privation might be one explanation. In eastern Nigeria, Cox (1963) found that the twinning rate was highest amongst poorer rural women despite the fact that this group also suffered the most from malnutrition. He suggested that riboflavine or protein deficiency, or both, might be of aetiological importance. However, these women also tend to belong to the Yoruba tribe and Nylander (1978) has suggested that certain plant foods which form a staple part of the non-urban Yoruba diet may contain hormone-like substances (see Chapter 3). In a preliminary report, Marinho *et al.* (1986) have implicated changes in dietary habits in halving the twinning rate in western Nigeria. Other authors have found no association between food privation and the twinning rate (Balard, 1924; Siemens, 1926; Eriksson, 1973).

Rates were generally stable in the late 1940s and the 1950s. The subsequent decline appears to have been virtually universal in developed countries.

Some of these phenomena appear to have been confined to specific age groups, in France and in USA black women aged 25 or more (Hemon *et al.*, 1981b; James, 1982a), in the USA women aged 30 or more (Jeanneret and MacMahon, 1962; James, 1982a) and in Denmark women aged 35 or more (Rachootin and Olsen, 1980). Hemon *et al.* (1981b) suggest that the recent decline is due to an increase in unrecognised spontaneous abortion which is positively associated with maternal age while James (1982a) suggests that the decline has been obscured in young women by the use of ovulation-stimulating agents.

Recently, the MZ twinning rate as estimated by Weinberg's rule in Great

Table 4.5. Summary of selected studies of twinning rates over the longer term (40 years or more)

Country or area	Period of study	Before First World War	Immediately after First World War	1920–1939	During Second World War	Immediately after Second World War	1946/7 onwards	Reference
Australia	1920–1969			Stable	Gradual increase	Suggestion of a peak in 1944 rather than 1945	Gradual increase until 1953, then decline	Brackenridge (1977)
Canada	1926–1970			Considerable decline	Decline continued	Small peak in 1945	Gradual increase until 1958, then decline	Elwood (1973)
Denmark	1931–1977			Decline apparent in mothers aged 35+	Fairly stable	Small peak for mothers aged 35+ in 1946	Steady decline	Rachootin and Olsen (1980)
Finland	1861–1960	Slight decline	Data presented in 10-year group	No change	Data presented in 10-year group	Data presented in 10-year group	Stable	Eriksson and Fellman (1973)
France	1901–1968	No consistent pattern in maternal age-specific rates	War years excluded	Decline apparent in mothers aged 25+	War years excluded	Data presented in 5-year group	Decline in mothers aged 25+	Hemon et al. (1981b)
Germany, Gorlitz	1611–1860	Twinning rates seem to have fluctuated secularly with a cycle of about 150 years						Richter et al. (1984)
Germany	1901–1939	Stable	Slight drop	Stable				Kruger and Propping (1976)
Hungary	1920–1981	Stable		Stable	Data incomplete	Peak?	Rates fairly stable until 1960, then decline until 1969	Metneki and Czeizel (1983)

Italy	1868–1977	Marked fluctuations in earliest years followed by relatively stable rates	Large peak in 1919	Stable in 1920s and 1930s. Marked changes between the 2 decades, probably an artefact	Fairly stable	No obvious peak	Steady decline	Parisi and Caperna (1981)
The Netherlands	1900–1971	Apparently stable	Data presented in 5-year group, no change	Steady decline	Low rate in 1945	No obvious peak	Rates fairly stable in 1950s, then declined	Hoogendoorn (1973)
Sweden	1861–1960	Stable	Data presented in 10-year group	Decline in 1930s	Data presented in 10-year group		Steady decline	Eriksson and Fellman (1973)
UK. Scotland	1856–1977[a]	Data incomplete but some evidence of a decline	Data presented in 5-year group	Data incomplete				⎫ MacGillivray (1981)
	1939–1977				Apparently stable	Small peak	Steady increase to 1958, then steady decline	⎭
USA. Utah	1820–1944	Data unreliable before 1860; downward trend to 1880, then increase	Slight peak in 1919	Stable in 1920s, decline in 1930s	Decline			Carmelli et al. (1981)
Virginia	1918–1977			⎱ fairly stable	Decline confined to southern and mountain regions		Largely stable through 1950s then decline	Mosteller et al. (1981)
whole country	1922–1958			⎰		Peak in 1946		Jeanneret and MacMahon (1962)

[a] = percentage of mothers who had multiple births.

Britain has been noted as having increased during the same period when the DZ rates were declining (James, 1980c; Emery, 1986). A similar pattern has been noted in Belgium, Denmark, the Netherlands, Norway and Switzerland, and there is evidence of an increase in the estimated MZ rate (Bressers *et al.*, 1986). It has been suggested that this trend is linked to increasing use of oral contraceptives (Bressers *et al.*, 1986; Emery, 1986). However, there is evidence of an increase in the estimated MZ twinning rate predating the introduction of oral contraception from the Aland Islands, Finland and from the Federal Republic of Germany (Bressers *et al.*, 1986). In addition a zygosity distribution had to be inferred by the Weinberg rule; in all of these countries all that is certain is that the overall twinning rate and the unlike-sex DZ rate declined. If the greater proportion of DZ pairs are of like sex, as James (1971) suggests, then the apparent increase in estimated MZ rate may be an artefact. A recent study in Aberdeen (Campbell *et al.*, 1987) shows no association between oral contraception use prior to pregnancy and either MZ or DZ twinning (see Chapter 3).

Clustering

Localised high twinning rates have been noted in Norwegian mountain villages (Bonnevie and Sverdrup, 1926), in the Finnish Aland Islands over the period 1750–1899 (Eriksson, 1962), in the Bola sub-district of New Britain (Scragg and Walsh, 1970), in the Romanian village of Eftimie Murgen during the period 1927–1977 (Schmidt *et al.*, 1983) and in Colonsay in the Inner Hebrides, Scotland between 1895 and 1960 (Sheets, 1986). The high rates are not explained by high proportions of older mothers. In isolated small communities such as these, inbreeding is a possibility, which would lead to an increase in the frequency of recessive traits. Bulmer (1970) noted that there was some evidence in favour of the hypothesis that DZ twinning has a sex-limited recessive mode of inheritance, but this has not been confirmed in a study in Nigeria (Nylander, 1970b). Moreover, a study of an isolated community in Quebec suggested that DZ twinning is a dominant trait (Philippe, 1981). Another possibility is that high degrees of out-migration leave a residual population of twin prone relatives. Finally, there may be locaslied environmental effects.

Kallen and Thorbert (1985) studied pregnancy outcome in three parishes in which the inhabitants had complained of air and water pollution consequent on the manufacture of phenoxy acid herbicides in a nearby chemical plant. The twinning rate was higher than expected from regional statistics. The perinatal mortality rate in the twins was higher than in the singletons, a finding consistent with a study of perinatal outcome in women working in laboratories during pregnancy (Ericson *et al.*, 1984). This suggests that twins are more vulnerable to environmental toxins than are singletons, but there are no data relating to prenatal loss.

There appears to be only one published report of temporo-spatial clustering of twinning. Zahalkova (1979) found that some 638 of 1025 twin pairs born in South Moravia, Czechoslovakia during the period 1972–1976 occurred closer together in space and time than would have been expected by chance.

Migrant Studies

It would be of particular interest to know of the twinning rates in migrants from areas of high incidence to areas of low incidence and vice versa.

So far as we are aware, there are no specific data on Nigerian migrants to Europe or North America but some data are available on American populations thought to have West African origins. Bulmer (1960a) concluded that the DZ twinning rate in West Africa is at least 20 per 1000 births; this estimate is based on booked admissions in the Gambia, Nigeria and Zaire in the 1950s. Rates in USA blacks tend to be higher than whites, but very much lower than the rates reported from West Africa, (Lilienfeld and Pasamanick, 1955; Jeanneret and MacMahon, 1962; Shipley et al., 1967; Heuser, 1967; Layde et al., 1980; Mosteller et al., 1981). Similarly, in Antigua Negroes the DZ rate is only 11.5 per 1000 (Bulmer, 1960a). In Salvador, Brazil, where most of the West African ancestry came from the Yoruba (Ramos, 1961), the frequency of dizygotic twins is only 13.6 per 1000 births (Pedreira et al., 1959).

In Nylander's (1971b) survey of deliveries in Ibadan, Nigeria, one twin pair was delivered in 63 maternities to women born in America and Europe, a rate of 15.9 per 1000. Within Nigeria, the twinning rate in the Yoruba resident in the cities of Lagos, Kaduna and Kano is about 30 per 1000 maternities, much lower than the 45 per 1000 maternities amongst those resident in Ibadan (Nylander, 1978). Nylander suggests that the difference is due to diet with the Yoruba migrants to cities other than Ibadan tending to follow a more 'European' diet.

There are data on twinning in Japanese migrants to California (Shipley et al., 1967), Canada, (Elwood, 1978) and Hawaii (Morton et al., 1967). In all three studies, the twinning rates were low, very similar to those in Japan. The peoples of Melanesia and Polynesia are thought to share close common ancestry with the peoples of mainland China and Japan (Pollard, 1985). The only data which would be expected to approximate the position in mainland China are from Taiwan, where twinning rates appear to be similar to those in Japan (Ping and Chin, 1967). Such data as are available from Melanesia and Polynesia suggest higher twinning rates (Pollard, 1985). In view of this observation, it is rather surprising that descendants of Indian immigrants who began to arrive in Fiji (Melanesia) in 1879 have twinning rates close to those of Japan (6.2 per 1000 live maternities) and about 40% lower than those of native Fijians (9.4 per 1000), even after standardising for maternal age, and apparently lower than the rates in the Indian subcontinent.

In Canada, Elwood (1978) found no significant differences between rates for Canadian born women whose families came from different countries in Europe. This contrasts with the differences between European countries, and suggests that the rates are modified by migration.

Modan *et al.* (1968) compared the twinning rate of Israeli-born women with that of immigrants to Israel who had been born in either Europe ('Occidental') or in Africa and Asia ('Oriental'). Maternal age-specific rates of MZ twinning did not differ but the DZ rate was higher in the Oriental group than in the other groups. The DZ rates in all three groups appear to be lower than those in Europe during the same period. It would be of considerable value to re-analyse the Israeli data by separating the groups of women born in African and Asian countries.

Higher Multiple Births

The highest naturally occurring multiple pregnancy recorded so far is nonuplets (Benirschke and Kim, 1973). However, if pregnancies following treatment of infertility by gonadotrophins or by drugs such as clomiphene are excluded, reports of quintuplets and higher multiple pregnancies are rare. Bulmer (1970) has considered combined data on quadruplets from national sources from England and Wales, France, Italy and the USA and reports a frequency of 1.7 per million maternities. This figure has been confirmed for Italy during the overall period 1868–1977, but peaks in excess of 2.6 quadruplet and quintuplet births per million maternities were reached in the periods 1930–1944 and 1970–1977 (Parisi and Caperna, 1981). In the rest of this section, triplets will be the focus of attention.

Hellin (1895) established empirically that the frequencies of the different orders of higher multiple births may be expressed as a power function of the twinning rate. Thus, if the twinning rate in a population is p, the frequency of triplets will be p^2 and of quadruplets p^3 and so forth. Hellin's rule would have biological validity if the conception of higher multiple pregnancies is regarded as a sequence of independent twinning events. In Hellin's formula, no account is taken of the different types of higher multiple—MZ, DZ (symmetrical and asymmetrical), trizygotic, tetrazygotic etc., which may occur. Moreover, no account is taken of variation in maternal age. Nevertheless, the formula appears to provide a rule of thumb for estimating the order of magnitude of rates of triplet and higher multiple pregnancy (Table 4.6). The most notable deviations observed are for Nigeria and Papua. Excesses of

Table 4.6. Summary of reports of frequency of triplets

County or area	Period of study	Twinning rate (per 1000)	Triplet sets				Reference
			Expected[a]		Observed		
			No.	Rate per 100000	No.	Rate per 100000	
Czechoslovakia, Prague	1929–62	10.4	26	10.8	29	12.1	Onyskowova et al. (1971)
Hungary	1960–71	9.9	168	9.8	156	9.1	Czeizel (1974)
Italy	1868–77	11.8		14.0		14.0	Parisi and Caperna (1981)
	1960–69	11.3		12.7		11.5	
	1970–77	9.6		9.2		9.1	
Japan	1951–59	6.4	730	4.1	987	5.6	Imaizumi and Inouye (1979)
	1960–68	6.4	672	4.1	915	5.5	
	1974	5.8	72	3.4	124	5.8	
The Netherlands	1960–71	11.2	366	12.6	270	9.3	Hoogendoorn (1973)
Nigeria, Igbo-Ora	1963–69	47.0	14	220.9	10	162.3	Nylander (1971c)
Ibadan	1967–69	66.5	97	442.2	39	177.8	
Nigeria, Katsina (Hausa)	1974–78	39.7	9	157.2	12	208.7	Rehan and Tafida (1980)
Nigeria, East (Igbo)	1974–78	33.7	26	113.7	18	79.4	Azubuike (1982)
Nigeria, Zaria — booked	1976–79	23.7	8	56.0	6	40.3	Harrison and Rossiter (1985)
unbooked		51.2	20	262.3	10	130.7	
Papua	1970–71	19.1	8	36.7	14	63.7	Archer (1973)
Poland	1949–71	11.5	2002	13.2	1473	9.6	Rola-Janicki (1974)
Singapore	1960–70	8.1	27	6.6	37	9.2	Tan et al. (1971)
Sweden	1921–50	13.5	586	18.1	402	12.4	Herrlin and Hauge (1967)
Taiwan	1956–65	6.0	20	3.7	39	7.2	Lin and Chen (1968)
UK, England and Wales	1938–49	12.2	1215	14.8	842	10.2	Record (1952)
	1971–75	9.8	334	9.6	353	10.2	Brown and Daw (1980)
Northern Ireland	1975–79	10.3	14	10.6	16	12.2	Appendix to Chapter 5
USA	1933–37	11.2	1201	12.6	986	10.3	Jeanneret and MacMahon (1962)
	1949–58	10.1	3473	10.2	2945	8.7	
	1964	10.4		10.9		10.0	Heuser (1967)

[a] On basis of Hellin's formula — square of the twinning rate.

observed to expected numbers of triplets were found in Papua, where the data were from national statistics (Archer, 1973) and Katsina in Nigeria, where excess of obstetric complications expected in a hospital series is thought to have been counterbalanced by a bias in favour of primigravidae in whom rates of multiple pregnancy are low (Rehan and Tafida, 1980). In all of the other instances, there are fewer triplets than expected. Nylander (1971c) suggests that there is under-ascertainment in these hospital series because certain complications of labour (e.g. obstruction) are less likely to occur in triplet and higher multiple pregnancies than in singleton and twin pregnancies because of the small size of the babies. If the rate of abortion in triplet conceptions was higher than in twins, this could also lead to the observed numbers of triplets being less than those expected from Hellin's rule, but adequate data are not available (Nylander, 1971c).

Whereas there are few large series of twins in which the determination of zygosity has been made directly, there appears to be only one series of triplets or higher multiples for which such data are available (Nylander and Corney, 1971). It is generally agreed that the most satisfactory indirect method is that of Allen (1960), which depends on the frequency of DZ triplets being twice the product of the MZ and DZ twinning rates (m and d respectively). This estimation of frequency is based on two assumptions: (1) the probability that two ova will be released is d, (2) the probability that either one of these ova will divide to produce DZ triplets is 2m. Estimation of the other types of triplets proceeds in a manner analogous to the Weinberg rule. All MZ triplets must be of the same sex. It is assumed that half of the DZ triplets will be like sexed and half of unlike sex and that one-quarter of the trizygotic (TZ) triplets will be like sexed and three-quarters of unlike sex. It then follows that the number of TZ triplets of unlike sex is equal to the number of triplets of unlike sex who are not DZ, and the total number of TZ triplets is 4/3 times this number. It further follows that the number of MZ triplets is the number of triplets who are not DZ or TZ.

Triplet rates by zygosity as estimated by Allen's method are presented for selected populations in Table 4.7. It was not possible, from the published data, to adjust for maternal age. The MZ triplet rate is below 3 per 100 000 maternities in all of the studies except Ibadan, which also differs from the other studies in being based on a hospital series rather than on national sources. The difference may therefore be due to bias and chance. The estimated DZ triplet rates in Ibadan are eight times, and the TZ rates sixteen times higher than the next highest rates in the table, a pattern of occurrence similar to, but more exaggerated than that for twinning. The estimated distribution in Ibadan was confirmed by direct determination of zygosity (Nylander and Corney, 1971). Amongst the other countries, the variation in DZ rates is fourfold and in TZ rates sixfold and may in part be due to differences in maternal age. As is the case for twinning, rates of polyovular

Table 4.7. Sex similarity and estimated zygosity distribution of triplets in different populations

Population	Total maternities	Triplet sets			Triplet rates per 100 000 maternities			Reference
		Like sex	Unlike sex	Estd DZ	MZ	DZ	TZ	
Australia, 1920–1969	8 524 000[a]	483	379	452	2.4	5.2	2.4	Brackenridge (1978)
Italy, 1933–1954	20 820 000	1 494	1 596	1 556	2.1	7.5	5.2	Bulmer (1970)
Japan, 1956	1 820 000	73	28	34	2.8	1.9	0.8	
1955–1967	23 652 790[a]	861	469	439	3.3	1.9	0.4	Imaizumi and Inouye (1984)
1974	2 127 000[a]	74	50	31	2.9	1.5	1.2	
Nigeria, Ibadan, 1967–1969	27 980	18	26	16	14.7	56.5	86.1	Nylander (1971c)
Sweden, 1921–1950	3 232 060	152	250	226	1.2	7.1	4.3	Herrlin and Hauge (1967)
UK, England and Wales								
1938–1962	17 700 000	931	999	1 092	1.3	6.2	3.4	Bulmer (1970)
1971–1975	3 468 020	154	199	153	1.1	4.4	4.7	Brown and Daw (1980)
USA, 1933–1937	9 657 199[a]	521	465	531	1.9	5.5	2.8	Jeanneret and
1952–1958	24 762 457[a]	1 992	945	1 164	2.0	4.7	2.0	MacMahon (1962)

[a] = estimated.

triplets in Japan are low. By contrast, rates of MZ triplets and quadruplets in Japan are the highest reported outside Nigeria (Imaizumi and Inouye, 1984).

In other respects, the descriptive epidemiology of triplet delivery resembles that of twinning. The relationship with maternal age has been noted to be an exaggerated form of that for twins (Rola-Janicki, 1974; Brackenridge, 1978). The frequency of MZ triplets does not vary appreciably with maternal age, whereas there is a marked progression in the dependence of DZ and TZ rates (Bulmer, 1970; Brackenridge, 1978). However, there appears to be no association between TZ rates and maternal age in Japan (Imaizumi and Inouye, 1984). James (1980a) identified a winter peak in triplet maternities in England and Wales. This seasonal pattern was similar to that for twin pairs of unlike sex but about double the amplitude.

In view of the decline in DZ twinning rates, a decline in triplet and higher maternities would be expected. Declines in DZ and TZ triplet rates have been reported in Italy since the late 1940s, with the MZ rates remaining roughly constant (Parisi and Caperna, 1981). A decline in the overall rate in the Netherlands and in Poland appears to have started in the late 1950s (Hoogendoorn, 1973; Rola-Janicki, 1974) and in the USA in the late 1940s (Jeanneret and MacMahon, 1962). Evidence from Hungary for the period 1960–1971 is less clear (Czeizel, 1974) and there appears to have been no change in rate in Japan over the period 1951–1967 and 1974 (Imaizumi and Inouye, 1979). In Japan, the rates of MZ and DZ triplets appear to have decreased slightly, while the rates of TZ triplets appear to have increased (Imaizumi and Inouye, 1984). A steady *increase* in the triplet rate in Australia has been reported over the 50 year period 1920–1969 (Brackenridge, 1978). This has been confined to the DZ and TZ types. Together, rates of these types of triplets have increased by 40% over the 50 year period, whereas mean maternal age has declined by 8.6%.

Parisi and Caperna (1981) note that the rate of quadruplet and quintuplet maternities in Italy increased in the 1970s, in contrast to the decline in twin and triplet rates, and the rate predicted on the basis of Hellin's rule. These authors suggest that the use of ovulation-stimulating preparations is likely to increase the probability of multple, not just double, ovulation. In turn, in conditions of low prenatal loss, the result would be an increase in the rate of higher multiple births while twin and triplet rates would remain largely unchanged. However, approximately 20% of pregnancies induced by clomiphene end in abortion while abortion rates of between 12% and 31% have been reported in gonadotrophin induced pregnancy (Schenker et al., 1981). Equally, multiple pregnancies of higher order than triplets may not be as susceptible to the effects of the factors responsible for the decline of twin and triplet rates, or these factors may be less powerful than ovulation-stimulation. Media reports appear to confirm the finding of an increase in quadruplets and higher multiples in other parts of the world (Schenker et al., 1981).

Bulmer (1970) described a theoretical model for multiple births based on the successive processes of multiple ovulation and division of the fertilised ovum into two, three or more embryos. He discussed this in relation to two empirical formulae:

1. the triplet rate = $1.36m^2 + 2md + 0.47d^2$ (MZ + DZ + TZ)
2. the quadruplet rate = $5.4m^3 + 3.7m^2d + 1.4md^2 + 0.72d^3$ (MZ + DZ + trizygotic + tetrazygotic)

where m is the MZ twinning rate and d the DZ twinning rate.

The results of applying Bulmer's formula to data more recently available are presented in Table 4.8. With the exception of data from Nigeria and from the USA for the period 1949–1958, the rates predicted by applying Bulmer's formula are less than those observed, but the agreement is reasonably close.

Bulmer found that the theoretical frequencies of trizygotic triplets and of tetrazygotic quadruplets are considerably greater than the numbers estimated by Allen's method. This is confirmed for triplets in further analysis of data from Nigeria (Nylander, 1971c) but not of data from England and Wales (Brown and Daw, 1980) and Japan (Imaizumi and Inouye, 1984). Again in these Japanese data the tetrazygotic quadruplet rate estimated by Allen's method is some ten times higher than that predicted from Bulmer's formula. Bulmer concluded that some control process reduced the number of higher multiple ovulations below that expected from the number of double ovula-

Table 4.8. Comparison of frequency of triplet sets with that estimated by Bulmer's formula (see text)

	Expected by Bulmer's formula		Observed		
	Number	Rate[a]	Number	Rate[a]	
Australia	793	9.3	862	10.3	Brackenridge (1978)
Hungary, 1960 and 1968	21	7.2	30	10.0	Czeizel (1974)
Japan, 1955–1967	1 041	4.4	1 330	5.6 ⎫	Imaizumi and Inouye
1974	79	3.7	124	5.8 ⎭	(1984)
Nigeria, 1967–1979	58	178.7	44	136.1	Nylander (1971c)
Sweden, 1921–1950	431	13.3	402	12.6	Herrlin and Hauge (1967)
Taiwan, 1956–1965	19	3.5	39	7.2	Lin and Chen (1968)
UK, England and Wales 1971–1975	275	7.9	353	10.2	Brown and Daw (1980)
USA, 1933–1937	950	10.0	986	10.3 ⎫	Jeanneret and
1949–1958	3 013	8.9	2 945	8.7 ⎭	MacMahon (1962)
1964		8.6		10.0	Heuser (1967)

[a] Per 100 000 maternities.

tions. It is tempting to speculate that the more recent findings in England and Wales and Japan reflect the use of ovulation inducing agents. It would be of considerable interest to know the distributions for higher multiple pregnancies achieved as a result of ovulation stimulation, which presumably alters this process of control. Consideration of division of the fertilised ovum to form MZ twin, triplet, quadruplet and higher order sets of embryos showed fair agreement between theory and observation for triplets (Bulmer, 1970). This is also the finding from the more recent studies in England and Wales and Japan, but the rate in Nigeria estimated by Allen's method (12.4/100 000) is some four times that expected from Bulmer's formula (3.0/100 000). The rate of MZ quadruplet pregnancies in pooled data analysed by Bulmer was more than five times, and in Japan during the period 1955–1967 two times, higher than predicted theoretically. Further evidence is required in order to understand further the process of conception of higher multiple sets of embryos and fetuses.

Twinning and Twins
Edited by I. MacGillivray, D. M. Campbell and B. Thompson
© 1988 John Wiley & Sons Ltd

CHAPTER 5

Factors affecting twinning

IAN MACGILLIVRAY

Department of Obstetrics and Gynaecology, University of Aberdeen, Aberdeen, UK

and

MIKE SAMPHIER

Medical Research Council Medical Sociology Unit, University of Glasgow, Glasgow, UK

and

JULIAN LITTLE

Department of Community Medicine and Epidemiology, University of Nottingham, Nottingham, UK

It is clearly established that the descriptive epidemiology of like-sex and unlike-sex twinning is very different. The like-sex twinning rate and, by inference, the MZ twinning rate, appears to remain fairly constant throughout the world. By contrast, there is marked variation in the unlike-sex twinning rate in different parts of the world, and there has been a substantial decline reported from many countries (Editorial, 1976). In this chapter, various factors reported to affect twinning will be reviewed.

Parity

Probably the first to recognise that twinning was more likely to occur in higher parity women was Matthews Duncan, a graduate of Aberdeen University, in his paper 'On the comparative frequency of twin bearing in different pregnancies' in 1865. His observations have been confirmed by many workers since (for example, Guttmacher, 1937; Anderson, 1956; Bulmer, 1959a; Eriksson and Fellman, 1967). However, a few authors have not been able to demonstrate any definite association with parity (Dahlberg, 1926; Lamy *et al.*, 1955; Gedda, 1961).

Nylander (1975b) found that twinning rates in the populations of both Ibadan (Nigeria) and Aberdeen (Scotland) increased with parity, but that the increase applied only to DZ twinning. The MZ twinning rates were similar

Table 5.1. Aberdeen City District (1951–1983): parity distribution of twins and singletons

Parity	1951–61		1962–72		1973–83		All years	
	Twins %	Singletons %	Twins %	Singletons %	Twins %	Singletons %	Twins %	Singletons %
0	39.0	38.8	29.8	39.9	44.8	45.4	37.1	40.9
1	27.0	30.4	36.2	31.8	36.9	36.9	32.4	32.6
2	16.0	16.1	19.6	16.7	12.3	13.2	16.4	15.6
3	8.9	7.9	9.2	7.2	5.2	3.3	8.2	6.4
4	5.5	3.8	2.5	2.8	0.4	0.8	3.3	2.7
5+	3.6	3.0	2.7	1.6	0.4	0.4	2.6	1.8
Total %	100.0	100.0	100.0	100.0	100.0	100.0	100.0	100.0
n	495	36 994	403	35 400	252	26 171	1 150	98 565
χ^2	6.6748		20.5248		3.3269		913.4609	
d.f.	5		5		5		5	
$p \leqq$	NS		0.001		NS		0.001	

and remained fairly constant (see Chapter 4). More recent data for north-east Scotland and Northern Ireland presented in the Appendix to this chapter confirm no association between like-sex twinning and parity. However, an association beween unlike-sex twinning and parity in Northern Ireland is not so apparent in north-east Scotland, this result being markedly affected by secular trends in childbearing towards smaller, planned families. Table 5.1 shows that for Aberdeen City District, the association of parity with twinning between 1951 and 1983 was highly significant, but was not a consistent feature over time. In each 11 year period, however, the twinning rate was highest in either parity 3 or 4 and over (Table 5.2). Table 5.3 shows that in the 15 year period for which zygosity was available only DZ twinning was significantly associated with higher parity ($p \leqslant 0.001$).

In Japanese data for 1974, the pattern of change in DZ *and* MZ twinning rates with increasing birth order was inconsistent between the different maternal age groups (Inouye and Imaizumi, 1981). No overall birth order effect was detected when analysis was performed using a linear regression model whereas an additive effect and an interaction with maternal age was identified when a quadratic model was used. Allen and Schachter (1970) suggested that women who have twins conceive with greater ease than other

Table 5.2. Aberdeen City District (1951–1983): twinning rates in three periods by parity, age and height

	1951–61	1962–72	1973–83	All years
Parity				
0	13.3	8.4	9.4	10.4
1	11.8	12.8	9.5	11.5
2	13.1	13.2	8.9	12.2
3	14.8	14.2	14.9	14.6
4+	17.6	13.3	6.3	15.3
Age				
−19	10.1	5.3	6.9	6.9
20–24	14.3	9.5	8.2	9.1
25–29	12.4	13.0	10.4	12.0
30–34	18.2	13.4	13.4	15.5
35+	14.6	18.1	9.3	15.0
Height				
Short	11.1	10.4	7.1	10.0
Medium	13.5	11.0	9.6	11.5
Tall	15.3	12.6	10.9	12.8
All	13.2	11.3	9.5	11.5

Table 5.3. Aberdeen City District (1969–1983): parity distribution by zygosity

Parity	Zygosity			All Twins %	Singletons %
	MZ %	DZ %	Not stated %		
0	45.3	32.7	43.2	38.5	44.4
1	35.8	38.7	43.2	38.0	35.6
2	14.2	17.1	10.9	15.4	14.0
3	3.4	8.5	2.7	6.0	4.2
4+	1.3	3.0	–	2.1	1.8
Total	100.0	100.0	100.0	100.0	100.0
n	148	199	37	384	38 184

All twins vs singletons $\chi^2 = 7.2899$, d.f. 4, not significant
MZ vs DZ $\chi^2 = 8.7731$, d.f. 4, not significant
MZ vs singletons $\lambda^2 = 0.4327$, d.f. 4, not significant
DZ vs singletons $\lambda^2 = 18.4856$, d.f. 4, $p \leqslant 0.001$

women. If this were true, then, in a society in which little birth control were practised, a parity effect could be an artefact of these women having more pregnancies than other women and forming a higher proportion of older mothers and of high-parity groups. In these circumstances, a specific parity effect could be demonstrated by investigating the order of delivery within sibships in which a twin birth had occurred. Allen (1978) performed an analysis of this type and found a parity effect which could account for most of the observed variation in population twinning rates with parity. Such a parity effect could be linked to Milham's gonadotrophin hypothesis (see Chapter 3).

Age

Matthews Duncan (Duncan, 1865) also found that the highest rate of twinning was in women from 35 to 39 years of age and that on each side of this 'climax of fertility' the tendency to twinning gradually diminished. The mean age of twin-bearing mothers was greater than that of other mothers and newly married mothers were more liable to have twins the older they were.

Duncan's observations were later confirmed by Guttmacher (1937) and McArthur (1952). Several authors have since shown that in Britain it is the DZ twinning rate that increases with maternal age to a maximum in the age group 35–39 years and decreases thereafter (Anderson, 1956; Registrar General for England and Wales, 1958; Bulmer, 1959a: Millis, 1959; Eriksson and Fellman, 1967). Nylander (1975c) in his studies in Aberdeen and Ibadan, Nigeria found a similar pattern, but in Ibadan the peak rate of twinning occurred earlier, in the 30–34 year age group.

It is now generally accepted that DZ Twinning rates in Europe, Canada, Japan and amongst USA whites increase markedly with maternal age to a peak in the late 30s and then decline (Bulmer, 1970; James, 1972; Wyshak, 1975; Elwood, 1978; Imaizumi and Inouye, 1979). In most studies the form of the curve describing this association is an inverted 'V'. One exception is the study of Myrianthopoulos (1970) which showed an increase to age group 30–34, a fall, and then an increase at ages of 40 or more. In USA blacks, twinning rates in the 30–34 age group are similar to those at ages 35–39, and there is a less marked fall in women aged 40 or more (Heuser, 1967), but this was not confirmed in data from Virginia (Mosteller et al., 1981). In data from California, there was no decline in DZ rates at maternal ages of 40 or more during the period 1940–1949, but the variation in age-specific rates in the period 1950–1959 resembled that described by Heuser (Shipley et al., 1967). A pattern similar to the Californian findings for 1940–1949 was observed for Mormon women who were themselves twins or sisters of twins (Carmelli et al., 1981).

The fall in twinning rates at the highest maternal ages has been explained as exhaustion of the Graafian follicles as the menopause approaches (Nylander, 1975c). The younger peak in the twinning rates in Nigeria as compared to Europe may be related to the earlier ages at which families are started, resulting in an earlier peak of ovarian activity. It would be interesting to compare maternal age effects between other areas with different ages at onset of childbearing.

Mosteller et al. (1981) suggested separate effects of birth order and maternal age might be due to quantum increases in pituitary gonadotrophin levels with parity added independently to steadily increasing levels due to maternal age. It may no longer be possible to establish a separate contribution of parity, in a population like Aberdeen where the two child family has become the norm (see below).

In Aberdeen City District from 1951 to 1983 women who delivered twins were significantly older than those who had a singleton birth and this applied in the three 11 year periods (Table 5.4) although to a lesser extent more recently. The mean age of primigravidae who delivered twins was always greater than that for those who delivered singletons in each quinquennium and also in the following three years, 1981–1983. The same applied to multigravidae with one minor discrepancy in 1976–1980. Table 5.2 shows that overall and for the extreme 11 year periods the highest twinning rate was in the 30–34 age group whereas it was highest in the older ages in the middle period. Data from 1969 to 1983 show that the mean age of mothers who had DZ twins was significantly greater than that of those who had singletons irrespective of parity (Table 5.5). Ages of mothers of MZ twins were similar to those of mothers of singletons. It may be noted that mothers of MZ twins with a monochorionic (MC) placenta were younger than those where the

Table 5.4. Aberdeen City District (1951–1983): maternal age distribution for twins and singletons

Year	1951–61		1962–72		1973–83		All years	
	Twins %	Singletons %	Twins %	Singletons %	Twins %	Singletons %	Twins %	Singletons %
−19	4.7	5.8	5.5	11.8	8.3	11.6	5.8	9.5
20–24	24.6	33.2	31.3	37.0	31.3	36.6	28.5	35.5
25–29	31.4	31.8	33.7	29.1	37.0	33.8	33.5	31.4
30–34	27.2	18.7	17.1	14.4	19.4	13.8	21.8	15.8
35+	12.1	10.5	12.4	7.7	4.0	4.2	10.4	7.8
Total %	100.0	100.0	100.0	100.0	100.0	100.0	100.0	100.0
n	471	36891	403	35381	252	26171	1126	98443
χ^2	29.9469		33.7240		10.6060		67.5380	
d.f.	4		4		4		4	
$p \leq$	0.001		0.001		0.05		0.001	

Table 5.5. Aberdeen City District (1969–1983): mean ages by parity for mothers of singletons and of twins by zygosity and placentation

	Mean age	SD	No.
Primiparae			
Singletons	22.97	4.37	16 946
Twins: MZ MC	23.82	4.95	34[a]
MZ DC	24.31	4.18	29[a]
DZ	26.03	5.21	65
Not stated	23.25	4.89	16
Multiparae			
Singletons	26.74	4.75	21 231
Twins: MZ MC	26.15	3.68	34[a]
MZ DC	26.80	4.32	45[a]
DZ	27.63	4.81	134
Not stated	25.14	4.09	21

Significant comparisons—all others not significant
Primiparae
Singletons *vs* DZ twins $\quad t = 5.63\ p \leqslant 0.01$
MZ *vs* DZ twins $\quad t = 2.03\ p \leqslant 0.05$
Multiparae
Singletons *vs* DZ twins $\quad t = 2.17\ p \leqslant 0.05$

[a]Excluding 3 MZ primigravidae and multiparae respectively because placentation uncertain.

placenta was dichorionic (DC), and in primigravidae they were significantly younger than mothers of DZ twins.

Bulmer (1959a) noted a small *paternal* age effect in twinning in data from the USA and Egypt, but not from New Zealand. He concluded that this effect was due, at least in part, to the increased parity of women whose husbands were older as compared to those who were older than their husbands. However, some authors have noted the possibility of a paternal effect in twinning (Greulich, 1934; Carmelli *et al.*, 1981; Parisi *et al.*, 1983: Schmidt *et al.*, 1983). Data on paternal age were available from Northern Ireland (see Appendix). Although there appears to be a small paternal age effect which persists after adjusting for maternal age and parity, this is not statistically significant.

Height

It was pointed out over a century ago (Tchouriloff, 1877) that tall women are more likely to produce twins than small women. This has been confirmed by

Table 5.6. Aberdeen City District (1951–1983): maternal height distribution for twins and singletons

Height	1951–61		1962–72		1973–83		All years	
	Twins %	Singletons %	Twins %	Singletons %	Twins %	Singletons %	Twins %	Singletons %
Short (under 155 cm)	26.3	30.9	23.9	25.6	15.0	20.1	23.0	26.2
Medium (155–163 cm)	55.5	53.7	53.5	54.4	56.1	55.0	54.9	54.2
Tall (164 cm and over)	18.2	15.4	22.6	20.0	28.9	24.9	22.1	19.6
Total %	100.0	100.0	100.0	100.0	100.0	100.0	100.0	100.0
n^*	483	36 623	398	35 227	246	25 886	1127	97 736
χ^2	6.0018		1.8563		4.7139		7.9370	
d.f.	2		2		2		2	
$p \leq$	0.05		NS		NS		0.02	

*Excluding height not recorded.

Table 5.7. Aberdeen City District (1969–1983): maternal height by twinning rates—crude and standardised for age and parity

Maternal height[a]	Zygosity			
	MZ	DZ	Not stated	All twins
Crude rates per 1000 maternities				
Short	3.53	3.40	0.88	7.81
Medium	3.98	4.88	1.09	9.95
Tall	3.50	7.01	0.64	11.15
Rates standardised for age and parity				
Short	3.5	3.6	0.8	—
Medium	4.0	4.9	1.0	—
Tall	3.5	6.7	0.5	—

[a]Short = Under 155 cm.
Tall = 164 cm and over.

many authors since then, for example (MacArthur, 1942; Anderson, 1956; Nylander, 1971a; Campbell *et al.*, 1974).

The most recent analysis of Aberdeen City District data for 1951–1983 shows an association between twinning and maternal height in favour of tall women (Table 5.6). The women were classified as short (under 155 cm), medium or tall (164 cm and over) as defined by Bernard (1952) after review of adult stature in Aberdeen. The association of twinning with increased height, however, was not statistically significant in the later periods when a secular increase in maternal height was taking place which resulted in fewer women of short stature (Illsley and Samphier, 1985). As an example of this secular change, primigravidae in 1984–1985 were on average nearly 3 cm taller than those in 1950–1951 (Thompson *et al.*, 1988). Table 5.2 shows, however, that in all periods twinning rates increased directly with height.

Nylander (1981) showed that in Ibadan, the marked gradient of twinning with maternal height persisted after standardisation for age and parity and that it was due to variation in the DZ twinning rate: the MZ twinning rate remained fairly constant. The 1969–1983 Aberdeen data give similar results (Table 5.7).

Social Class

Reports on variation in twinning rates by social class are often conflicting and difficult to interpret because the methods of defining social class differ. In a study based on information from vital records in Austria, Hungary and New

Zealand, and from the National Child Development Study in the UK, Golding (1986a) found associations between increased twinning rates and low educational attainment, or where either parent had worked in agriculture; twinning rates were lower in the professional occupations. Myrianthopoulos (1970) found higher twinning rates in the upper socioeconomic groups in whites and blacks in the USA and this has been confirmed for DZ twinning in Hawaii (Morton *et al.*, 1967). Again, in the USA, Lilienfeld and Pasamanick (1955) found that MZ twinning rates were highest in the upper socioeconomic groups whereas the converse applied for DZ twinning rates. However, this observed pattern may be an artefact of the use of the Weinberg rule to estimate zygosity distributions (see Chapter 4). In Taiwan, overall twinning rates have been reported as higher in both 'well to do' and 'poor' families than in the 'moderately well off' women. In the families of twins this assessment was made by interviewers whereas in the families of the control group it was made by schoolteachers (Lin and Chen, 1968). There is no marked variation in the DZ twinning rate by the occupation of the head of the household in Japan, the highest rate being for those who work in agriculture only (2.13 per 1000) and the lowest (1.75 per 1000) for blue collar workers (Imaizumi *et al.*, 1980). There is even less variation in MZ twinning rates. No association has been identified in studies in France (Hemon *et al.*, 1979a).

Nylander (1981) found a higher DZ twinning rate in Ibadan amongst women in the lowest social class with a gradient related to increasing height.

In the UK social class is usually based on occupations as classified by the Registrar General. Some changes in the classification of certain jobs may be made and new occupations added when the revised Classification of Occupations is issued every 10 years to coincide with the National Census. Over time the occupational class composition has changed reflecting an increase in professional, administrative, managerial and technological jobs and a decline in manufacturing industry.

Daley (quoted by Anderson, 1956) found no relationship between social class and twinning rates. However, Smith (1966) analysed the figures for Scotland in the years 1962–1964 and showed an inverse association of DZ twinning with social class in each maternal age group, i.e. women in the lowest social class had the highest twinning rate, which he speculated was probably due to their higher parity. The data presented in the Appendix to this chapter show no statistical association between social class (six categories) and unlike-sex twinning in Northern Ireland and north-east Scotland in the period 1975–1979. A marginal association with like-sex twinning for north-east Scotland only is likely to be an artefact.

Recent analysis of Aberdeen City District data 1951–1983 highlights some of the problems in dealing with social classification of women. Social class is usually based on men's occupations and customarily on those of the husbands of maternity patients. This means that only married women (legitimate

Table 5.8. Aberdeen City District (1951–1983): husband's/partner's occupation—Distribution for twins and singletons

Occupation	1951–61		1962–72		1973–83		1951–83	
	Twins %	Singletons %	Twins %	Singletons %	Twins %	Singletons %	Twins %	Singletons %
Non-manual	18.4	26.0	24.1	28.5	34.5	31.7	23.9	28.3
Skilled manual	41.4	44.3	40.7	39.5	35.3	34.4	39.9	40.0
Other manual	35.6	27.0	31.0	26.8	25.4	25.9	31.7	26.7
Not stated	4.6	2.7	4.2	5.2	4.8	8.0	4.5	5.0
Total %	1000.0	100.0	100.0	100.0	100.0	100.0	100.0	100.0
n	495	36 994	403	35 400	252	26 171	1 150	98 565
χ^2	25.1244		5.4754		0.4465		19.0106	
d.f.	2		2		2		2	
Excluding 'not stated' $p \leqslant$	0.001		NS		NS		0.001	

births) can be included and they have formed a decreasing proportion of the maternity population over time (Pritchard and Thompson, 1982; Thompson et al., 1988). For example, in the early 1980s about one-fifth of Aberdeen primigravidae were unmarried, a fourfold increase in 30 years. Many of the women having illegitimate babies (whatever their marital status) were co-habiting and the partners registered the births and it seems appropriate to consider them as husbands for present purposes. Thus, in Table 5.8 the occupations of husbands and partners have been combined. Over the whole period, twinning was significantly associated with women whose husbands/partners were manual workers but this applied only in the first period. Table 5.9 shows a marked secular trend in twinning by social class—the twinning rate increased slightly in each 11 year period in the non-manual occupational group, but it decreased steadily and was almost halved in the 'other manual' group. Thus, whereas twinning was associated with manual workers in the first two 11 year periods, the twinning rate was highest in the upper social classes in the last period.

A recent research project on the social, dietary and obstetric characteristics of Aberdeen primigravidae has shown that the woman's own usual occupation is becoming more discriminating than that of husband's (Thompson et al., 1988). However, the conventional classification of occupations is not

Table 5.9. Aberdeen City District (1951–1983): Crude Twinning rates (per 1000 maternities) in three 11 year periods by occupation

	1951–61	1962–72	1973–83	All years
(a) Husbands'/partners' occupation				
Non-manual				
(I, II, III non-manual)	9.4	9.5	10.4	9.7
Skilled manual				
(III manual)	12.4	11.6	9.8	11.5
Other manual (IV and V)	17.3	13.0	9.4	13.7
Not stated	22.7	9.2	5.7	10.5
(b) Women's usual occupation				
Professional and technical	11.5	10.9	14.0	12.3
Clerical	11.7	10.5	8.0	10.1
Distributive and skilled				
manual	9.6	10.2	9.5	9.8
Other manual	13.3	12.8	8.6	12.0
Remainder	39.7	22.1	8.0	26.1
Total rate	13.2	11.3	9.5	11.5
Twins (*n*)	495	403	252	1 150
Singletons (*n*)	36 994	35 400	26 171	98 565

Table 5.10. Aberdeen City District (1951–1983): woman's own usual occupation—distribution for twins and singletons

Occupation	1951–61		1962–72		1973–83		All years	
	Twins %	Singletons %	Twins %	Singletons %	Twins %	Singletons %	Twins %	Singletons %
Professional and technical	5.6	6.5	11.2	11.6	25.8	17.5	12.0	11.3
Clerical	18.4	20.7	26.8	28.7	25.8	30.9	23.0	26.3
Distributive and skilled manual	26.7	36.8	31.0	34.2	23.0	23.2	27.4	32.2
Other manual	29.9	29.7	26.1	23.0	20.3	22.3	26.4	25.3
Remainder[a]	19.4	6.3	4.9	2.5	5.1	6.1	11.2	4.9
Total %	100.0	100.0	100.0	100.0	100.0	100.0	100.0	100.0
n	495	36 994	403	35 400	252	26 171	1150	98 565
Excluding remainder								
λ^2		7.5700		3.0348		12.2120		10.0857
d.f.		3		3		3		3
$p \leqslant$		NS		NS		0.01		0.02

[a]Mainly never worked or category of skill uncertain.

appropriate for women's occupations because they are so heavily concentrated in certain categories of jobs, e.g. clerical. Thus, a modified classification has been used in the analysis of Aberdeen data since the late 1940s. It
must be noted that over time there has been a marked increase in employ-
ment opportunities for women with a rapidly expanding labour market
associated with technological and economic advances. Table 5.10 shows that
the association of twinning with the woman's own usual occupation, in
contrast to the finding based on the husband's/partners occupation, was only
significant in the last 11 years. The twinning rates show a similar pattern to
that already described for husbands/partners, with a marked increase in the
highest occupational group in recent years (Table 5.9). The assessment of the
effect of social class on the incidence of twinning is difficult. It will be noted
that twinning was significantly associated with the husband's/partner's
occupation in 1951–1961, with the wife's own usual occupation in 1973–1983,
but with neither of their occupations in the middle period. Given the
consistent finding of associations between social position and a variety of
health outcomes (Department of Health and Social Security, 1980) it seems
reasonable to investigate this in more detail. The present Aberdeen analysis
and the apparently contradictory findings reported in other studies would
seem to indicate secular changes and/or cross cutting effects which partially
conceal any social class association. For example, Carr-Hill and Pritchard
(1985) have reported that maternal height decreases and weight-for-height
increases with decreasing social class.

The Concurrent Effects of Parity, Age, Height, and Social Class

The Aberdeen City District data for the 1951–1983 period, with its consistent
recording of measures of parity, age, height, and occupational status affords
an opportunity to explore the relationships between these variables and the
incidence of twinning. (Note that zygosity is not recorded for the full period.)
Linear Logit models have been utilised to test the significance of and the
interrelationship between these four variables and time period in the prediction of the distribution of twin births. The statistical package SPSS-X was
used for these analyses (SPSS-X, 1983).

Table 5.11 shows the categories used, the partial likelihood ratio chi square
and level of significance, and the parameter estimates for each variable. The
models used demonstrate a significant and independent effect of age and
height, and confirmed the direction of the associations described above.
Similarly, time period has a significant effect reflecting the secular decline in
the incidence of multiple births. However, it is important to recognise that
time period may act as a surrogate for other secular changes, such as variation
in the proportions of MZ and DZ twins, as described in Chapter 4.

The parity distribution shown in Table 5.1 indicates a highly significant

Table 5.11. Aberdeen City District (1951–1983): significance of independent contribution of different factors to twinning

Factor	Parameter estimate	Partial likelihood ratio chi square	d.f.	p
Parity		0.03	2	NS
0	−0.012			
1	0.007			
2	0.031			
3+	−0.026			
Maternal age		69.1	4	0.001
<=19	0.229			
20−24	0.089			
25−29	−0.057			
30−34	−0.162			
35+	−0.099			
Maternal height		7.2	2	0.05
short (<=154 cm)	0.060			
medium (155−163)	−0.003			
tall (164+ cm)	−0.057			
Time period		8.2	2	0.02
1951–1961	−0.040			
1962–1972	−0.035			
1973–1983	0.075			
Husbands/partner's occupation		67.1	3	0.001
non-manual	0.148			
skilled manual	0.132			
unskilled manual	0.019			
not stated	−0.299			
Woman's own occupation		41.0	4	0.001
prof/technical	0.004			
clerical	0.180			
skilled manual	0.048			
unskilled manual	−0.115			
remainder	−0.117			

Negative values indicate a higher propensity to twinning.

Table 5.12. Aberdeen City District (1951–1983): parameter estimates for social class based on the woman's own occupation

Occupation	1951–1961	1962–1972	1973–1983
Professional and technical	0.094	0.156	−0.238
Clerical	0.200	0.154	0.186
Distributive and skilled manual	−0.038	0.117	0.065
Other manual	−0.123	−0.160	−0.062
Remainder	−0.133	−0.267	0.049

Negative values indicate a higher propensity to twinning.

association with twinning, overall, but this is not confirmed by the linear Logit analysis. Only the extreme parity 0 and 3+ showed a higher propensity to twinning.

The two alternative measures of occupational status, based on the husband/ partner and on the woman herself were tested, and both exhibited a significant inverse relationship with twinning.

The interaction of these factors was then considered. The significance of parity vanished once the age variable was added, indicating that the apparent association between parity and twinning is a concealed age effect. The woman's own occupational status, but not that of the husband/partner, showed a significant secular trend ($p \leq 0.01$). However, in the earliest period the high proportion in the 'remainder' category (Table 5.10), i.e. women who had never worked or for whom information was incomplete, presented problems in interpretation. A consistent gradient, associating twinning with lower social status was only found in the middle period. In the final 11 years, women in professional and technical occupations were most likely to have twins (Table 5.12).

These analyses illustrate some of the problems in unravelling the real association of different factors with twinning, a comparatively rare event which is showing a marked secular decline in a changing situation of marital and family life and of revolutionary development in economic and environmental conditions.

Seasonal Variations

The marked geographical variations in twinning in different parts of the world have led to consideration of possible climatic and related factors being involved in the aetiology. Thus, some workers have considered seasonal variations in twinning. However, so far as we are aware, the report of

Kendler and Robinette (1983) is the only published analysis of seasonal variation in MZ and DZ twinning rates in a series in which zygosity was determined directly. These authors found no significant seasonal variation using the comparatively insensitive method of basing a chi-square statistic on the monthly totals, but re-analysis by the Walter–Elwood technique shows a significant sinusoidal variation in the ratio of DZ pairs to controls, maximal in May (Little and Elwood, 1987). However, the study of Kendler and Robinette was based not on births but on adult males who had been born during the period 1917–1927. The study is, therefore, difficult to interpret because of a variety of possible selection factors. For example, there was substantial seasonal variation in infant mortality rates during this period (Hare et al., 1981) and patterns of infant mortality are known to differ as between twins and singletons. Analysis of data for Aberdeen City District 1969–1983 showed little variation in either DZ or MZ twinning by month of last menstrual period.

Reports of seasonal variation in twinning rates where zygosity distributions have been estimated by the Weinberg rule in populations of births are available from Canada (Elwood, 1978), Japan (Imaizumi et al., 1980), Taiwan (Cheng et al., 1986) and the UK—England and Wales (James, 1980a) and north-east Scotland and Northern Ireland (Little and Elwood, 1987). In all of these populations except Northern Ireland and Taiwan, there was a peak in DZ twinning rates around November–December. Little and Elwood found that, within each population, peaks in MZ and DZ rates were 6 months apart, suggesting that the apparent seasonal patterns are artefacts of the determination of zygosity by an indirect technique such as the Weinberg rule. The seasonal trends were significant only in Canada and in England and Wales (Little and Elwood, 1987), but very large numbers are required to detect seasonal variations of the magnitude described by James (1980a). Imaizumi et al. (1980) noted substantial variations in monthly rates of MZ twinning, the highest rate being coincident with that for DZ twinning, while James also found evidence of seasonality in MZ twinning, peaking in November. In addition to these studies, there have been reports of seasonal variation in the overall twinning rate in Cuba (Golding, 1986b), Denmark (Kappel et al., 1986), Liverpool, England (Edwards, 1938), Finland (Timonen and Carpen, 1968), Germany (Richter et al., 1984), Budapest (Czeizel et al., 1979) and Hungary as a whole (Golding, 1986b), Japan (Kamimura, 1976; Miura et al., 1984), New Zealand (Golding, 1986b), Nigeria (Knox and Morley, 1960; Cox, 1963; Nylander, 1975c; Rehan and Tafida, 1980), Singapore (Lin and Chen, 1968), Sweden and the USA (Golding, 1986b), but these are inconsistent. For example, Nylander (1975c) noted that, as in previous studies, based on hospital series in Nigeria (Knox and Morley, 1960; Cox, 1963), the twinning rate in the Ibadan hospitals was higher during the rainy season than during the dry season. However, the seasonal pattern in the total population study in Igbo-Ora was the reverse of that found in the hospital series. The pattern observed in the hospital series may reflect varying utilisation of hospital facilities at different times of the year. Nylander suggests that women expecting twins and therefore more likely to experience obstetric complications will endeavour to enter hospital whatever the weather or difficulties of transport, whereas other women may be more easily deterred from entering hospital during the rainy season. Reports from Scotland (Smith, 1966), New York State (Selvin and Janerich, 1972), Czechoslovakia (Zahalkova, 1974), and Italy (Gedda *et al.*, 1986) report no seasonal pattern. As publications tend to favour positive results it may be that other negative findings have not been reported.

Seasonal trends have to be interpreted in the context of temporal variation in the longer term. Firstly, a systematic long-term decline or increase in twinning rates would produce an apparent minimum or maximum respectively in the winter months. The decline in rates which started in the late 1950s may have led to the under-estimation of the extent of a winter peak in the studies from Canada (Elwood, 1978), England and Wales (James, 1980a) and north-east Scotland (Little and Elwood, 1987). Secondly, there may be large variations in seasonal trends between years. For example, seasonal variations in the MZ twinning rate in north-east Scotland for the overall period 1975–1979 show a sinusoidal pattern but analysis for single years does not reveal any consistent pattern (Little and Elwood, 1987). Similar fluctuations have been noted in Japan (Miura *et al.*, 1984) and in Gorlitz, Germany (Richter *et al.*, 1984). In the German study of parish records over the 250 year period 1611–1860, the twinning rate was relatively constant in spring and autumn, but variable in winter and summer, so that there would be peaks when the overall twinning rate was high, and troughs when it was low.

The seasonal evidence is inconclusive, but in view of the geographical variation, some interest has focused on nutrition and related factors.

Nutrition

It is well known that in animals the higher the level of nutrition, the greater the litter size (Wallace, 1951; Hammond, 1952). It might be expected that as height and body weight are partly determined by nutrition the higher twinning rates found in tall and obese women might be related to their greater dietary intake. However, it was found in a dietary survey carried out in Aberdeen that a group of women having twin pregnancies did not have any greater intake of energy or protein than women with singleton pregnancies (Campbell *et al.*, 1982). Indeed, the women expecting twins were taking a lower average energy intake than that recommended by the Department of Health and Social Security (1979). Nevertheless, they produced babies with combined birthweights much heavier than the birthweights of singletons to comparable mothers. It is possible, however, that these heavier women did have a higher dietary intake, especially in the earlier years of life, but this was not sustained once their pattern of body build had been established.

Although twin pregnancies are not associated with a higher nutritional intake, nevertheless acute nutritional deprivation may lead to a lowering of the twinning rate by decreasing fertility as discussed in Chapter 4.

Smoking

It is known that smoking depresses appetite but that women who smoke do not have a lower intake of the main nutrients than non-smokers (Thompson *et al.*, 1988). Smokers also tend to be shorter and of lower social class (Carr-Hill and Pritchard, 1985). There has been a marked increase in women smokers over the years and Table 5.13 shows that in Aberdeen in 1969–1983 nearly half the pregnant women smoked. There was, however, no significant association between twinning and whether the woman smoked or not—although smokers had higher rates for both MZ and DZ twinning.

Weight

It was found in Aberdeen by Campbell *et al.* (1974) that in primigravidae with twin pregnancies there were only 10% in the lower quartile of weight for

Table 5.13. Aberdeen City District (1969–1983): distribution and rates of twinning for smokers and non-smokers

	Non-smokers	Smokers	Not stated	Total
Twins — total	173	179	32	384
Zygosity MZ	67	67	14	148
DZ	90	93	16	199
Not stated	16	19	2	37
Singletons	17 946	16 516	3717	38 179

Excluding zygosity and smoking 'not stated'
All twins *vs* singletons $\lambda^2 = 1.0817$, d.f. 1, not significant
MZ *vs* DZ $\lambda^2 = 0.0009$, d.f. 1, not significant
MZ *vs* singletons $\lambda^2 = 0.5006$, d.f. 1, not significant
DZ *vs* singletons $\lambda^2 = 0.1546$, d.f. 1, not significant

Twinning rates: none significant for smoking

All twins	9.6	10.8
MZ	3.7	4.1
DZ	5.0	5.6

height, this group counterbalanced by an excess of about 7% in both the normal and obese groups. The primigravidae were divided into thin, normal and obese groups at mid-pregnancy according to the weight for height centile categories based on an Aberdeen population (Kemsley *et al.*, 1962). It is not clear whether this reduced twinning rate in thin women could be related to a different production of gonadotrophins in the normal and obese groups compared with small, thin women. Wyshak (1981) found that mothers of twins are heavier and they also have slightly earlier menarche and meno-pause. Mothers of twins were reported to be heavier in France (Hemon *et al.*, 1981a); in Ibadan (Nylander, 1981) and in Oxford (Corney *et al.*, 1981). These findings might reflect nutritional factors in childhood or an interaction between gonadotrophin levels and weight.

Fecundability and Fertility

In view of the lack of clear evidence of environmental effect it has been hypothesised that women who produce twins are more fecund than other women, i.e. that they conceive more easily, possibly due to their ovulating more regularly and more often releasing two ova. This may be expressed in higher fertility affecting the twinning rates. Testing this hypothesis is bedevil-led by restrictions in family size and differential use of efficient contraception.

Bulmer (1959a) reported that women who conceived within 3 months of marriage were more likely to have twins than women who became pregnant later in marriage. Similar findings were reported in Australia (Pollard, 1969).

Jeanneret and MacMahon (1962) found a striking peak in twin births in the USA in 1946. Allen and Schachter (1971) suggested that conceptions had coincided with husbands being discharged from military service after the Second World War and that this peak in twins occurred a few months earlier than that for total births. They attributed it to the higher fecundability of twin-prone mothers. It can be argued, however, that more frequent sexual intercourse in the first few months of marriage or on return of the husband after prolonged absence, might also account for the increased DZ twinning rate. More frequent coitus could result in the fertilisation at different times of two ova of a double ovualtion (see Chapter 3).

Schmidt *et al.* (1983) found an extremely high twinning rate between 1927 and 1977 in an isolated Romanian village compared with other villages comparable in such factors as age, parity, nutrition and a high degree of inbreeding. The data showed that mothers of twins were more fertile than other mothers and review of pedigrees of six to eight generations supported the hypothesis of a genetic predisposition to twinning in this village. Similar findings and explanations have been made for rural Scandinavia (Eriksson and Fellman, 1973) reinforced by the report of a decrease in DZ twinning rates following the opening up of the Aland Islands of Finland (Eriksson,

1962, 1973). Hemon *et al.* (1981b), however, after considering the genetic hypothesis in a comparison of secular changes in DZ twinning rates in different parts of France relative to changes in factors affecting isolation concluded that the differential fecundability hypothesis was a more likely explanation.

Support for the theory of high fecundability and twin proneness comes from data on illegitimate and pre-nuptially conceived pregnancies. From records Dahlberg (1952) showed that over 60 years ago in Denmark mothers of illegitimate children, although mainly primigravidae, had a twinning rate as high as married mothers of the same age group. Eriksson and Fellman (1967) from analysis of official statistics and church records in Scandinavia reported a significantly higher twinning rate in illegitimate than in legitimate maternities, especially in mothers aged 25–39 years. The high incidence of twinning in illegitimate as well as legitimate pregnancies conceived before marriage (Bulmer, 1959a) might indicate that these women were more fecund and, therefore, were less able to avoid becoming pregnant.

Recent data from Aberdeen City District of twinning rates for illegitimate and legitimate maternities by parity and age are given in Table 5.14. The data are given in three 11 year cohorts and show changes over time. In the first period 1951–1961 the twinning rate for illegitimate maternities was not only

Table 5.14. Twinning rates for illegitimate and legitimate maternities by age and parity for three 11 year cohorts

	Primiparae			Multiparae		
Age group	1951–61	1962–72	1973–83	1951–61	1962–72	1973–83
Illegitimate						
–19	14.3	6.8	6.4	—	—	10.4
20–24	13.5	12.8	9.7	17.6	9.3	6.2
25–29	9.5	39.6	—	15.7	10.2	11.7
30–34	—	—	37.0	38.6	47.9	—
35+	115.4	—	—	67.6	—	—
All ages	16.1	10.6	7.7	21.6	13.7	6.9
Legitimate						
–19	10.5	6.7	6.6	3.4	2.9	8.3
20–24	8.5	7.1	6.7	9.9	11.2	9.5
25–29	9.1	9.3	12.1	13.5	14.2	9.9
30–34	19.2	10.2	20.0	16.6	12.9	11.8
35+	14.1	23.4	22.6	12.9	18.6	7.2
All ages	10.3	7.7	9.7	14.5	13.2	9.4
Total maternities						
No.	14 319	14 423	12 012	23 557	21 830	14 443
% Illegitimate	6.1	10.4	17.4	3.9	4.3	8.1

higher overall, but also higher in all age groups for both primiparae and multiparae compared with the corresponding legitimate maternities. This still applied to primiparae in 1962–1972, but in multiparae the illegitimate twinning rate was only markedly higher in the 30–34 year age groups and slightly higher overall. In the last 11 years the overall illegitimate twinning rate was lower than the twinning rate for legitimate maternities for both primiparae and multiparae, although it was higher in some age groups. Over the three periods, however, total maternities had fallen in primiparae by 16% and in multiparae by 39%; the proportion of illegitimate maternities had almost trebled in primiparae and more than doubled in multiparae. These data reflect the problems of applying a legal concept to a biological phenomenon in a changing situation of social behaviour in respect of sex, marriage and use of contraception.

Eriksson and Fellman (1967) suggested that mothers with illegitimate maternities 'comprise an elite from a standpoint of fertility and reproduction and that they may become pregnant more easily owing to an increased tendency to polyovulation and a low frequency of anovulatory cycles including the possibility of superfecundation and superfetation'. However, the evidence for superfecundation in human multiple births is as yet unconvincing. As ovulation has been reported to occur during pregnancy and twins may be conceived at different times superfetation is a possibility, but it must be regarded as a rare phenomenon (see Chapter 3).

Record et al. (1978) discussed the problems of measuring the fertility of mothers of twins relative to that of other mothers. They analysed data on a decade of births in Birmingham (England) taking account of age and parity. They found that the survival of both twins had an inhibiting effect on further reproduction in contrast to the enhancing effect if both twins died. Both the sex of the twins and zygosity made little difference to fertility.

Mothers of DZ twins are much more likely to have twins again than women who have not previously had twins (Weinberg, 1909; Greulich, 1934; Dahlberg, 1952; Bulmer, 1958; Wyshak and White, 1965; Nylander, 1970b). Mothers of MZ twins, however, do not appear to have any greater frequency of twinning in later pregnancies than women who have not had twins.

In their extensive studies of data for Salt Lake City, White and Wyshak (1964) observed that women who had twins, if they had twinning in their background, tended to have larger families than those with no such history. They later speculated (Wyshak and White, 1969) that the increased fertility of twin producers might be due to increased secretion of pituitary gonadotrophin affecting both fertility and DZ twinning (see Chapter 3).

Familial Tendencies

It is well known that there is a tendency to twinning in some families, but it is not clear whether this applies to both MZ and DZ twinning, and whether both maternal and paternal influences are implicated. Data on the familial tendency to twinning are available in the main from isolated case reports of individual families usually from the collection of information on twin pregnancies such as the Register of the Mendel Institute in Rome (Parisi *et al.*, 1983), or rarely, from archives relating to total populations such as those of the Church of Jesus Christ and the Latter Day Saints in Salt Lake City (White and Wyshak, 1964). Unfortunately, there are deficiencies in most collections of data in that there may be under-reporting, particularly of twin births if one of the twins was born dead or died soon after and of singleton births on the paternal side.

As noted previously, the MZ twinning rate in different races and in different parts of the world is remarkably constant and it has been argued that MZ twinning is not under hereditary control (see Chapter 4). Some studies, however, have shown that a tendency to MZ twinning is transmitted through the maternal line (Gedda, 1951; Lil'in and Gindilis, 1976; Parisi *et al.*, 1983). However, other studies have shown transmission through the paternal line in certain families with recurrent MZ twinning (Harvey *et al.*, 1977; Michels and Riccardi, 1978; Shapiro *et al.*, 1978). Parisi and co-workers (1983) considered that paternal transmission was rare, but possibly due to single gene effects, resulting in early developmental anomalies, and thus directly or indirectly related to MZ twinning.

There is no doubt that there is a familial tendency to DZ twinning, but some authors believe that it is inherited only in the maternal line (Weinberg, 1909; Danforth, 1916; Wehefrith, 1925; Dahlberg, 1926; Lenz 1933; White and Wyshak, 1964; Bulmer, 1970). For example, in the studies of the church records at Salt Lake City, White and Wyshak (1964) found that the twinning rate in the offspring of women who were themselves DZ twins was 17.1 per 1000 maternities, compared with 11.6 per 1000 maternities for the general population, but the twinning rate in the offspring of males who were themselves DZ twins was only 7.9 per 1000 maternities. There have, however, been isolated case reports of men with more than one wife, each of whom had produced multiple births. Browne (1946) quotes the cases of two Russian peasants who were both married twice and had 87 and 64 children respectively by their two wives, including quadruplets, triplets and twins.

The high incidence of twinning and the practice of polygyny among the Yoruba in western Nigeria allowed Nylander (1970b) an excellent opportunity to study the effect of maternal and paternal influences on dizygotic twinning. He studied 977 twin maternities (83 MZ and 894 DZ) and concluded that:

1. Women whose husbands are themselves twins have similar twinning rates to women whose husbands are not twins.
2. Women whose husbands have had twins by other wives have similar

twinning rates to women whose husbands have not had twins by other wives.
3. Women whose fathers are twins have a twinning rate not significantly higher than for women whose fathers are not twins.
4. Women whose fathers have had twins by other wives have similar twinning rates to women whose fathers have not had twins by other wives.

His findings suggest that there is no paternal contribution to dizygotic twinning. In a study of white–black inter-racial crossing in the USA, Khoury and Erickson (1983) found that black mothers had a higher rate of unlike-sex twinning than white mothers, but black fathers did not have a higher rate of unlike-sex or like-sex twinning than white fathers. This finding indicates that the high rate of DZ twinning in blacks is associated with the maternal and not the paternal ethnic group. On the other hand, Parisi *et al.* (1983), in a review of the families of 950 unselcted twin pairs of determined zygosity (323 MZ and 627 DZ) concluded that a propensity to DZ twinning could be inherited through both the maternal and paternal line. They suggested that there is a relationship between the two types of twinning on the basis of a significantly increased frequency of DZ twins among maternal relatives of MZ twins.

If twinning were in part genetically determined, it would be expected that mothers who themselves were twins would be more likely to have twins than other mothers. This has been reported, for example, by Weinberg (1909) and by White and Wyshak (1964). However, the results of at least one study (in Nigeria) do not show this (Nylander, 1970b), but the very high rate of DZ twinning among the Yoruba may be due to other factors obscuring the contribution of genetic factors.

To sum up, it seems that there is a familial tendency to DZ twinning through the maternal line, but transmission through the paternal line seems less clear. Any familial tendency to MZ twinning is rare, and the available evidence would be consistent with transmission through the maternal or paternal lines or both.

Blood Groups

Several authors have suggested that there is an association between the incidence of twinning and blood groups (Osborne and De George, 1957; Gedda, 1961; Bolognesi and Milani-Comparetti, 1970) and it has been postulated that mothers who belong to group O have a higher incidence of twinning. Hemon *et al.* (1981a) found that mothers of twins were more likely to be of blood group O or A. The high twinning rate in areas of France with high group B frequency (Vallois, 1949; Bulmer, 1960a) is probably a reflection of ethnic differences due to migration. Nylander (1981) reported no significant association between twinning and blood groups in either Ibadan or

Table 5.15. Aberdeen City District (1969–1983): distribution of ABO blood groups for mothers of twins by zygosity and of singletons

| | Twins | | | | |
Blood group	MZ %	DZ %	Not Known %	Total %	Singletons %
A	36.5	40.2	59.0	40.6	35.1
B	9.5	10.6	2.6	9.4	10.5
AB	3.4	3.5	5.1	3.6	3.1
O	49.3	44.7	30.8	45.1	50.9
Not stated	1.3	1.0	2.5	1.3	0.4
Total	100.0	100.0	100.0	100.0	100.0
n	148	199	37	384	38 182

Excluding blood group not stated
Total twins vs singletons $\quad \lambda^2 = 6.7069$, d.f. 3, not significant
MZ vs DZ $\quad \lambda^2 = 0.7928$, d.f. 3, not significant
MZ vs singletons $\quad \lambda^2 = 0.3268$, d.f. 3, not significant
DZ vs singletons $\quad \lambda^2 = 3.0779$, d.f. 3, not significant

Aberdeen. Recent analysis for the total population of Aberdeen City District shows that the distribution of ABO blood groups is very similar for mothers of MZ twins and of singletons whereas mothers of DZ twins are more likely to be of blood group A at the expense of O. However, neither MZ nor DZ twinning is significantly associated with ABO blood group (Table 5.15).

De George (1970b), in a case control study, concluded that the Rh negative

Table 5.16. Aberdeen City District (1969–1983): distribution of RH factor for mothers of twins by zygosity and of singletons

| | Twins | | | | |
Rh factor	MZ %	DZ %	Not known %	Total %	Singletons %
Positive	78.4	82.4	81.1	80.7	81.6
Negative	19.6	16.6	16.2	17.7	17.9
Not stated	2.0	1.0	2.7	1.6	0.5
Total	100.0	100.0	100.0	100.0	100.0
n	148	199	37	384	38 182

Excluding Rh not stated
All twins vs singletons $\quad \lambda^2 = 0.0023$, d.f. 1, not significant
MZ vs DZ $\quad \lambda^2 = 0.3952$, d.f. 1, not significant
MZ vs singletons $\quad \lambda^2 = 0.2707$, d.f. 1, not significant
DZ vs singletons $\quad \lambda^2 = 0.1247$, d.f. 1, not significant

blood type, especially in blood group O mothers, was associated with DZ twinning, particularly of unlike-sex pairs.

Nylander (1981) found no association between twinning and Rh factor in Ibadan or Aberdeen. Recent data confirm this finding for Aberdeen (Table 5.16).

Factors Affecting Twinning

All the evidence considered in this chapter indicates that some of the factors are associated with twinning, whereas others can reasonably be discounted and in some cases the interpretation of findings is equivocal. Any association is usually with DZ twinning.

Maternal age is clearly related to twinning, although the peak age may vary; a paternal age effect is doubtful. The role of parity remains somewhat obscure. Taller women are more likely to have twins and evidence suggests that this also applies to heavier women. However, the limited amount of data available indicates that daily intake of the main nutrients is not a factor, although there is some speculation that certain item(s) in diet may help to explain some geographical or ethnic differences in twinning. It is generally agreed that there is a familial tendency to DZ twinning through the maternal line, but transmission through the father is uncertain. The findings on ABO blood groups and Rh blood type are conflicting, but these factors are probably not involved, nor is smoking. There is no convincing evidence of a seasonal component in twinning. The interpretation of data depending on social behaviour of illegitimate births or on social categorisation by social class, is confused. Consideration of some of the factors leads to speculation about the possible contribution of gonadotrophin levels, for example, in affecting adult stature and fertility.

It must be recognised that making definitive conclusions is bedevilled by secular trends, inadequate population data, variations in methods and in analysis and in the determination of zygosity, as well as by differences in social behaviour and environmental conditions.

Some factors affecting twinning in north-east Scotland and Northern Ireland

JULIAN LITTLE

Introduction

In this study, the descriptive epidemiology of twinning was investigated in north-east Scotland and Northern Ireland, two populations which are considered to be particularly suitable for epidemiological comparison on the basis of their similarity in ethnic composition (Kidd et al., 1967).

Materials and methods

The study was based on records of maternity and child health services, the same as used in the study of seasonal variation by Little and Elwood (1987). As the organisation of these services differs between the two areas, different methods of collation of data had to be adopted.

Data on pregnancies ending in birth in north-east Scotland during the period 1975–1979 were obtained in computerised form from the Scottish Medical Records maternity discharge scheme, known as SMR2. As the scheme is based on maternities, identification of twins is built into the system.

Data on births (live and still) delivered in Northern Ireland during the period 1975–1979 were obtained from the Child Health System, which includes statutory notification of birth and information collected by the health visitor during the first effective visit after birth. Individual birth records coded as twins were linked in pairs by computerised comparison of variables such as district and date of birth, maternal and paternal age, and previous medical history of the parents. From 2876 records of individual twins, 2712 (94%) were successfully linked in pairs.

For both populations, MZ and DZ twinning rates were estimated by Weinberg's differential rule.

Table 5A.1. Associations between twinning and maternal age parity and social class in north-east Scotland and Northern Ireland, 1975–1979 — crude rates and ratio of rates (RR)

	Dizygotic twinning				Monozygotic twinning			
	North-east Scotland		Northern Ireland		North-east Scotland		Northern Ireland	
	Rate per 1000	RR (95% CI[a])	Rate per 1000	RR (95% CI[a])	Rate per 1000	RR (95% CI[a])	Rate per 1000	RR (95% CI[a])
(a) Maternal age								
<19	3.1	baseline	1.4	baseline	2.3	baseline	4.3	baseline
20–24	3.6	1.1 (0.7–1.9)	4.0	2.0 (1.5–5.0)	4.3	1.9 (1.1–3.5)	3.4	0.8 (0.5–1.1)
25–29	6.9	2.2 (1.3–3.6)	6.4	4.4 (2.5–7.9)	2.4	1.1 (0.6–2.0)	4.3	1.0 (0.7–1.5)
30–34	8.9	2.9 (1.7–4.0)	9.9	6.9 (3.9–12.3)	5.0	2.2 (1.2–4.2)	3.0	0.7 (0.5–1.0)
35–39	14.3	4.6 (2.5–8.5)	11.1	7.7 (4.3–13.9)	0.6	0.3 (0.0–2.0)	3.7	0.9 (0.6–1.4)
40+	0.0	0.0	11.0	7.7 (4.0–14.6)	5.7	2.5 (0.6–11.1)	3.9	0.9 (0.5–1.7)
NK[b]	—		23.3	16.2 (6.1–43.6)	—		0.0	0.0
	$\chi^2_{(5)} = 58.7; p < 0.001$		$\chi^2_{(6)} = 175.9; p < 0.001$		$\chi^2_{(5)} = 23.4; p < 0.001$		$\chi^2_{(6)} = 12.4; p < 0.025$	

(b) Parity (*rates are crude, RRs are adjusted for maternal age*)

	rate	baseline	rate	baseline	rate	baseline	rate	baseline
0	4.4	baseline	3.5	baseline	4.0	baseline	4.3	baseline
1	5.7	1.1 (0.8–1.4)	6.7	1.6 (1.3–1.9)	3.6	0.9 (0.6–1.2)	3.9	0.9 (0.7–1.2)
2	8.5	1.4 (1.0–1.9)	8.7	1.8 (1.5–2.3)	1.4	0.4 (0.2–0.7)	2.8	0.6 (0.5–0.9)
3	8.9	1.3 (0.8–2.2)	8.5	1.6 (1.3–2.2)	1.5	0.3 (0.1–1.0)	4.5	0.9 (0.7–1.3)
4	7.2	1.0 (0.4–2.7)	14.1	2.6 (1.9–3.5)	3.6	1.1 (0.3–3.6)	0.7	0.5 (0.3–0.8)
5+	14.5	1.9 (0.7–5.4)	12.4	2.2 (1.6–2.9)	0.0	0.0	2.6	0.5 (0.3–0.8)
NK[b]	0.0	0.0	7.0	1.5 (0.0–2.9)	0.0	0.0	3.5	0.9 (0.4–2.1)
	$\chi^2_{(6)} = 4.8$; NS		$\chi^2_{(6)} = 52.7$; $p < 0.001$		$\chi^2_{(6)} = 17.8$; $p < 0.01$		$\chi^2_{(6)} = 19.6$; $p < 0.005$	

(c) Social class (*rates are crude, RRs are adjusted for maternal age*)

	rate	baseline	rate	baseline	rate	baseline	rate	baseline
I	4.3	baseline	9.5	baseline	3.7	baseline	3.0	baseline
II	8.0	2.0 (1.1–3.5)	8.9	1.1 (0.7–1.6)	1.4	0.4 (0.2–0.9)	3.8	0.8 (0.5–1.4)
III	5.6	1.7 (1.0–2.8)	6.0	1.0 (0.7–1.4)	4.3	1.1 (0.6–1.9)	3.8	0.9 (0.6–1.3)
IV	5.0	1.6 (0.9–2.8)	6.1	0.8 (0.6–1.0)	3.5	1.0 (0.5–1.8)	3.5	0.9 (0.6–1.2)
V	4.2	1.5 (0.7–3.1)	5.7	0.8 (0.6–1.1)	3.5	1.1 (0.5–2.4)	3.5	0.8 (0.5–1.2)
NC[c]	6.3	2.1 (1.2–3.0)	6.6	0.8 (0.6–1.2)	2.2	0.7 (0.4–1.5) }	4.5	0.8 (0.5–1.2)
NK[b]			7.6	1.0 (0.7–1.4)			2.6	0.6 (0.4–1.1)
	$\chi^2_{(5)} = 0.4$; NS		$\chi^2_{(6)} = 10.8$; NS		$\chi^2_{(5)} = 13.1$; $p < 0.025$		$\chi^2_{(6)} = 3.1$; NS	

[a]Confidence interval.
[b]Not known.
[c]Not classified.

Seasonal variation was investigated first by the standard chi-square test for departures from uniform proportions. However, this technique does not test for a regular trend. For this reason, therefore, the method of Walter and Elwood (1975) was applied in order to test for sinusoidal departures from uniformity. The results of the application of these tests to the data from north-east Scotland as a whole and Northern Ireland for the period 1975–1979 have been described elsewhere (Little and Elwood, 1987). All other analysis was performed by logistic multiple regression using the Generalised Linear Interactive Modelling (GLIM) package (Baker and Nelder, 1978). The other variables considered are maternal age, parity, social class, and for Northern Ireland only, paternal age.

Results

In north-east Scotland, 455 sets of twins were delivered amongst a total of 50 246 maternities, a rate of 9.1 per 1000. This rate is somewhat lower than the 10.3 per 1000 observed in Northern Ireland. This represents 1356 twin maternities of known multiplicity out of a total of 131 576 maternities.

One hundred and forty-three twin pairs of unlike sex were delivered in north-east Scotland, 438 such pairs in Northern Ireland. MZ and DZ twinning rates as estimated by Weinberg's method were 3.3 and 5.7 respectively per 1000 in north-east Scotland and 3.7 and 6.7 in Northern Ireland.

The results of the analysis of associations with maternal age, parity and social class are presented in Table 5A.1. In the case of parity and social class, the relative risks (ratios of rates in particular categories to a baseline) are adjusted for maternal age. Data on paternal age and twinning in Northern Ireland, adjusted for maternal age with and without further adjustment for parity, are presented in Table 5A.2.

The association reported elsewhere for maternal age is confirmed. There is no association between MZ twinning and parity. In Northern Ireland, there does seem to be an association between DZ twinning and parity, but this is not apparent in the data from north-east Scotland. No consistent association with social class was identified. The association with paternal age, if it exists, is weak and does not achieve statistical significance.

Discussion

Because MZ and DZ rates are estimated, the associated error variances are greater than if a diagnosis of zygosity had been made by a direct method (Bulmer, 1970; James, 1980a). No allowance has been made for this in the logistic multiple regression analysis and hence the chi-square statistics relating to variation in twinning rates by zygosity are over-estimates. Thus, associations in these data with social class appear to be unlikely. In addition, no

Table 5A.2. Associations between twinning and paternal age in Northern Ireland, 1975–1979

Paternal age	Dizygotic twinning RR (95% CI) adjusted for		MZ twinning RR (95% CI) adjusted for maternal age only
	maternal age only	maternal age and parity	
< 19	baseline	baseline	baseline
20–24	2.2 (0.6–8.7)	2.2 (0.5–8.8)	1.3 (0.5–3.0)
25–29	2.7 (0.7–10.6)	2.5 (0.6–10.3)	1.4 (0.6–3.2)
30–34	2.7 (0.7–10.4)	2.4 (0.6–9.7)	1.7 (0.7–4.1)
35–39	2.7 (0.7–10.5)	2.3 (0.6–9.5)	1.6 (0.7–4.0)
40–44	3.2 (0.8–12.8)	2.8 (0.7–11.5)	1.3 (0.5–3.2)
45+	3.3 (0.8–13.4)	2.8 (0.7–12.0)	1.9 (0.7–5.1)
NK	0.2 (0.0 → ∞)	0.1 (0.0 → ∞)	0.0
	$\chi^2_{(7)} = 7.6$; NS	$\chi^2_{(7)} = 5.6$; NS	$\chi^2_{(7)} = 7.7$; NS

account was taken in the analysis of the possible flaw in the Weinberg method, but it is not certain that proposed adjustments for both the additional error variance and the inequality in the sex distribution of DZ pairs are appropriate (Allen, 1981).

The clear dependence of DZ twinning on maternal age is confirmed, but the association with MZ twinning differs between the populations. The differences in the relationship between DZ twinning and parity between north-east Scotland and Northern Ireland may be related to different patterns of reproduction. It may be noted that in Aberdeen City District and suburbs, there was a clear association with parity in the 1950s and 1960s.

From the analysis of the Northern Ireland data, it appears that women who conceive with a husband or partner aged under 20 are less likely to have twins than other women. There is a suggestion of a dose–response relationship with DZ rates increasing steadily with paternal age at ages over 20, but this is not statistically significant. Further work is required to confirm or refute this effect.

Twinning and Twins
Edited by I. MacGillivray, D. M. Campbell and B. Thompson
© 1988 John Wiley & Sons Ltd

CHAPTER 6

Physiological changes and adaptation

DORIS M. CAMPBELL

Department of Obstetrics and Gynaecology, University of Aberdeen, Aberdeen, UK

In the animal world, litter size is determined by the requirements for survival, and the smaller the animal the greater is the litter size. Also it is interesting to note that the combined weight of the offspring or babies is proportional to the size of the mother: thus the individual offspring of a small animal will each weigh less than the singleton offspring of a large one. Relatively large size at birth appears to be an evolutionary advantage and multiple pregnancy in the human has even been considered to be an atavistic reversion.

The maternal physiological adaptation to single pregnancy is considerable and an even greater response is necessary in twin pregnancy to ensure good sized, healthy babies. It is not surprising, then, that twinning rates in humans are greater in the woman who is healthy, tall, well-built, and has had good nutrition (refer to Chapter 5). In the animal kingdom this is illustrated in the sheep where well-nourished ewes produce two or three lambs compared with only one produced by the poorly nourished ewe (Owen, 1976). It has been suggested that in physiological terms such women are better reproducers than those with singleton pregnancies, and might be termed 'super mums' (MacGillivray, 1984).

Endocrine Changes

The trigger to maternal physiological response is hormonal, there being an increased production of both steroid and protein hormones from the feto-placental unit during twin pregnancy. Urinary oestriol excretion has been shown to be increased in twin pregnancy by many authors, (for example, Kellar *et al.*, 1959; Coyle and Brown, 1963; Beischer *et al.*, 1968; MacGillivray *et al.*, 1971). A similar increase applies to the plasma oestriol (Masson, 1973) up to 36 weeks gestation, after which there is a very rapid rise in twin pregnancies to more than double the singleton mean. Progesterone production

Table 6.1. Mean maternal serum SP_1 and hPL in twin
pregnancies

	SP_1	hPL
Twins	184.3 ± 69.9	9.8 ± 3.2
Singletons	140.5 ± 35.4	6.0 ± 1.5
	($t = 2.68$)	($t = 5.13$)
	($p < 0.01$)	($p < 0.0005$)

is also increased in twin pregnancies compared to singletons (Van der Molen, 1963; TambyRaja and Ratnam, 1981).

The trophoblast proteins, human placental lactogen (hPL) and Schwangerschafts protein 1 (SP_1) are also increased in twin pregnancy compared with singletons (Table 6.1) and have proved useful in the early diagnosis of twin pregnancy (Grennert et al., 1976; Jandial et al., 1979). A raised alpha-fetoprotein level often alerts the clinician to the possibility of a multiple pregnancy, although it may indicate abnormality. In Aberdeen, Thom and co-workers (1984) showed that there is a difference in the production of alpha-fetoprotein in monozygotic compared with dizygotic twin pregnancies. This difference may be related to the differences in placentation.

Weight Gain

Weight gain is a relatively easily measured and good indicator of the maternal response to pregnancy. Mean total weight gain in twin pregnancies is greater than in singletons, 14.6 kg compared with 11.1 kg by 36 weeks gestation and the pattern is different. The maximum weekly weight gain in twin pregnancies occurs in both early and late weeks of gestation (Table 6.2) in contrast to singleton pregnancy (Campbell et al., 1974) when the maximum rate of gain is in mid-pregnancy.

Table 6.2. Mean weekly rate of weight gain (kg/week) in twin pregnancies in primigravidae (1950–1969)

Gestation (weeks)	Twin			Singleton mean[a]
	No.	Mean	SD	
13–20	79	0.60	0.23	0.42
20–30	153	0.55	0.24	0.47
30–36	146	0.64	0.33	0.40

[a]From Hytten and Leitch (1971).

Table 6.3. Weight gain in twin pregnancy (1969–1983): total Galton Series

		Primigravidae	Multigravidae
(a) 12–20 weeks (kg)			
	MZ	3.78 ± 2.06 (23)	4.56 ± 1.74 (25)
	DZ	4.02 ± 2.21 (37)	4.24 ± 2.04 (37)
	NS	4.16 ± 2.16 (8)	3.09 ± 1.73 (12)
Total		3.96 ± 2.13 (68)	4.16 ± 1.94 (74)
Rate/week		0.50	0.52
(b) 20–30 weeks (kg)			
	MZ	6.21 ± 2.20 (48)	5.87 ± 2.30 (56)
	DZ	6.30 ± 2.80 (65)	5.25 ± 2.32 (90)
	NS	6.83 ± 3.96 (8)	5.36 ± 2.27 (23)
Total		6.30 ± 2.65 (121)	5.47 ± 2.27 (169)
Rate/week		0.63	0.55
(c) 30–36 weeks (kg)			
	MZ	4.01 ± 1.94 (46)	3.26 ± 1.82 (57)
	DZ	3.38 ± 2.00 (50)	3.34 ± 2.35 (115)
	NS	5.72 ± 1.78 (4)	3.36 ± 1.78 (15)
Total		3.99 ± 1.98 (100)	3.31 ± 2.15 (187)
Rate/week		0.67	0.55

NS: not stated.

Table 6.3 examines the weight gain by zygosity and parity for more recent years. There are no significant differences noted when monozygotic twin pregnancies are compared with dizygotic at any of the intervals studied either in primigravidae or multigravidae. Our findings with respect to the effect of zygosity on weight gain are different from that reported by Papiernik *et al.* (1976), but only a small sample of twin pregnancies from a population were included in the French study and zygosity was not accurately determined.

There is obviously an increased weight of products of conception in twin pregnancies and it is likely that all of the constituents of weight gain as defined by Hytten and Leitch (1971) are also increased. It is not certain, however, that breast tissue and uterine musculature are increased more during twin than singleton pregnancies. The total body water retention as measured using deuterium oxide is increased in twin pregnancies, particularly in primigravidae with twin pregnancies (Table 6.4). There is a relationship between total body water and birthweight in singleton pregnancies in primigravidae, but not in multiparae (Campbell and MacGillivray, 1972). A similar relationship is evident in twin pregnancies (Table 6.5) suggesting that an increased maternal physiological response is associated with a good outcome in a twin pregnancy.

Table 6.4. Mean (± SD.) total body water (litres) in normal twin and singleton pregnancies

	Gestation (weeks)	Twins	Singletons
(a) Primigravidae	30	39.2 ± 7.01 (11)	38.5 ± 6.3 (43)
	34	43.5 ± 8.23 (11)	40.6 ± 7.4 (49)
	38	50.5 ± 5.76 (4)	41.6 ± 7.8 (46)
(b) Multiparae	30	38.6 ± 6.26 (25)	35.4 ± 6.59 (19)
	34	41.0 ± 5.95 (29)	37.4 ± 4.46 (19)
	38	43.0 ± 8.34 (17)	39.4 ± 5.36 (19)

Numbers in brackets indicate numbers in each group.

Although no direct measurement has been made of total body fat in twin pregnancy, it is likely that there is an increase in stored fat to be utilised as an energy source during late pregnancy, and for fetal growth and lactation in twin pregnancy (MacGillivray *et al.*, 1971).

Nutrition and Metabolism

Although the dietary food intake during pregnancy is not increased in women expecting twins over and above intakes of those expecting singletons (Table 6.6) fetal weight is greater in twin pregnancies indicating that absorption of nutrients from the diet and utilisation of energy, is enhanced to optimal levels in twin pregnancies. In both twin pregnancies and singleton pregnancies energy intake is lower than recommended (Department of Health and Social Security, 1979) although protein intake is satisfactory. Little is known about the absorption of nutrients across the intestinal mucosa during pregnancy except for iron, which is known to be absorbed more readily in situations of the increased demand of twin pregnancy. However, mineral intake from the diet is the same in women irrespective of whether they are expecting twins or

Table 6.5. Relation between birthweight (g) and total body water (litres) at 34 weeks in primigravidae and 38 weeks in multiparae

Primigravid twins	$y = 0.00609x + 14.68$	
	$r = 0.73$	d.f. 7, $p < 0.05$
Multiparous twins	$y = 0.00310x + 26.10$	
	$r = 0.27$	d.f. 16, NS

(Where x is total body water and y is combined birthweight of twins)

Table 6.6. Mean daily energy and protein intake in twin pregnancy

	Energy intake		Protein intake (g)
	(MJ)	(kcal)	
Twins (40)	8.55 ± 2.26	2036 ± 538	70.31 ± 15.26
Singletons (57)	8.92 ± 1.79	2124 ± 426	75.48 ± 17.9
DHSS recommended	10.0	2400	60

Numbers in brackets indicate numbers in each group.

singletons (Campbell *et al.*, 1982). The indications are that most Western diets are quite sufficient in nutrients for the increased fetal growth in twin pregnancies.

The altered carbohydrate metabolism which occurs in pregnancy is influenced by many factors, including placental hormones such as human placental lactogen, oestrogen and progesterone, all of which increase in twin pregnancies. This has been shown to lead to a slower rate of glucose disposal after a glucose load in twin pregnancies compared with singletons, although the levels of fasting plasma glucose remain unchanged (Campbell and Mac-Gillivray, 1979). Different standards of abnormality require to be determined before considering such women as diabetic, and it could be that the insulin response to glucose load may be more exaggerated in twin pregnancies, or that insulin sensitivity may be changed.

Blood and Cardiovascular Changes

The haemostatic mechanism was also studied in twin pregnancies in Aberdeen (Condie and Campbell, 1978) and it was found that plasma fibrinogen was considerably elevated in mothers of twins, while other parameters showed no clear-cut change. This could represent a rebound phenomenon secondary to a degree of fibrin deposition, or an oestrogenic enhancement of the synthesis of fibrinogen.

The more dramatic physiological adaptation of women to pregnancy occurs in the cardiovascular system. The cardiac output is markedly increased in singleton pregnancies, but only slightly more so (Rovinsky and Jaffin, 1966). However, when posture was taken into account when these measurements were being made, Campbell and co-workers (1985) found no difference in either stroke volume or cardiac output using a non-invasive technique with repeated measurements between women expecting singletons or twins. However, total peripheral resistance is likely to be lowered even further in a twin pregnancy on account of a greater production of progesterone and

Table 6.7. Distribution of diastolic blood pressure at 20 weeks gestation in primigravid twin and singleton pregnancies (% rate)

Diastolic BP (mmHg)	<70	70–79	80–89	≥90
Twin pregnancies				
($n = 171$)	24.6 (42)	49.7 (85)	23.4 (40)	2.3 (4)
Singleton pregnancies				
($n = 4215$)	22.4 (944)	43.6 (1838)	28.4 (1197)	5.6 (236)

Numbers in brackets indicate numbers in each group.
$p < 0.05$.

possibly prostaglandins leading to vasodilatation with a lowering of the diastolic blood pressure. Lower diastolic blood pressure was found in mid-pregnancy in women expecting twins (Table 6.7) (Campbell and Campbell, 1985), but this did not apply to the systolic blood pressure. In twin pregnancy there was a greater fall from the non-pregnant levels in the diastolic pressure by mid-pregnancy, and a greater rise of diastolic pressure by delivery. The pulse rate, which is increased in singleton pregnancies, is further slightly increased in twin pregnancies.

Other related changes are concerned with the volume and constituents of the blood. There are marked increases in plasma volume and red cell volume

Table 6.8. Plasma volume in normal twin and singleton pregnancies (mean and SD)

(a) Twin				
Gestation	Primigravidae		Multiparae	
20	3050	(1)	3647 ± 424	(4)
22–24	3951 ± 516	(5)	3823 ± 772	(13)
26–28	4318 ± 853	(9)	4085 ± 557	(12)
30–32	4311 ± 672	(20)	4498 ± 603	(46)
34–36	4156 ± 610	(20)	4591 ± 756	(43)
37–38	4522 ± 591	(6)	4567 ± 540	(22)
39–40	4455	(2)	4574 ± 455	(9)
(b) Singleton				
	First pregnancy		Second pregnancy	
12	2590 ± 178	(7)	2646 ± 167	(5)
16	2700 ± 259	(10)	2866 ± 224	(7)
20	3062 ± 222	(10)	3153 ± 237	(10)
25	3313 ± 527	(11)	3481 ± 439	(11)
30	3671 ± 628	(12)	3929 ± 288	(12)
34	3831 ± 695	(12)	3861 ± 388	(10)
38	3780 ± 523	(12)	3817 ± 632	(10)

Numbers in brackets indicate numbers in each group.

Table 6.9. Mean (± SD) plasma volume (ml) by combined birthweight centiles in primigravid twin pregnancies

	Birthweight centiles				
	<25	25–<50	50–<75	50–<75	≥75
Normotensive and mild pre-eclampsia (78)	3769 ± 481 (28)	4049 ± 643 (12)	4013 ± 439 (17)		4175 ± 566 (21)
Proteinuric pre-eclampsia (30)	3952 ± 661 (14)	4092 ± 278 (4)	4240 ± 468 (5)		4112 ± 307 (7)
All (108)	3830 ± 547 (42)	4060 ± 574 (16)	4065 ± 446 (22)		4159 ± 573 (28)

Numbers in brackets indicate numbers in each group.

in twin pregnancies compared with singleton pregnancies. Rovinsky and Jaffin (1965) found a mean value of 4 litres of plasma volume in singleton pregnancies between 37 and 40 weeks compared to a mean of 4.7 litres at the same gestation in seven twin pregnancies, but these authors did not differentiate their subjects into primigravidae and multigravidae. In singleton pregnancies, there is a difference between the plasma volume expansion in first compared with second pregnancies (Campbell and MacGillivray, 1972) and this has also been demonstrated in twin pregnancies (Table 6.8) (Campbell and MacGillivray, 1977). The maximum increase in primigravid twin pregnancies did not occur until 36–38 weeks, whereas the maximum plasma volume in multipara twin pregnancies was achieved by 30–32 weeks gestation.

The serum volume correlated with the babyweight in both first and second pregnancies (Campbell and MacGillivray, 1984). It was found that the combined birthweight of twins related to the expansion of the plasma volume

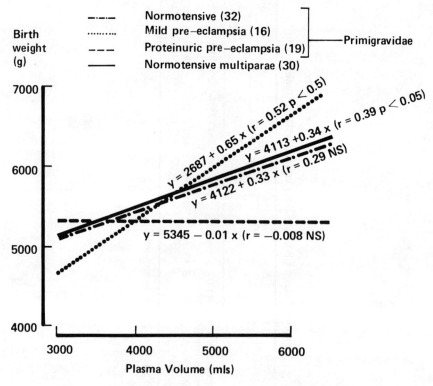

Figure 6.1. Maternal plasma volume after 30 weeks and combined birthweight: twin pregnancies born after 37 weeks.

Table 6.10 Mean (± SD) total red cell volume (ml) in twin and singleton pregnancy

	Gestation (weeks)	Twins	Singletons
(a) Primigravidae	30	1910 ± 293 (20)	1732 ± 328 (43)
	34	1973 ± 335 (20)	1694 ± 323 (46)
	38	2172 ± 246 (6)	1797 ± 351 (45)
(b) Multiparae	30	1864 ± 258 (45)	1612 ± 281 (20)
	34	2082 ± 451 (42)	1710 ± 283 (19)
	38	2072 ± 393 (21)	1677 ± 291 (18)

Numbers in brackets indicate numbers in each group.

in both primigravidae and in multiparae, as happens with singleton pregnancies (Table 6.9) (Figure 6.1). A very marked increase in the red cell mass in twin pregnancy was reported by Rovinsky and Jaffin (1965) and this was confirmed in Aberdeen (MacGillivray et al., 1971; Campbell and MacGillivray, 1977) (Table 6.10). This is indicative of a markedly increased oxygen carrying capacity required for the oxygen transfer to the two fetuses. The increase in the red cell mass, however, is not relatively as great as that in the plasma volume, so that there is, as a consequence, a marked haemodilution. This leads to water soluble substances such as folate being markedly decreased in concentration in serum or plasma.

Haemoglobin concentration as measured in the standard manner is low from early pregnancy (Table 6.11). Women with twin pregnancies had an average haemoglobin concentration of approximately 10 g/dl from 20 weeks onwards. However, the mean cell haemoglobin concentration and the mean cell volume did not alter in those women who did not receive any iron or folic acid supplements in pregnancy (Hall et al., 1979). Only 15% of them showed any evidence of iron deficiency in the peripheral blood film by the end of pregnancy.

Table 6.11. Haemoglobin in twin pregnancy by gestation

Gestation (weeks)	No.	Mean Hb ± SD (g/dl)
20–23	13	10.4 ± 1.1
24–27	15	10.1 ± 1.7
28–31	29	10.4 ± 1.4
32–34	26	10.9 ± 1.2
36–37	16	10.5 ± 3.1
38–40	13	11.8 ± 1.1

Table 6.12. Macrocytosis in singleton and twin pregnancies

	Definite macrocytosis %	Equivocal macrocytosis %
Twins (123)	2.4	4.1
Singletons (2024)	1.9	5.2

Numbers in brackets indicate numbers in each group.

The total amount of circulating folate is unchanged during pregnancy, although as mentioned earlier, the concentration of folate in serum falls remarkably in twin pregnancies (Hall *et al.*, 1976). The red cell folate concentration was found to be unchanged, although a very large scatter of values made this of little diagnostic use (Hall, 1987).

The presence of macrocytosis with hypersegmentation of neutrophil polymorphs in the peripheral blood is usually considered to be indicative of developing megaloblastic anaemia. The incidence of this complication has been found to be the same in singleton as in twin pregnancies in a total population in Aberdeen (Table 6.12). (See Chapter 7).

The white blood cell count is increased in normal pregnancy and is further increased in twin pregnancies. Similarly, the erythrocyte sedimentation rate shows a greater increase than in singleton pregnancies.

The concentration of the total proteins in twin pregnancies falls from 6.1 g/100 ml in singletons to 5.5 g/100 ml in twin pregnancies, but the total intravascular mass of proteins was found to be greater in twin than in singleton pregnancies (MacGillivray *et al.*, 1971). The serum concentration of sodium, potassium and chloride and serum osmolality did not differ between twin pregnancies and singleton pregnancies (Campbell and MacGillivray, 1977).

There have been few studies of blood and cardiovascular changes in triplet or higher multiple pregnancies, but in a study of a quadruplet pregnancy (Fullerton *et al.*, 1965) there was a very considerable increase in plasma volume up to 5990 ml at 34 weeks and a red blood cell volume increase to 2795 ml.

Renal, Respiratory and Liver Function

Renal function is altered to a greater extent in twin pregnancy compared to singleton, as for example, the increased glomerular filtration rate demonstrated by Swapp and Gomez (1975).

The respiratory function also shows greater change in twin pregnancy than in singleton, as a greater increase in the tidal volume was found by Templeton and Kelman (1974).

Hepatic function also shows a greater change in uncomplicated multiple pregnancies than in singleton pregnancies, as exemplified by the bromsulph- thalein test (Beazley and Tindall, 1966). Using a modification of this test (Barber-Riley *et al.*, 1961) it was found in a small number of twin pregnancies that both the rate of transfer of the dye from plasma to liver and that from liver to plasma were increased (Fotheringham, 1974). These changes resulted firstly from an increased amount of blood passing through the liver and, secondly, an alteration in the binding of proteins by pregnancy steroid hormones leading to a greater return of unbound dye to the plasma. There have been no measures of other changes in the alimentary system, but it is probable that in multiple pregnancies, oesophageal reflux, hypochlorhydria, reduced gastric motility and constipation are even greater than in singleton pregnancies.

Women pregnant with multiple births, therefore, have in many respects an exaggerated maternal response to the pregnancy which, as well as being of importance for fetal growth of the twins, is also of relevant clinical import- ance. The physiological changes can raise suspicion and aid in a diagnosis of multiple pregnancies. Different standards of normality have to be accepted for multiple pregnancies compared with singleton pregnancies, and allowance must also be made for more frequent occurrence of abnormalities in twin pregnancies.

Twinning and Twins
Edited by I. MacGillivray, D. M. Campbell and B. Thompson
© 1988 John Wiley & Sons Ltd

CHAPTER 7

Management of twin pregnancies

IAN MACGILLIVRAY and DORIS M. CAMPBELL

*Department of Obstetrics and Gynaecology, University of Aberdeen,
Aberdeen, UK*

The diagnosis of multiple pregnancy as early as possible is important, not only because of the greater frequency and earlier onset of complications compared with a singleton pregnancy, but also to assist in the accurate assessment of gestational age. Early diagnosis is also important so that arrangements can be made for booking for delivery in a centre equipped to deal with twin pregnancies. Failure to diagnose multiple pregnancy can lead to serious problems for both mother and babies. For example, in the management of labour, if twins are undiagnosed and an oxytocic drug is given at the time of delivery resulting in a reduced uteroplacental blood flow and thus excessive uterine contractions, the oxygen supply to the second baby is decreased; in addition, closure of the cervix will make delivery of twin two more difficult. It used to be relatively common for twin pregnancies not to be diagnosed until late in pregnancy or even at delivery. In a London study (Law, 1967) only 45.6% of twin pregnancies were diagnosed before the 32nd week although 86% were diagnosed before the start of labour. With the advent of ultrasonic scanning, twin pregnancies are frequently confirmed much earlier. For example, in the Scottish Twin Study of a total population of 650 twin pregnancies in 1983 (Patel *et al.*, 1984) 69% were diagnosed by a first scan before 20 weeks gestation and overall 95% were diagnosed antenatally. Although altogether 559 of the twin pregnancies (86%) were confirmed by ultrasound, 44 of these were not identified at the first scan. When the ultrasound scan was carried out before 12 weeks, 28 out of 128 twin pregnancies (21.9%) were not diagnosed, whereas when the scan was after 20 weeks, only two out of 68 (2.9%) were missed. Routine ultrasonic scanning at booking has been advocated for all pregnant women, but this is unlikely to detect all multiple pregnancies as the gestation at time of scanning/booking will not be optimum for the diagnosis of twin pregnancy. It is still important, therefore, to look out for other clinical evidence of multiple pregnancies.

The most notable feature is the greater size of the uterus with multiple pregnancy compared to singleton pregnancy. Some multiparae themselves may note and comment that they feel larger than they did in a previous singleton pregnancy. It is best to measure the fundal height in centimetres above the symphysis pubis. In singleton pregnancy the fundal height is approximately 20 cm at 20 weeks' gestation, whereas in a twin pregnancy it will be greater, e.g. ± 24 cm. The abdominal circumference can also be of some value in indicating a twin pregnancy, but is more reliable in the later weeks of pregnancy. In a singleton pregnancy the circumference increases by about 1 inch (2.5 cm) per week from 34 to 40 weeks, when the circumference is usually about 40 inches (102 cm) at the umbilicus. Circumferences greater than this should arouse suspicion of either multiple pregnancy or some abnormality such as polyhydramnios or tumours. Increased weekly weight gain can also be a useful indicator of multiple pregnancy, as the rate of weight gain is greater than in a singleton pregnancy, although marked variations can occur. The average weight gain between 13 and 20 weeks in a multiple pregnancy is about 600 g compared with about 400 g in a singleton pregnancy (see Chapter 6). Also abdominal palpation may reveal a suspiciously large number of small fetal parts although care is needed to avoid confusion with limbs in an occipito-posterior position. Four fetal poles of the two fetuses cannot usually be palpated, but three can often be identified. If a head is clearly felt which seems to be small in relation to the size of the uterus, a multiple pregnancy should be suspected, as this is much more likely than a microcephalic fetus.

Some assistance in diagnosis can be obtained from listening for two fetal hearts, but this poses problems. The two fetal hearts must be auscultated simultaneously by two different observers, and there must be a difference of 10 beats per minute between the two fetal hearts. Standard auscultation by one person is usually considered to be useless in the diagnosis of a twin pregnancy. If the detection of cardiac blood flow is by the Doppler principle, twin pregnancy may be more reliably diagnosed. When the first fetal heart is detected and the rate recorded, the direction of the ultrasonic probe is changed to find the other fetal heart. If the rates are discrepant or the angle of the ultrasonic beam has been altered by more than 90° twins can confidently be diagnosed. It is preferable to use two separate machines simultaneously so that the direction of the probes can easily be determined.

Multiple fetuses can readily be shown by radiography from 20 weeks onwards. In the case of greater multiples, ultrasonic scanning may not detect all the fetuses because of their mobility, and in late pregnancy because of shadowing of one fetus by another; in such cases radiography may be employed not only to show the number of fetuses, but also to detect any bony abnormalities which might be present.

Complications of Multiple Pregnancies

It is generally believed that a twin pregnancy places a greater strain on the mother than a singleton pregnancy as evidenced by James Matthews Duncan

(1865) who stated that 'the rarity of plural births in women and increased danger to mother and offspring in these circumstances renders such an event in a certain limited sense a disease or abnormality'. In the first half of pregnancy there is little difference between a twin and a singleton pregnancy apart from a greater tendency to abortion. In the second half of pregnancy, however, as the uterus becomes larger 'mechanical' discomfort becomes more noticeable with an increased frequency of backache and lower abdominal pain. As a result of the increased intra-abdominal pressure, the frequency of micturition, constipation, varicose veins and oedema are all increased. As the pregnancy advances towards term, it becomes difficult for a women expecting twins to be comfortable in any position of rest, and walking is difficult, due partly to locomotor difficulties and partly to breathlessness as the diaphragm is pushed upwards and splinted.

Abortion

It is difficult to determine the frequency of twin pregnancy abortions as they are often not recognised, particularly in early gestation (see Chapter 4). However, ultrasound scanning studies increasingly provide evidence of the phenomenon known as 'the vanishing twin'. In nine studies documenting this phenomenon, 'disappearance' rates ranged form 0% to 78%, depending on patient population and the timing of ultrasonography (Landy *et al.*, 1982). The only relevant complication reported was vaginal bleeding, i.e. diagnosed as threatened abortion, with subsequent singleton birth.

The threatened abortion rate of women who delivered twins was significantly higher in the 1983 Scottish Twin Study (Patel *et al.*, 1984), 11% compared with 3% in women who delivered singletons. It was previously

Table 7.1. Incidence of threatened abortion in Aberdeen City District 1951–1983

	Twins			Singletons		
	No. of threatened abortions	Total no.	%	No. of threatened abortions	Total no.	%
1951–55	7	235	2.98	362	16 157	2.24
1956–60	12	211	5.69	656	17 394	3.77
1961–65	8	210	3.81	726	17 275	4.20
1966–70	38	176	21.59	2 189	15 623	14.01
1971–75	34	132	25.76	1 990	13 237	15.03
1976–80	31	118	26.27	2 171	11 436	18.95
1981–83	18	68	26.47	1 523	7 443	20.47
Total	148	1 150	12.87	9 617	98 565	9.78

reported from Aberdeen for the years 1958–1965 (Nylander and MacGillivray, 1975) that threatened abortion was not particularly common in women who delivered twins. On examining the incidence of this complication over a longer time period (Table 7.1) it is evident that in keeping with the Scottish 1983 data, threatened abortion occurs significantly oftener in pregnancies resulting in twins ($z = 3.50$, $p < 0.001$). However, the incidence of threatened abortion has increased in recent years, in both twin and singleton pregnancies, at least partly due to women's increased awareness and reporting. The only 5 year period when threatened abortion was not commoner in pregnancies which ended in the birth of twins was 1961–1965, the main years of the earlier study by Nylander and MacGillivray (1975).

Hydatidiform Mole

A hydatidiform mole within a twin pregnancy may go undetected until it is delivered alongside a normal infant. With frequent ultrasound scanning moles are less likely to remain undetected. However, early detection of asymptomatic molar twin pregnancies will mean that obstetricians must carefully balance the dangers of allowing the pregnancy to continue against the loss of a wanted fetus.

Some authors advocate immediate termination of the pregnancy on the grounds of the risk of malignant change in the hydatidiform mole (James and Lauersen, 1975; Yee et al., 1982; Sande and Eyjolfsson, 1985) whereas others contend that there is no evidence that continuing the pregnancy increases the risk or accelerates the rate at which malignant change occurs (Suzuki et al., 1980; Davis and Fuentes, 1984).

If the pregnancy is allowed to continue the patient must be closely monitored for early signs of fulminating pre-eclamptic toxaemia—a frequent complication of hydatidiform mole—or of vaginal bleeding.

Antepartum Haemorrhage

It is generally considered that antepartum haemorrhage is likely to occur more frequently in twin than in singleton pregnancies on account of the greater incidence of pre-eclampsia and possibly placental abruption and also the larger area of placental tissue with a likelihood of placenta praevia. A higher incidence of placenta praevia was found in twin pregnancies by Munnell and Taylor (1946), but Bender (1952) found an incidence of 0.6% in twin pregnancy compared with 0.9% in singleton pregnancy. Paintin (1962) found the same total incidence (3%) of all types of antepartum haemorrhage in both twin and in singleton pregnancies. In the 1983 Scottish Twin Study (Patel et al., 1984) the rate of antepartum haemorrhage was found to be 4% in both twin and singleton pregnancies.

Table 7.2. Incidence of antepartum haemorrhage in Aberdeen City District 1951–1983

	Twins (1 150) %		Singletons (98 565) %	
Placenta praevia (PP)	0.70	(8)	0.42	(413)
Abruptio	0.09	(1)	0.14	(139)
Antepartum haemorrhage of unknown origin (APHUO)	5.22	(60)	4.14	(4 078)
None	94.00	(1 081)	95.30	(93 935)

Numbers in brackets are total numbers in each group.

In the earlier study from Aberdeen, Nylander and MacGillivray (1975) found no difference in the incidence of all antepartum haemorrhage between twin and singleton pregnancies or between monozygotic and dizygotic twin pregnanices. However, our recent analysis of the Aberdeen data of the total population from 1951 to 1983 shows an overall incidence of antepartum haemorrhage in twin pregnancies (6%) to be significantly greater ($z = 2.07$, $p \leq 0.05$) than the rate in singleton pregnancies (4.7%) (Table 7.2). Table 7.3 shows an increasing incidence of antepartum haemorrhage (excluding placenta praevia) in both singleton and twin pregnancies (probably due to increased reporting of vaginal bleeding) and a considerably greater rate in twin pregnancies in recent years. In contrast Table 7.4 shows the corresponding figures for placenta praevia which have remained fairly steady. In twin pregnancies there are no significant differences in the rates of antepartum haemorrhage by zygosity or placentation (Table 7.5).

Table 7.3. Incidence of antepartum haemorrhage (APH) excluding placenta praevia in Aberdeen City District 1951–1983

	Twins % APH		Singletons % APH	
1951–55	1.70	(235)	2.67	(16 157)
1956–60	3.79	(211)	2.89	(17 394)
1961–65	2.86	(219)	3.09	(17 275)
1966–70	4.55	(176)	4.61	(15 623)
1971–75	7.58	(132)	5.08	(13 237)
1976–80	14.41	(118)	6.73	(11 436)
1981–83	11.76	(68)	7.87	(7 443)

Numbers in brackets are total numbers in each group.

Table 7.4. Incidence of placenta praevia (PP) in Aberdeen
City District 1951–1983

	Twins % PP		Singletons % PP	
1951–55	0.43	(235)	0.10	(16 157)
1956–60	—	(211)	0.35	(17 394)
1961–65	1.43	(219)	0.60	(17 275)
1966–70	1.70	(176)	0.54	(15 623)
1971–75	—	(132)	0.39	(13 237)
1976–80	0.85	(118)	0.48	(11 436)
1981–83	—	(68)	0.56	(7 443)

Numbers in brackets are total numbers in each group.

The management of antepartum haemorrhage in twin pregnancies does not
differ from that in singleton pregnancies.

Polyhydramnios (Hydramnios)

The incidence of polyhydramnios in twin pregnancies has been reported as
3.6–10.6% by McClure (1937) Guttmacher (1939), Munnell and Taylor
(1946), Potter and Fuller (1949) and Bender (1952). Much of the variation is
no doubt due to the differences in diagnostic criteria. In Aberdeen, Nylander
and MacGillivray (1975) found that the incidence of hydramnios was 2.4% in
twin pregnancies compared with 0.4% in singleton pregnancies, figures

Table 7.5. Incidence of antepartum haemorrhage in Aberdeen City District
1969–1983: singleton pregnancy and twin pregnancies by zygosity and placentation

	% Rates								
	Total	PP		Abruptio		APHUO		All APH together	
MZ MC	(68)	—	(0)	—	(0)	7.35	(5)	7.35	(5)
MZ DC	(74)	—	(0)	—	(0)	10.81	(8)	10.81	(8)
MZ (NS)	(6)	—	(0)	—	(0)	16.67	(1)	16.67	(1)
All MZ	(148)	—	(0)	—	(0)	9.46	(14)	9.46	(14)
DZ DC	(199)	0.5	(1)	0.5	(1)	9.55	(19)	10.55	(21)
NK	(32)	2.7	(1)	—	(0)	10.81	(4)	13.51	(5)
Singleton	(38 186)	0.49	(186)	0.31	(117)	5.82 (2 224)		6.62 (2 527)	

NS: not stated; NK: not known.
Numbers in brackets are numbers in each group.

Table 7.6. Incidence of hydramnios Aberdeen City District
1951–1983

	Twins %		Singletons %	
1951–55	1.70	(235)	0.09	(16 157)
1956–60	0.95	(211)	0.25	(17 394)
1961–65	5.24	(219)	0.42	(17 275)
1966–70	1.70	(176)	0.33	(15 623)
1971–75	0.76	(132)	0.37	(13 237)
1976–80	4.24	(118)	1.05	(11 436)
1981–83	4.41	(68)	1.05	(7 443)
All	2.52	(1 150)	0.44	(98 565)

Numbers in brackets are numbers in each group.

similar to those for the extended period 1951–1983 (hightly significant $z = 10.37, p < 0.0001$). However, there has been an increase in the diagnosis of hydramnios since the mid-1970s, particularly affecting twin pregnancies (Table 7.6).

The incidence of hydramnios in the 1983 Scottish Twin Study (Patel *et al.*, 1984) was high at 6% in twin pregnancies compared with 0.3% in singleton pregnancies, but no consistent definition was used in all centres participating.

A fairly similar incidence of hydramnios was found in monozygotic and dizygotic twin pregnancies by Guttmacher (1939) and Aberdeen data confirmed this (Nylander and MacGillivray, 1975). However, a higher incidence of acute hyramnios was found in single ovum twins by Gaehtgens (1936). The acute and chronic forms of polyhydramnios were not differentiated in any of the other studies.

The management of polyhydramnios is similar to that in singleton pregnancy. However, if hydramnios in twins is associated with a fetal abnormality it may in certain circumstances be possible to stop the hydramnios by feticide of the affected twin and allow the pregnancy of the normal twin to continue. Management of particularly acute hydramnios may include amniocentesis, but this is fraught with the risk of preterm labour. Diuretics are not of value in the management and bedrest along with symptomatic treatment is only of value to relieve the woman's discomfort.

Pre-eclampsia

It is well known that there is a greater frequency of pre-eclampsia in twin pregnancy compared with singleton pregnancy, although the actual incidence reported from different centres varies. This is in part due to the different criteria and definition of the condition and in part to differences in the populations under review (MacGillivray, 1983). As this condition is commoner in primigravidae it is particularly important to control for parity. Guttmacher (1939) found that the condition occurred about three times as often in viable twin pregnancies, and Bender (1952) agreed. In Aberdeen primigravidae, MacGillivray (1958) found that the incidence of proteinuric pre-eclampsia was five times greater in twin than in singleton pregnancies. The incidence of gestational hypertension, i.e. a rise in diastolic pressure to 90 mmHg or more in the second half of pregnancy, was only increased from 18% in singleton pregnancies to 25% in twin pregnancies. Nylander and MacGillivray (1975) examined the incidence in Ibadan using the same definition as in Aberdeen. The incidence of proteinuric pre-eclampsia in twin pregnancies of all parities was 4.5% compared with 6% in singletons. However, when they looked at first pregnancies only, the rates were 5.9% and 1.1% for twin and singleton pregnancies respectively, emphasising the importance of parity.

The recent Scottish Twin Study (Patel *et al.*, 1984) showed a significant increase in both proteinuric pre-eclampsia and gestational hypertension in twin pregnancies. This also applied in Aberdeen over the period 1951–1983 (Table 7.7). The increase is particularly marked for proteinuric pre-eclampsia in multiparae. Although the incidence of pre-eclampsia fluctuates with time with an apparent rise in singleton pregnancies in recent years, it is always greater in twin pregnancies (Table 7.8).

Pre-eclampsia was reported to be more common in women with unlike-sex twins (Stevenson *et al.*, 1971) and by implication dizygotic rather than

Table 7.7. Pre-eclampsia in singleton and twin pregnancies in Aberdeen City District 1951–1983 by parity

(a) Primigravidae	Twins (376) %		Singletons (39 820) %	
Eclampsia	2.93	(11)	0.12	(68)
Proteinuric pre-eclampsia	21.01	(79)	6.05	(2 409)
Gestational hypertension	31.38	(118)	26.08	(10 385)
None	44.68	(168)	67.70	(26 958)
(b) Multiparae	Twins (774)		Singletons (58 745)	
Eclampsia	0.26	(2)	0.05	(27)
Proteinuric pre-eclampsia	10.59	(82)	1.45	(850)
Gestational hypertension	19.12	(148)	14.05	(8 254)
None	70.03	(542)	84.46	(49 614)

Numbers in brackets are numbers in each group.

Table 7.8. Proteinuric pre-eclampsia in Aberdeen City District in twin and singleton pregnancies

	Primigravidae twins %	Multiparae twins %	Primigravidae singletons %	Multiparae singletons %
1951–55	27.12 (16)	8.52 (15)	5.48 (333)	1.14 (115)
1956–60	15.49 (11)	11.43 (16)	4.76 (316)	1.19 (128)
1961–65	16.13 (10)	8.11 (12)	4.04 (255)	1.13 (124)
1966–70	27.27 (15)	10.74 (13)	4.42 (280)	1.21 (112)
1971–75	23.26 (10)	10.11 (9)	7.04 (411)	1.22 (90)
1976–80	22.81 (13)	14.75 (9)	7.44 (382)	2.00 (126)
1981–83	13.79 (4)	20.51 (8)	12.40 (432)	3.92 (155)

Numbers in brackets are numbers in each group.

monozygotic twinning (Stevenson *et al.*, 1976). However, MacFarlane and Scott (1976) reported no difference in pre-eclampsia between monozygotic and dizygotic twin pregnancies when zygosity was estimated from Weinberg's formula. In the Aberdeen series, it was found on the basis of accurate zygosity determination at birth by blood grouping and placental enzymes that the incidence of proteinuric pre-eclampsia was similar in monozygotic and dizygotic twin pregnancies (Campbell *et al.*, 1977). Table 7.9 shows that this applies for both primigravidae and multigravidae.

The increased frequency of severe pre-eclampsia and its association with growth retardation makes this a very serious condition for the mother and babies. There is need for special vigilance over mothers expecting twins with frequent routine blood pressure checking and urine testing in order to detect the condition as early as possible. The management of pre-eclampsia and eclampsia in twin pregnancies is similar to that in singleton pregnancies, but the decision on the optimum timing of delivery is even more difficult. As the condition may progress rapidly, even women with apparently mild pre-eclampsia should be admitted for observation so that the mother's condition can be balanced against fetal intrauterine growth retardation and the difficulty of adequate fetal monitoring of two babies. Hormone assays are not of value and there are more problems with cardiotocography and its interpretation than in singleton pregnancies. No special diet is required and salt restriction unnecessary. The use of diuretics is contraindicated except for the management of acute pulmonary oedema and congestive cardiac failure and in renal failure. Hypotensive therapy may be used judiciously, particularly in labour to avoid life threatening rises in blood pressure. Anticonvulsant therapy should be used as in singleton pregnancies. Having decided on the optimum time of delivery, caesarean section may be necessary if induction of

Table 7.9. Percentage incidence of hypertensive disease of pregnancy in Grampian Region twin pregnancies (1969–1983) by parity, zygosity and placentation

Zygosity and placentation		Severe pre-eclampsia	Mild pre-eclampsia	Normotensives
(A) Pregnancy No. 1				
MZ MC	(57)	26.3	31.6	42.1
MZ DC	(53)	11.3	26.4	62.3
MZ Not stated	(5)	—	40.0	60.0
DZ DC	(136)	13.9	23.5	62.5
Not stated	(29)	13.8	13.8	72.4
Total	(280)	15.7	25.0	59.3
(B) Pregnancy No. ⩾ 2				
MZ MC	(97)	11.3	18.6	70.1
MZ DC	(88)	9.1	19.3	71.6
MZ Not stated	(6)	—	33.3	66.9
DZ DC	(333)	10.5	19.8	69.7
Not stated	(63)	12.7	15.9	71.4
Total	(587)	10.6	19.3	70.2
Pregnancy No. 1				
All MZ	(115)	18.3	29.6	
All DZ	(136)	13.9	23.5	
Not stated	(29)	13.8	13.8	
Pregnancy No. ⩾ 2				
All MZ	(191)	9.95	19.4	
All DZ	(333)	10.5	19.8	
Not stated	(63)	12.7	15.9	

Numbers in brackets are numbers in each group.

labour might be difficult, even though the presentations of the babies may be favourable.

Anaemia

The greater expansion of plasma volume compared with red cell volume results in a lowering of the haemoglobin concentration which is greater in twin than singleton pregnancies (see changes detailed in Chapter 6). This may give a false impression that anaemia is more common in twin than in singleton pregnancies, and might be expected because of the greater demands of two fetuses on maternal stores. The haemoglobin concentration and packed cell volume, therefore, are unreliable indicators. More reliance should be placed on the mean corpuscular haemoglobin concentration, which does not change.

Using haemoglobin concentration as an indicator, Guttmacher (1939) found that the proportion of patients with twin pregnancies with a level below 70% was much higher than in singleton pregnancies.

In a study of anaemia, defined as packed cell volume of less than 27%, in Ibadan, Nigeria, Nylander and MacGillivray (1975) found that the incidence was the same in both singleton and in twin pregnancies, being 10.6 and 10.4% respectively. However, most of the anaemia in the Nigerian population is due to folic acid deficiency and haemolytic anaemia rather than iron deficiency. Harrison (1969) found that 92% of pregnant women in Ibadan had folic acid deficiency anaemia, mostly associated with haemolysis. Hall (1970), in a study of a total antenatal population in Aberdeen, found that the incidence of macrocytosis (folic acid deficiency), both definite and equivocal, in the peripheral blood was similar in twin and singleton pregnancies, namely 2.4% and 1.9% in respectively.

Anaemia defined as haemoglobin concentration less than 9.5 g/dl was found to be not significantly different in twin pregnancies (6%) than in singleton pregnancies (5.1%) in the 1983 Scottish Twin Study (Patel et al., 1984). Hall et al. (1979) examined all 123 twin pregnancies in the Grampian Region of Scotland for a defined period, February 1975 until May 1977., Eighteen women (15%) showed definite evidence of iron deficiency on peripheral blood film examination and a further eight (7%) had equivocal changes. Of the 27 women in this study who had sternal marrow aspiration, eleven (40%) showed reduced iron stores. With respect to folic acid deficiency, eight (29.6%) women showed megaloblastic haemopoiesis in the sternal marrow. This incidence is higher than the 13% reported for singleton pregnancies (Chanarin et al., 1968). Of the eight women with megaloblastic change in the marrow, only two had anaemia and six had low red cell folate levels. It was considered that the incidence of clinically significant anaemia was low, and explained by any deficiency being of a transient and self-limiting nature. They suggested that because of past findings of the uncertainties of women taking routine prophylactic iron/folic acid, this should not be recommended. Specific treatment should be given where there was evidence of significant anaemia.

Fetal Abnormalities

Prenatal diagnosis is one of the most significant recent developments. When major congenital abnormalities are detected antenatally in both fetuses (a relatively rare occurrence—see Chapter 11), it is usual to offer termination of the pregnancy to the parents. However, if a severe abnormality/disorder is detected using prenatal diagnostic techniques in one twin and the other appears normal, a third possibility of management exists. Selective feticide may be carried out on the affected twin by injection of air through a fetoscope into a large fetal vessel (Rodeck, 1984). The risks of this procedure for the healthy twin have not been fully evaluated, but if the affected twin is likely to be severely handicapped the parents usually prefer to accept the risk. The finding of a dead twin at delivery should lead to a search for malformations caused by a vascular disturbance in the living co-twin. Furthermore, zygosity should be determined in twins with gonadal dysgenesis.

Rhesus Incompatability

It is possible when rhesus isoimmunisation occurs in multiple pregnancies to attempt to assess fetal blood groups and the degree of haemolysis in each of the fetuses. This is now easier than previously with the introduction of fetoscopy and fetal blood sampling and the use of ultrasound scanning during amniocentesis to aid in sampling fluid from both sacs. This was a problem in the past, partially resolved using dyes and x-ray techniques (Nylander and MacGillivray, 1975). In the management of an individual case with rhesus isoimmunisation when one baby only or both may be equally affected, decisions about the optimum timing of delivery and the need for intrauterine transfusion have to be considered in the light of such factors as previous history, gestation, and growth of the babies. Fortunately, rhesus isoimmunisation is now a rare problem.

Preterm Labour

The incidence of preterm labour in twin pregnancies is reported as ranging from 20 to 50% compared with 5 to 10% in singleton pregnancies. The gestation at onset of labour in twin and singleton pregnancies for the

Table 7.10. Gestation at delivery in twin and singleton pregnancies in Aberdeen City District 1951–1983—all cases

Weeks	Twins %		Singletons %	
<24	0.17	(2)	0.02	(18)
25–27	2.00	(23)	0.10	(121)
28–30	4.52	(52)	0.50	(440)
31–33	8.09	(93)	1.00	(1 011)
34–36	23.96	(264)	3.30	(3 277)
37–39	43.57	(501)	24.10	(23 749)
40+	15.65	(180)	70.60	(69 590)
Not known	3.04	(35)	0.40	(359)
Total	1 150		98 565	

Numbers in brackets are numbers in each group.

Table 7.11. Gestation at delivery in twin and singleton pregnancies in Aberdeen City District 1951–1983—certain gestations only

Weeks	Twins (946) %		Singletons (83 853) %	
<24	—		0.01	(11)
25–27	2.0	(19)	0.10	(81)
28–30	4.2	(40)	0.40	(331)
31–33	8.1	(77)	0.90	(745)
34–36	24.0	(227)	2.90	(2 442)
37–39	44.7	(423)	23.70	(19 909)
40+	16.9	(160)	72.00	(60 334)

Numbers in brackets are numbers in each group.

Aberdeen series (1951–1983) is shown for all pregnancies (Table 7.10) and for those with certain gestation only (Table 7.11). The importance of including cases of uncertain gestation in population studies has been emphasised for singleton pregnancies (Hall and Carr-Hill, 1985) when uncertainty of gestation itself may be identified as an adverse feature. Over the whole time period gestation was more likely to be uncertain in mothers expecting twins than singletons (Table 7.12), but in recent years due to more frequent ultrasonic scanning in early pregnancy this difference has largely disappeared.

The data for twins in the Aberdeen City District for 1969–1983 was analysed for gestation length by zygosity and placentation (Table 7.13). The preterm rate, that is delivery before 37 completed weeks, for the series of 384 twin pregnancies was 40.4%. Preterm labour occurred in 34.2% of the DZ

Table 7.12. Incidence of uncertain gestation in Aberdeen City District in twin and singleton pregnancies

	Twins (1 150) %		Singletons (98 565) %
1951–55	9.36	(22)	9.88 (1 597)
1956–60	14.22	(30)	10.55 (1 835)
1961–65	14.76	(31)	9.30 (1 606)
1966–70	7.39	(13)	9.33 (1 458)
1971–75	15.15	(20)	9.25 (1 224)
1976–80	10.17	(12)	6.98 (798)
1981–85	2.94	(2)	2.57 (191)
Total	11.30	(130)	8.84 (8 709)

Numbers in brackets are numbers in each group.

Table 7.13. Gestation at delivery in twin pregnancies in Aberdeen City District 1969–1983 by zygosity and placentation

	MZ MC (68)		MZ DC (74)		DZ DC (199)		Total (384) including not stated	
≤24	—		—		—		—	
25–27	1.47	(1)	—		—		1.56	(6)
28–30	—		4.05	(3)	5.03	(10)	4.43	(17)
31–33	11.76	(8)	6.76	(5)	7.54	(15)	8.59	(33)
34–36	35.29	(24)	28.38	(21)	21.61	(43)	25.78	(99)
37–39	48.53	(33)	47.30	(35)	49.75	(99)	46.88	(180)
40–42	1.47	(1)	10.81	(8)	11.56	(23)	9.38	(36)
Not known	1.47	(1)	2.70	(2)	4.52	(9)	3.39	(13)

Numbers in brackets are numbers in each group.

Table 7.14. Preterm deliveries by zygosity and placentation in Grampian Region of Scotland 1969–1983

	Preterm %		Term %		All %	
(a) Primigravidae						
MZ MC	69.0	(40)	31.0	(18)	100	(58)
MZ DC	66.7	(36)	33.3	(18)	100	(54)
DZ DC	53.1	(68)	46.9	(60)	100	(128)
Not known	21.7	(10)	78.3	(36)	100	(46)
Total	53.9	(154)	46.1	(132)	100	(286)
(b) Multigravidae						
MZ MC	40.2	(39)	59.8	(58)	100	(97)
MZ DC	27.3	(24)	72.7	(64)	100	(88)
DZ DC	26.5	(83)	73.5	(230)	100	(313)
Not known	10.5	(10)	89.5	(85)	100	(95)
Total	26.3	(156)	73.7	(437)	100	(593)
(c) All						
MZ MC	51.0	(79)	49.0	(76)	100	(155)
MZ DC	42.3	(60)	59.7	(82)	100	(142)
DZ DC	34.2	(151)	65.8	(290)	100	(441)
Not known	14.2	(20)	85.8	(121)	100	(141)
Total	35.3	(310)	64.7	(569)	100	(879)

Numbers in brackets are numbers in each group.

DC, in 39.2% of the MZ DC, and 48.51% of the MZ MC twin pregnancies. These preterm delivery rates are similar to those for the Grampian Region of Scotland (Table 7.14) and both are statistically significant when examined by zygosity and placentation, suggesting that both zygosity and placentation are significant with respect to early delivery.

The records of the 879 twin pregnancies in the Grampian Region of Scotland have been scrutinised to determine the mode of onset of preterm labour and divided into those with spontaneous occurrence of labour with uterine contractions, those with spontaneous rupture of the membranes before labour, and those in whom labour had been induced or elective caesarean section performed. Results showed that the rate of preterm deliv-

Table 7.15. Type of preterm delivery in 310 twin pregnancies by zygosity and placentation 1969–1983

	Elective %		Spontaneous rupture of membranes %		Contraction and retraction %		Total %	
(a) Primigravidae								
MZ MC	35.0	(14)	30.0	(12)	35.0	(14)	100	(40)
MZ DC	5.6	(2)	58.3	(21)	36.1	(13)	100	(36)
DZ DC	16.2	(11)	39.7	(27)	44.1	(30)	100	(68)
Not known	20.0	(2)	30.0	(3)	50.0	(5)	100	(10)
Total	18.8	(29)	40.9	(63)	40.3	(62)	100	(154)

$\chi^2 = 14.25$, d.f. 6, $p < 0.05$.

	Elective %		Spontaneous rupture of membranes %		Contraction and retraction %		Total %	
(b) Multigravidae								
MZ MX	10.3	(4)	56.4	(22)	33.3	(13)	100	(39)
MZ DC	12.5	(3)	54.2	(13)	33.3	(8)	100	(24)
DZ DC	10.8	(9)	39.8	(33)	49.4	(41)	100	(83)
Not known	10.0	(1)	30.0	(3)	60.8	(6)	100	(10)
Total	10.9	(17)	45.5	(71)	43.6	(68)	100	(156)

$\chi^2 = 5.4$ d.f. 6, NS

	Elective %		Spontaneous rupture of membranes %		Contraction and retraction %		Total %	
(c) All								
MZ MC	22.8	(18)	43.0	(34)	34.2	(27)	100	(79)
MZ DC	8.3	(5)	56.7	(34)	35.0	(21)	100	(60)
DZ DC	13.3	(20)	39.7	(60)	47.0	(71)	100	(151)
Not known	15.0	(3)	30.0	(6)	55.0	(11)	100	(20)
Total	14.8	(46)	43.2	(134)	41.9	(130)	100	(310)

$\chi^2 = 12.64$, d.f. 6, $p < 0.05$

numbers in brackets are numbers in each group.

ery was highest in MZ MC and lowest in DZ DC twin pregnancies, for both primigravidae and multigravidae (Table 7.14)., Significant differences in type of onset of preterm labour by zygosity and placentation are seen for twins overall (Table 7.15), although this is due mainly to the differences seen in primigravidae. In dizygotic twins there was a slight preponderance in the onset of contractions rather than spontaneous rupture of the membranes in contrast to monozygotic twins. There was no significant difference between monochorionic and dichorionic placentation in the types on onset of preterm labour except for the higher induced delivery in monozygotic, monochorionic twins in primigravidae.

In a preliminary Aberdeen study some interesting observations on the effect of zygosity, placentation and fetal sex on the type of onset of preterm labour were made by MacGillivray *et al.* (1982). An altered sex ratio, namely increased number of males, had previously been shown for singleton pregnancies ending in preterm labour (Hall and Carr-Hill, 1982).

There was a marked preponderance of boys over girls in the monozygotic twins delivered preterm, but this was not found in the dizygotic twins (Table 7.16). The reasons for these differences in the onset of preterm labour in the monozygotic and dizygotic twin pregnancies are not clear, but they may have some significant bearing on the problem of preterm labour. Very high incidences of preterm labour in triplet pregnancies of 75% (Syrop and Varner, 1985) and 78% (Itzkowic, 1979) have been reported.

Management of Twin Pregnancies

It has been shown in an extensive study in Aberdeen (Hall *et al.*, 1980) that much of present-day antenatal care is unnecessary and can be time-consuming, both for the women and the medical staff. It is, however, essential that all pregnant women should be seen early in pregnancy to enable care to be concentrated on those at high risk of complications. Obviously women with multiple pregnancies fall into this category and should be seen more frequently for antenatal care. Women expecting twins will need more support and more advice and usually have more questions to be answered than women with singleton pregnancies. It is not necessary that they should be undressed and examined abdominally any more frequently than singletons, provided they are feeling adequate fetal movement. Antenatal care should concentrate on detection of the commonly occurring problems.

Because of the greater incidence and earlier onset of pre-eclampsia, it is essential that the blood pressure measurement and urine analysis should be performed more frequently. It is generally accepted that relative to singleton standards of birthweight for gestation, twin babies show intrauterine growth retardation (see Chapter 9), although the growth and weight of twins is considered to be the same as singletons up to 32 weeks. Regular weighing of

Table 7.16. Sex ratio at birth in preterm twin deliveries in Grampian Region of Scotland 1969–1983, by zygosity and placentation

(a) Primigravidae (154)

	MZMC (40)			MZDC (36)			DZDC (68)					NK (10)			
	BB	GG	Sex ratio	BB	GG	Sex ratio	BB	GG	BG	Sex ratio	Ratio of BB:GG	BB	GG	BG	Sex ratio
Elective	7	7	100	1	1	100	3	4	4	83	75:100	1	1	—	100
Spontaneous rupture of membranes	6	6	100	12	9	133	8	6	13	116	133:100	—	3	—	—
Contraction	7	7	100	9	4	225	10	8	12	114	125:100	4	1	—	400
All preterm	20	20	100	22	14	157	21	18	29	109	117:100	5	5	—	100

(b) Multigravidae (156)

	MZMC (39)			MZDC (24)			DZDC (83)					NK (10)			
	BB	GG	Sex ratio	BB	GG	Sex ratio	BB	GG	BG	Sex ratio	Ratio of BB:GG	BB	GG	BG	Sex ratio
Elective	2	2	100	2	1	200	5	1	3	260	500:100	—	1	—	—
Spontaneous rupture of membranes	13	9	144	11	2	550	8	10	15	89	80:100	—	3	—	—
Contraction	11	2	550	4	4	100	10	9	22	105	111:100	1	5	—	20
All preterm	26	13	200	17	7	243	23	20	40	108	115:100	1	9	—	11

(c) Total (310)

	MZMC (79)			MZDC (60)			DZDC (151)					NK (20)			
	BB	GG	Sex ratio	BB	GG	Sex ratio	BB	GG	BG	Sex ratio	Ratio of BB:GG	BB	GG	BG	Sex ratio
Elective	9	9	100	3	2	150	8	5	7	135	160:100	1	2	—	50
Spontaneous rupture of membranes	19	15	127	23	11	209	16	16	28	100	100:100	—	6	—	—
Contraction	18	9	200	13	8	163	20	17	34	109	118:100	5	6	—	83
All preterm	46	33	139	39	21	186	44	38	69	108	106:100	6	14	—	43

Sex ratio at birth is number of males born for every 100 females.
B: boy; G: girl.

the mother antenatally may be of value as poor weight gain (see Chapter 6) may indicate those at greatest risk of poor fetal growth.

The fetal growth of the twins can be assessed approximately by measuring the fundal height and abdominal girth of the mother. Charting of these has been reported to be of value (Leroy *et al.*, 1982; and Schneider *et al.*, 1978).

Regular assessment of fetal growth by ultrasound scanning has been advocated in twin pregnancies (D'Alton and Dudley, 1986), but parameters of normal fetal growth in twins have not been established, although it is suggested that singleton growth curves may be appropriate up until 28 weeks gestation. Ultrasonic scanning, however, may be of value in detecting twins with discordant intrauterine growth when substantial differences in measurements between the twins are noted. This may be useful in alerting medical staff to the possibility of twin to twin transfusion.

Predicting those at risk of preterm labour or the impending onset of preterm labour has proved difficult. Weekes *et al.* (1977) found that low maternal age, low parity and monozygosity were significantly related to preterm labour in twin pregnancy. This was confirmed by the Aberdeen work with respect to parity and zygosity (see above). Unfortunately, it is not possible while the twins are in utero to readily determine monozygosity; of course dizygosity will be certain if the babies can be identified as of opposite sex.

Low socioeconomic status has been found to be of value as a high risk factor for preterm delivery in singleton pregnancy (Fedrick and Anderson, 1976), but this is not the case for twin pregnancies (Table 7.17).

Threatened preterm labour may be detected by weekly routine examination of the cervix from about 28 weeks gestation onward as advocated by Houlton *et al.*, (1982) in Durban. A cervical score is determined by subtracting the dilatation from the length in cm. There was a significant association between this score and the onset of labour within the next 14 days. Sixty per cent of cases of preterm labour would have been predicted with a false positive rate of 20%. When multiparae were excluded, the predictive value was 80% and the false positive rate was less than 5%. Neilson *et al.* (1986) found in a controlled trial of 172 patients with twin pregnancies that a 'Durban cervical score' of less than −2 before 34 weeks predicted spontaneous delivery with a sensitivity of 42%, specificity of 84% and predictive value of 71%. Cervical screening has also been found to be of value by Saunders *et al.* (1985) but O'Connor *et al.* (1981) did not find that either cervical assessment or measurement of uterine activity was helpful in predicting preterm labour.

In a recent study of results in Aberdeen (Table 7.18) it was found that in 45 cases in which the cervix was assessed between 28 and 32 weeks, preterm labour occurred in six out of 32 women who had a long, closed cervix. On the other hand, nine out of twelve women with a cervix partly effaced and dilated

Table 7.17. Gestation at delivery in twins by social class in Aberdeen City District 1969–1983 (% by column)

Social class	Total	Gestation (weeks)						
		−27	28–30	31–33	34–36	37–39	40 +	Not known
I, II, IIIa	32.29 (124)	50 (3)	47.06 (8)	24.24 (8)	34.34 (34)	32.22 (58)	30.56 (11)	15.38 (2)
IIIb, IIIc	35.94 (138)	16.67 (1)	29.41 (5)	51.52 (17)	38.38 (38)	36.67 (66)	30.56 (11)	—
IV and V	23.70 (91)	16.67 (1)	5.88 (1)	21.21 (7)	21.21 (21)	22.78 (41)	33.33 (12)	61.54 (8)
Single, widowed	3.13 (12)	16.67 (1)	5.88 (1)	—	2.02 (2)	2.22 (4)	2.78 (1)	23.08 (3)
Not known	4.95 (19)	—	11.76 (2)	3.03 (1)	4.04 (4)	6.11 (11)	2.78 (1)	—
Total	100 (384)	100 (6)	99.99 (17)	100 (33)	99.99 (99)	100 (180)	100.01 (36)	100 (13)
% Delivery <37 weeks by social class								
I, II, IIIa	42.74							
IIIb, IIIc	44.20							
IV and V	32.97							
Single, widowed	33.33							
Not known	36.84							
Total	40.36							

Numbers in brackets are numbers in each group.

Table 7.18. State of cervix between 28 and 32 weeks

Gestation at delivery (weeks)	Closed < 36	Closed ≥ 36	< 2 cm Dilated < 36	< 2 cm Dilated ≥ 36	> 2 cm Dilated < 36	> 2 cm Dilated ≥ 36	Total
Primigravidae	3	12	0	2	0	0	17
Multigravidae	3	14	3	7	1	0	28
All	6	26	3	9	1	0	45

up to 2 cm delivered at 36 weeks or later. The remaining woman whose cervix was dilated to 4 cm at 29 weeks delivered at 30 weeks. Although a closed cervix does not ensure that preterm labour will not occur, dilatation to more than 2 cm at 28–38 weeks gestation indicates that preterm labour is fairly likely and admission to hospital for rest should be considered. In two women when the cervix was noted to be dilated to more than 2 cm at 33–35 weeks, the pregnancy continued for another 4 weeks.

While it may be possible to predict some of the women with twin pregnancies who will go into preterm labour it is doubtful whether bedrest or any other measure will prevent it. It is, however, essential that those women with threatened preterm labour are admitted to a suitably equipped and staffed hospital so that the preterm babies receive the appropriate care.

Beta-sympathomimetic drugs have been used prophylactically to try to prevent preterm labour. Marivate et al. (1977) in a controlled trial using fenoterol, a stimulant with predominantly β_2 effect, found no significant difference between the two groups given fenoterol or placebo respectively in the rate of fetal growth or the gestation at onset of labour, or the rate of change of cervical score. In another controlled trial Cetrulo and Freeman (1976) gave oral ritodrine. The placebo or ritodrine was started as soon after 20 weeks as the diagnosis of multiple pregnancy as made. In 30 twin pregnancies no difference was found in gestational age, birthweight or perinatal mortality. TambyRaja et al. (1978) showed that both mean gestation length and mean birthweight were significantly greater in the 42 women with twin pregnancies treated with 2 mg of ritodrine three times daily compared with 42 controls. The perinatal mortality was also lower in the treated group. This, however, is the only study claiming a beneficial effect and the cases were not matched other than for age and parity. O'Connor et al. (1979) carried out a double blind trial in which 25 women expecting twins were given 40 mg ritodrine daily orally and 24 women were given a placebo. They also found that ritodrine did not prolong gestation or increase birthweight, but there was a high incidence of side effects. Prescott (1980) critically examined this latter double blind trial and showed that the results were inconclusive as the trial was not sensitive enough to differences in gestation length or twin birthweight which might be clinically important and advocated a further larger study. Another study using orally administered terbutaline (Skajaerris and Aberg, 1982) with 25 women treated and 25 controls given a placebo, again showed no difference in preterm deliveries or in birthweights of the twins. The majority of the evidence at present does not seem to provide any clear indication of benefit of prophylactic administration of beta-adrenergic stimulants to women with twin pregnancies.

In the belief that cervical incompetence is a factor in the aetiology of preterm labour in multiple pregnancies cervical cerclage has been recommended. Weekes *et al.* (1977) in a review of different consultants' management of twin pregnancies, showed no differences in the onset of spontaneous preterm labour, mean gestation at delivery, or mean birthweights of the twins, in three groups of women; in one group a cervical suture was inserted routinely as soon as possible after the diagnosis, the second group was treated by bedrest, and the third group had no specific treatment. Sinha *et al.* (1979) attempted to compare those who had a cervical suture inserted prophylactically in the first trimester with a matched control group and found that preterm labour was more likely to occur in those cases where a cervical suture had been inserted. In this group they also noted that 53.4% of the women had cervical damage and concluded that cervical cerclage was possibly harmful in twin pregnancies. Cervical suture appeared to be of no value in prolonging gestation in ten patients with triplet pregnancies (Itzkowic, 1979).

The crude indicator of perinatal mortality is of very doubtful value in assessing the efficacy or otherwise of bedrest, but it was on this basis that claims were made for the beneficial effects of bedrest in twin pregnancies. It was also believed that bedrest would reduce the incidence of pre-eclampsia, improve fetal growth and prevent preterm labour. It was suggested at the beginning of the century (Ballantyne, 1902) that rest would encourage fetal wellbeing and would be beneficial in the last month of pregnancy. Bedrest, preferably in hospital, from 36 weeks onwards was claimed by Hirst (1939) to encourage fetal growth and to prolong multiple pregnancies to 38 weeks. It was suggested by Russell (1952) that the lower perinatal mortality rate in twins born to middle class women in Aberdeen was due to their having more rest than working class women, and, therefore, producing larger babies which survived. Russell, therefore, advocated that all women with twin pregnancies should be admitted to hospital at the 30th week for rest. Bender (1952) also advocated bedrest as a result of his observations in Liverpool, but without any controlled trial. It became fashionable thereafter for British obstetricians to recommend bedrest for patients in the third trimester of twin pregnancy. Anderson (1956) after reconsidering the Aberdeen experience, felt that although antenatal rest in hospital appeared to help to prolong the pregnancy, the effect was probably very slight. Guttmacher and Kohl (1958) from America considered that the likelihood of postponing the onset of labour until the end of the 35th week was probably increased by hospitalisation and bedrest beginning at the 30th to 32nd week, but again no trial was carried out.

Table 7.19. Bedrest beneficial — 1960s

Study; Years	Groups	Selection	Numbers	Mean gestation at delivery	Perinatal mortality per 1000	Birthweight
Bruns and Cooper (1961; 1952–58)	A—rested for an average of 13 days	Diagnosed	27	—	90	—
	B—not rested	Undiagnosed	43	—	220	—
MacDonald (1962; 1953–58)	A—rested	Unspecified	186	12.9% < 36 weeks	89	—
	B—not rested		314	35.0% < 36 weeks	146	—
Browne and Dixon (1963; 1950–60)	A—rested at least 7 days between 30 and 36 weeks	Unspecified	215	—	40	37.2% < 2500 g
	B—not rested		157	—	61	50.7% < 2500 g
Robertson (1964; 1956–62)	A—admitted before 36 weeks for rest	Unspecified	152	—	151	Mean 2577 g
	B—admitted after 36 weeks for rest		61	—	16	Mean 2758 g
Barter et al. (1965; 1954–64)	A—bedrest at home	Unspecified	37	—	108	35.5% < 2500 g
	B—undiagnosed or not rested		225	—	217	52.4% < 2500 g

MacGillivray (1986) reviewed the literature on clinical trials of bedrest in twin pregnancies. The results of various studies are shown for the 1960s, 1970s and 1980s according to whether the authors thought bedrest was beneficial (Tables 7.19–7.24). It appears that the consensus of opinion is that there is no obstetrical advantage to be gained by admitting women expecting twins for routine rest in hospital, as it is unlikely to affect preterm labour, pre-eclampsia, perinatal mortality or birthweight.

There is considerable disadvantage in adopting such a policy because of the disruption which this causes in the life of the woman and her family (Powers and Miller, 1979; Editorial, 1981; Tresmontant et al., 1983). There is also a very considerable financial cost involved in this type of management. The 1983 Scottish Twin Study (Patel et al., 1984) attempted to assess the cost and calculated that bedrest average £2491 per admission.

It is essential, however, that women with twin pregnancies should be admitted to hospital when there are any specific indications, such as the development of pre-eclampsia, antepartum haemorrhage or threatened preterm labour. Indeed, it may be necessary to admit some women with twin pregnancies to hospital from agout 30 weeks onwards because of the distances that they reside from a central hospital. In this way babies will be delivered under the best circumstances and receive any urgent paediatric care which might be required.

Following admission for pregnancy complications, monitoring the condition of the mother and babies is essential.

Assessment of fetal lung maturity is very seldom necessary if gestational age has been determined early in pregnancy, but may be of occasional value. Discrepancies between the results from the two amniotic sacs have been noted. Dobbie et al. (1983) showed that the concordance for lecithin/sphingomyelin, phosphatidyl glycerol/sphingomyelin and phosphatidyl inositol/sphingomyelin ratios was higher in monozygotic than dizygotic pregnancies and discrepancies were much less for phosphatidyl glycerol than for lecithin/sphingomyelin ratios. Fetal movement charts are of value, but it has to be remembered that the movements are greater in twin pregnancies than in singleton pregnancies, and even greater in triplets (Samueloff et al., 1983).

Antepartum fetal heart-rate monitoring is possible in multiple pregnancies, but is obviously more difficult than in singleton pregnancies. Bailey et al. (1980) found non-stress cardiotocography to be of value in 50 cases of multiple pregnancy. They found that of five cases in which one of a pair of twins showed a non-reactive pattern, four of these babies died (two intrauterine deaths and two neonatal deaths) and all were growth retarded at birth. They also found that the non-stress cardiotocography was better than serial oestrogens assays or serial biparietal diameter measurements in multiple pregnancies, and this was confirmed in 27 cases of twins by Lenstrup (1984).

Most obstetricians believe that postmaturity poses a risk to singleton

Table 7.20. Bedrest not beneficial — 1960s

Study	Groups	Selection	Numbers	Mean gestation at delivery	Perinatal mortality per 1000	Birthweight
Dunn (1961; 1953–58)	A—rested at least 7 days between 30 and 36 weeks	Unspecified	60	267 days	234	Mean 2581 g
	B—not rested		64	264 days	167	Mean 2496 g
Jonas (1963; 1954–61)	A—rested at least 48 hours before end of 36th week	Unspecified	Prims. 27 Multips. 80	37% < 37 weeks 26% < 37 weeks	70 40	54% < 2500 g 35% < 2500 g
	B—not rested		Prims. 17 Multips. 74	41% < 37 weeks 39% < 37 weeks	30 50	62% < 2500 g 70% < 2500 g
	C—Undiagnosed		Prims. 15 Multips. 36	87% < 37 weeks 58% < 37 weeks	430 230	97% < 2500 g 70% < 2500 g

Table 7.21. Bedrest beneficial — 1970s

Study	Groups	Selection	Numbers	Mean gestation at delivery	Perinatal mortality per 1000	Birthweight
Komaromy and Lampé (1977)	A—agreed to be hospitalised from 32 weeks	Unspecified	242	37.4 weeks	54	Mean 2581 g
	B—not hospitalised		249	35.0 weeks	217	Mean 1972 g
Persson and Grennert (1979)	A—hospitalised between 28 and 36 weeks	Unspecified 1973–77	86	34.6 weeks	6	44% <2500 g
	B—non acceptors or not detected	1973–77	24	33.5 weeks	105	62% <2500 g
	C—not rested	1963–65	93	33.8 weeks	59	49% <2500 g

Table 7.22. Bedrest not beneficial — 1970s

Study	Groups	Selection	Numbers	Mean gestation at delivery	Perinatal mortality per 1000	Mean birthweight
Jeffrey et al. (1974)	A—hospitalised between 30 and 37 weeks	Unspecified but gestation < 30 weeks excluded	41	36.2 weeks	61	2273 g
	B—no bedrest		31	37.7 weeks	115	2321 g
	C—not diagnosed		42	37.5 weeks	57	2173 g
Weekes et al. (1977)	A—hospitalised from 28 to 34 weeks onwards	Consultant's choice	60	259 days	67	I—2550 g II—2610 g
	B—not hospitalised		36	261 days	56	I—2520 g II—2350 g

Table 7.23. Bedrest beneficial — 1980s

Study	Groups	Selection	Numbers		Mean gestation at delivery		Perinatal mortality Per 1000		Mean birthweight	
			Prims.	Multips.	Prims.	Multips.	Prims.	Multips.	Prims.	Multips.
Van der Pol et al. (1982)										
	A—hospitalised from 32 weeks	1975–79	33	30	246.6 (days)	259.3 (days)	0	0	2415 g	2488 g
	B—not rested	1969–74	39	46	260.3 (days)	202.2 (days)	26	33	2251 g	2510 g
Kappel et al. (1985)	A—hospitalised at least 2 weeks from 29 to 36 weeks		37		35.1 < 37 weeks		14		2734 g	
	B—bedrest at home	Refused hospitalisation	31		54.8% < 37 weeks		32		2624 g	
	C—not rested		34		82.2% < 37 weeks		103		2150 g	

Table 7.24. Bedrest not beneficial—1980s

Study	Group	Selection	Numbers	Mean gestation at delivery (weeks)	Perinatal mortality per 1000	Birthweight
Hartikainen-Sorri and Jouppila (1984)	A—hospitalised	Odd year of birth	28	36.7	71.0	17% < 1500 g
	B—not rested	Even year of birth	45	37.4	11.0	22% < 1500 g
Saunders et al. (1985)	A—hospitalised from 32 weeks	Randomised trial	105	37.3	38.1	36.2% < 2500 g
	B—controls		107	37.9	23.4	43.0% < 2500 g
Hartikainen-Sorri (1985)	Special out-patient care	1982–83 Consecutive twin pregnancies <24 weeks gestation	100	37.4	20.0	3% < 1500 g

fetuses when the gestation is greater than 42 weeks. In twin pregnancies many will not allow the pregnancy to progress beyond term. As discussed above, assessment of at risk fetuses is difficult and early induction of labour, e.g. at 38 weeks, may be the management of choice, particularly if there is evidence of intrauterine growth retardation.

Management of twin pregnancies

With E. M. BRYAN

Counselling

Careful counselling is essential for all parents before they embark on prenatal testing for fetal anomalies. With a multiple pregnancy it is vital that both the couple and the obstetrician are aware of the additional considerations that may arise (Bang *et al.*, 1975; Hunter and Cox, 1979: Harper, 1981; Meir and Saunders, 1982).

The parents must be made clearly aware of the options available to them if one fetus is found to be abnormal, that is the continuation of the pregnancy, the termination of the pregnancy, or selective feticide.

Prenatal diagnosis by ultrasonic scanning and amniocentesis is now widely available and other methods such as fetal blood sampling, chorionic villus sampling and fetoscopy are provided in a few specialist centres.

As discussed in Chapter 11 the risks of a particular abnormality may differ in a multiple pregnancy. The risks and difficulties of any procedure are greater than with a single pregnancy.

Even when satisfactory specimens are obtained, the results may pose a far greater dilemma for parents of twins than singletons as the chances of both twins being abnormal are small (Jassani *et al.*, 1980). Concordance for neural tube defects even in MZ twins is unusual and Down's syndrome, although usually concordant in MZ twins, rarely affects both of a DZ pair.

Many parents who would not hesitate to have a pregnancy terminated for a single abnormal fetus could not agree if it meant the sacrifice of a normal baby at the same time. Yet the stress of knowingly carrying an abnormal fetus for the remainder of the pregnancy may have a terrible effect on the mother. For other parents, their decision may depend on whether the affected child is likely to die at, or soon after, birth or survive for years as a burden to himself, his twin and his family.

Selective intrauterine killing of the abnormal fetus, otherwise known as selective feticide or selective birth, removes the horror of aborting a normal fetus. On the other hand, the thought of a dead fetus lying by the side of their living baby may be very distressing to some parents (Rodeck, 1984). Others may object to the particular techniques available (Filkins *et al.*, 1984). Yet for many this may be the first chance of a normal baby after many failures (Redwine and Petres, 1984). For these parents selective feticide may well seem the best alternative.

The reasons for selective feticide have included twins discordant for trisomy 21 (Beck *et al.*, 1981; Kerenyi and Chitkara, 1981; Rodeck, 1984); Tay–Sachs disease (Petres and Redwine, 1981; Redwine and Petres, 1984); Hurler's syndrome (Aberg *et al.*, 1978); Turner's syndrome (Gigon *et al.*, 1981); haemophilia (Mulcahy *et al.*, 1984; Rodeck, 1984); microcephaly, spina bifida, Duchenne muscular dystrophy, and epidermolysis bullosa letalis (Rodeck, 1984). The methods employed vary.

A hysterotomy and removal of the affected fetus has been successfully carried out (Beck *et al.*, 1981: Gigon *et al.*, 1981). The advantage of this method is that the mother avoids the psychologically distressing experience of carrying a dead baby and the theoretical risk of disseminated intravascular coagulation resulting from a macerated fetus. However, some would consider that this degree of uterine disturbance created an unacceptable risk of preterm labour (Rodeck, 1984).

Rodeck (1984) has successfully used the method of umbilical vein catheterisation and injection of air on several occasions. Under fetoscopic vision the umbilical vein of the affected fetus is punctured and a blood sample aspirated.

Cardiac puncture with exsanguination of the fetus (Aberg *et al.*, 1978; Kerenyi and Chitkara, 1981) and an intracardiac injection of formaldehyde (Philip, 1981) have also been used to effect intrauterine death.

The great majority of twins discordant for fetal anomalies will be dizygotic so intravascular coagulopathy in the survivor, which can occur in monochorionic (and therefore MZ) twins, should not be a hazard. In the rare case of MZ discordancy (e.g. neural tube defects, Turner's or Down's syndromes) selective feticide cannot be considered unless there is dichorionic placentation (Redwine and Hays, 1986).

Before accepting the option of selective feticide, parents must be aware of the potential risks attached to the procedure, those of precipitating an abortion or preterm labour, the incorrect selection of the fetus when no anatomical markers are available, maternal infection or coagulopathy. All such parents will need a great deal of support and counselling throughout the pregnancy and sometimes for years after.

Twinning and Twins
Edited by I. MacGillivray, D. M. Campbell and B. Thompson
© 1988 John Wiley & Sons Ltd

CHAPTER 8

Management of labour and delivery

DORIS M. CAMPBELL and IAN MACGILLIVRAY

Department of Obstetrics and Gynaecology, University of Aberdeen, Aberdeen, UK

Labour is more hazardous in multiple pregnancies, partly because of the frequency of complications of pregnancy, also because of possible malpresentation and malposition of the fetuses and in particular because of the high rate of preterm labour. Early diagnosis and avoiding action are most likely to improve the prognosis for mother and babies.

Gestation

Twins are usually born at the same length of gestation. Exceptionally, the second twin has deliberately been allowed to remain alone in utero and to become more mature, but this should only be considered if the first twin has been aborted. The birth of the second twin then becomes comparable to that of a singleton.

A major problem with twins is the high rate of preterm labour which can result in increased mortality and morbidity. For example, the delivery of small preterm babies, particularly if presenting by the breech, may be precipitate after a labour so rapid that the mother could not be admitted to hospital in time. This has been advanced as an argument for the routine admission of all women with multiple pregnancies from 28 weeks gestation, but this should be unnecessary if the mother is within easy reach of appropriate hospital services.

Just as there is doubt about the efficacy of bedrest and/or beta-sympathomimetic drugs in the prevention of preterm labour (see Chapter 7), there is doubt about their value once preterm labour has become established. Labour is not likely to be arrested by either measure (Berger *et al.*, 1981), but it is necessary that the woman expecting twins who goes into labour be admitted to hospital. Although the value of beta-sympathomimetic drugs is limited once labour is established, it may be advisable that they be given to buy time for the action of corticosteroids such as betamethasone to enhance

Table 8.1. Induction and Caesarean section rates in Aberdeen City District (1951–1983) in twin and singleton pregnancies

	Twins (1 150)		Singletons (98 565)	
	%	No.	%	No.
Elective caesarean section	3.48	40	2.35	2 316
Induced	26.35	303	27.93	27 534
Not induced, i.e. spontaneous labour	69.83	803	69.69	68 690
Not known	0.35	4	0.03	25

the maturity of the fetal lungs, particularly when the gestation is less than 32 weeks.

On account of pregnancy complications, in particular proteinuric pre-eclampsia, labour may have to be induced preterm.

Induction of labour may also be necessary if the pregnancy is 'prolonged', but this is unlikely to occur in twin pregnancies. There is controversy about the hazards of prolonged pregnancy in twin pregnancies, particularly about the length of pregnancy which should be considered prolonged. It is usual to consider a singleton pregnancy as prolonged if it lasts for 42 weeks. In a twin pregnancy the dangers of postmaturity probably occur earlier and it would seem reasonable that all twins should be delivered by the end of 40 completed weeks gestation. If it were possible to detect impending fetal distress from postmaturity by such tests as amnioscopy, amniocentesis, cardiotocography, hormone assays, fetal movement counts or combinations of these the obstetrician would be in a better position to judge the risks of letting the pregnancy continue indefinitely without intervention. However, these tests are difficult enough to interpret in singleton pregnancies and they are much more difficult to apply and to interpret in multiple pregnancies (see Chapter 7). Thus, an arbitrary decision has to be made regarding the risks of postmaturity in twin pregnancy, hence the suggestion that all twin pregnancies should be delivered by the end of 40 weeks. The induction and elective caesarean section rates for Aberdeen City District for the period 1951 to 1983 for all parities are given in Table 8.1. The induction rate increased in both singletons and twins up to 1975 and since then has diminished (Table 8.2), the overall induction rate in twins being comparable to that in singletons throughout the time period studied.

Elective Caesarean Section

An elective caesarean section may be necessary in some cases where the mother, whether expecting twins or a singleton, develops certain complica-

Table 8.2. Induction (% rate) Aberdeen City District twin and singleton pregnancies by time

Years	Twins		Singletons	
	%	No.	%	No.
1951–55	20.40	48	16.02	2 589
1956–60	16.59	35	20.48	3 562
1961–65	26.19	58	22.73	3 926
1966–70	27.84	49	36.76	5 743
1971–75	43.94	58	41.10	5 441
1976–80	31.36	37	34.85	3 985
1981–83	30.88	21	30.74	2 288

tions such as proteinuric pre-eclampsia or antepartum haemorrhage and her life is at risk; in such circumstances gestation length is irrelevant. Other circumstances in which an elective section may be carried out include if the mother is an older primigravida, or has had a previous caesarean section for a recurring cause, or marked fetal growth retardation of one or both twins is suspected.

Elective section for fetal reasons in twin pregnancy is a highly controversial topic. Two main factors dominate this argument, namely length of gestation, in particular short gestation, and malpresentation of either twin. Protagonists of caesarean section, mainly from North America (Farroqui et al., 1973; Taylor, 1976; Kelsick and Minkoff, 1982; Cetrulo et al., 1980), have suggested that caesarean section should be performed for all twin pregnancies where the presentation is other than cephalic/cephalic, particularly if the gestation length is less than 34 weeks; such a policy has resulted in sections being performed in about 80% of deliveries at 34 weeks or less, and in 64% at 35 weeks or more (Cetrulo, 1986). It is claimed that such intervention results in improved fetal outcome (see Chapter 10). Most obstetricians in Europe and the UK would prefer to aim for vaginal delivery unless there is a clear contraindication such as the development of fetal distress or obstructed labour. Such an approach does not appear to have resulted in poorer outcomes (MacGillivray and Campbell, 1981; Rydhstrom and Ohrlander, 1985; Olofsson and Rydhstrom, 1985). Some obstetricians in North America consider the caesarean section rate to be excessive and are advocating more vaginal deliveries in twins (Bell et al., 1986; Chervenak, 1986).

The elective caesarean section rate in Aberdeen was significantly higher for twins than for singletons (Table 8.1). The elective caesarean section rate in 5 year periods between 1951 and 1983 shows a marked increase from 1976 in the twin pregnancies, but only a slight increase in singleton pregnancies (Table 8.3).

Table 8.3. Elective caesarean section (% rate) in Aberdeen
City District in twin and singleton pregnancies by time

	Twins		Singletons	
Years	%	No.	%	No.
1951–55	1.70	4	1.18	190
1956–60	2.37	5	1.29	224
1961–65	3.81	8	2.21	382
1966–70	1.14	2	2.63	411
1971–75	1.52	2	2.62	347
1976–80	10.17	12	3.86	442
1981–83	10.29	7	4.30	320

Management of Labour

The length of labour in twin pregnancy is about the same as that in a singleton pregnancy (Bender, 1952; Ross and Phillpott, 1953; Law, 1967), but unless there is interference, the second stage of labour can be prolonged. Law (1967) suggested that the duration of the second stage should be between one and two hours, but nowadays it would usually be shorter. Oxytocin stimulation is frequently given when the first stage of labour is not progressing quickly enough and also for the second stage. It is useful to have an intravenous infusion of 5% dextrose running before the end of the first stage which allows oxytocin to be added to the infusion as required to stimulate contractions during the second stage. This can be particularly helpful after the birth of the first baby and in the management of the third stage (see below). The mother's condition should be carefully monitored and the progress of labour recorded graphically on a partogram as in singleton pregnancy.

It is desirable that the condition of the babies should be monitored by cardiotocography with instrumentation as available. Phonocardiography is possibly better than electrocardiography, but this depends on the expertise of users. It is usual practice in major centres to apply an electrode to the presenting part of twin I and to monitor twin II externally. Technical difficulties encountered may lead to problems of misinterpretation of tracing on occasions. Fehrmann (1980) described an occasion on which the electro-cardiogram of a live second twin was detected through the scalp electrode attached to the dead first twin. Realtime B scan has been found to be of value in locating the fetal hearts for antepartum monitoring even in a triplet pregnancy (Powell-Phillips *et al.*, 1979). In situations where sophisticated instrumentation is not available, the condition of both babies should be recorded as accurately as possible with Pinard stethoscopes by two observers together, each listening to a fetal heart.

In advanced maternity centres an anaesthetist, usually one with a particular interest and expertise in obstetric anaesthesia, is routinely available for all twin deliveries. Epidural anaesthesia has become very popular for pain relief in all stages of labour and in twin pregnancy it has an additional advantage over traditional methods. Once epidural analgesia has been established it will allow the necessary manipulations or caesarean section required for the delivery of both twins and the placenta without further additional anaesthesia. It also ensures by minimising the mother's desire to 'push', that the cervix will be fully dilated prior to delivery which is particularly important if the first baby is presenting as a breech.

Pudendal nerve block analgesia for operative vaginal delivery of the first baby may be used as an alternative. If a pudendal block is used, however, the patient should be fully prepared for general anaesthesia in case this becomes necessary for delivery of the second baby. Such an emergency, where the general anaesthetic has to be given in a hurry, is potentially hazardous and is best avoided.

Mode of Delivery

A decision regarding the type of delivery will most likely have been made before the onset of labour (see earlier section). In some cases, however, malposition or malpresentation of the first twin may only be detected after labour has started. When this happens obstetric intervention will be the same as if the problem had arisen in a singleton delivery. For example, if there is a face, brow or shoulder presentation of twin 1, delivery will generally be by caesarean section.

If fetal distress of either twin is detected during the first stage of labour, a caesarean section will usually be performed. However, such intervention will depend on various factors such as the degree of dilatation of the cervix and the length of gestation, e.g. at very early gestation (< 26 weeks) it is unlikely to improve fetal outcome, but may be harmful to the mother.

Several studies (Table 8.4) have shown that about half of the cases of twin pregnancies have cephalic presentation in both twins. Only Ross and Phillpott (1953) report a lower incidence. In about three-quarters of twins the presentation of the first twin is cephalic—Portes and Granjon (1946) reported 74.9%; Danielson (1960) 77.8%; Ross and Phillpott (1953) 68.8%; and in our Aberdeen series it was 75.3%.

The indications for caesarean section in Aberdeen (1951–1975) (Table 8.5) were different in twin and singleton pregnancies. In singletons, dysfunction/disproportion and fetal distress were commoner reasons compared with abnormal presentation which was significantly greater in twin pregnancies.

The choice of caesarean section for malpresentations will depend on the individual obstetrician's preference. Some will limit vaginal delivery to cases

Table 8.4. Presentation at delivery (%) in twin pregnancy

	Portes and Granjon (1946)	Ross and Philpott (1953) Primiparae	Ross and Philpott (1953) Multiparae	Guttmacher and Kohl (1958)	Danielson (1960)	Aberdeen City District (1967–1983)
Cephalic/cephalic	44.3	34.5	37.1	46.9	53.3	48.6
Cephalic/breech ⎫ Breech/cephalic ⎭	38.4	30.9 5.5	33.1 12.4	37.0	24.5 11.9	24.5 9.9
Breech/breech	9.9	14.5	7.4	8.7	9.6	11.0
Cephalic/other ⎫ Other/cephalic ⎭	5.3	3.4 —	5.7 —	4.9	0.7 —	2.2 0.4
Breech/other ⎫ Other/breech ⎭	1.4	— —	— —	1.9	— —	0.4 0.2
Other/other	0.2	10.9	4.1	0.6	—	2.8

Table 8.5. Indications for caesarean section in twin and singleton pregnancies in Aberdeen City District (1951–1975)

Indications	Twins (46)		Singletons (3 945)	
	%	No.	%	No.
Dysfunction/disproportion	23.91	11	32.42	1 279
Placenta praevia	6.52	3	7.66	302
Fetal distress	2.17	1	16.98	670
Abnormal presentation	32.61	15	14.88	587
Maternal age, previous obstetric history, gynaecological disorder	21.74	10	21.50	848
Maternal disease	4.35	2	2.94	112
Pre-eclampsia	8.70	4	2.23	88
Antepartum haemorrhage other than placenta praevia	—	0	1.50	59

where both twins are presenting as cephalic, but others will be willing to deliver vaginally if the first is presenting as cephalic irrespective of the presentation of the second twin. Some will be willing to attempt vaginal delivery if the first twin is presenting by the breech, depending on his or her attitude to delivery of the singleton breech. Brow or face presentation of the first baby is not an absolute indication for elective caesarean section, but most obstetricians would favour such action. Some, however, might wish to wait and see what progress and conversion took place in a trial of labour.

Delivery of twins by caesarean section is not without risk to the babies, e.g. respiratory distress syndrome at early gestation may be increased following caesarean section. There can also be a risk of trauma to the second baby, especially at the extremes of size either large or small when there is a difficult breech extraction through the lower uterine segment incision.

Where the small transverse incision in the lower segment seems likely to be inadequate the classical or upper segment incision or a De Lee incision may be considered. The classical incision is made vertically in the midline through the peritoneum and the upper segment after the correction of dextrorotation of the uterus. The De Lee incision is a low longitudinal uterine incision two-thirds of which is in the lower segment and one-third in the upper segment. The visceral peritoneum is opened transversely and reflected as high up and as low down as possible before making the verticle incision in the uterus. It may be useful in transverse lies and in breech presentations. Unfortunately, the strongest case for delivering breeches by caesarean section is in primigravidae in whom it is undesirable to perform a classical or even a De Lee incision.

When labour is allowed to proceed with a breech presentation, the condition of the baby is monitored carefully, preferably with an electrode on the buttocks. The delivery may be either spontaneous or assisted, but a breech extraction should be avoided if at all possible. It is preferable to do a caesarean section if the breech does not show at the perineum with maternal bearing down efforts.

Prolapse of the cord is more likely to occur with twin pregnancies than singletons particularly if there is hydramnios. If the cervix is fully dilated, vaginal delivery should be effected as quickly as possible; otherwise a caesarean section should be performed.

Delivery of the Second Twin

After the delivery of the first twin, the lie of the second twin should be checked by abdominal palpation and corrected to longitudinal if necessary. This should be done as soon as the first twin is delivered and the fetal heart of twin II has been checked. The membranes should be ruptured within a few minutes of the delivery of the first baby when the lie is longitudinal and the uterus has started to contract again. If the uterus does not contract after a few minutes, an oxytocin infusion should be started to stimulate the uterus.

Spontaneous delivery of twin II occurred in 48.1% in the British Perinatal Mortality Survey 1958 (Butler and Alberman, 1969) and in 39.2% in the Aberdeen City District Survey of 1951–1983 (Table 8.6).

Unintentional retention of the second twin is now only likely to occur where there is no medical supervision of labour. Adeleye (1972) in Nigeria,

Table 8.6. Type of delivery in twin and singleton pregnancies in Aberdeen City District (1951–1983)

| | Twins (1 150) | | | | Singletons (98 565) | |
| | I | | II | | | |
	%	No.	%	No.	%	No.
Spontaneous vaginal delivery	56.43	649	39.22	451	80.61	79 454
Caesarean section	7.13	82	7.65	88	5.92	5 835
Forceps	18.70	215	17.13	197	11.38	11 218
Assisted breech	16.96	195	32.52	374	1.72	1 693
Vacuum extraction	0.26	3	0.61	7	0.34	340
Destructive	—	—	0.09	1	0.009	9
Other	—	—	0.09	1	0.005	5
Not known	0.52	6	2.70	31	0.001	11

reviewing 168 records of the retention of twin II, defined as a delivery interval between the twins of 30 minutes or more, found that the perinatal mortality in the booked hospital delivery group was 23.5% compared with 50.4% in the emergency admission group. The patients admitted to hospital as emergencies after delivery of twin I must have experienced delay before twin II was born for a much longer period than half an hour, and it is not surprising that the perinatal mortality rate was higher. The main causes of retention of twin II were malpresentations and uterine inertia. Active intervention reduced the length of the retention and consequently perinatal mortality.

Recently some obstetricians (Depp et al., 1986) have been advocating applying an electrode to the presenting part of twin II once the membranes are ruptured and allowing labour and delivery to progress more slowly if there is no evidence of fetal anoxia. It seems unnecessary, however, to wait for fetal compromise when delivery of twin II can easily be achieved and there is no evidence to justify such a delay. Avoidance of undue haste or undue delay in the delivery of twin II would appear to be the best policy.

Prolapse of the umbilical cord of the second twin is not uncommon, but as the cervix is fully dilated there is usually no problem in delivering the second twin before asphyxia develops. If it has been necessary to correct the transverse lie and the baby then presents as a breech, the cord may become entangled with the baby's legs. In such a situation if there is undue tension on the cord, it can be cut before the baby is delivered.

Forceps delivery of the second twin may be necessary if fetal distress develops or if the mother's efforts in bearing down are inadequate. Obstetric forceps are used when the position is direct occipito-anterior or posterior, but rotation and application of Kielland's forceps may be necessary if the head is lying in the transverse position. Application of forceps to a high head above the pelvic brim is dangerous and should not be attempted. The uterus can usually be made to contract and with some manual pressure on the head from above it should come into the pelvis and forceps can be applied. Some obstetricians prefer to use the ventouse or vacuum extractor and this may be useful when the head remains high above the brim. It is, however, preferable to avoid application of the ventouse to small immature babies as the vacuum cap has to raise a 'chignon' which might result in scalp damage.

Caesarean section is seldom required for delivery of the second twin unless there has been no antenatal care and medical supervision of labour, e.g. in parts of Africa. It may be indicated if the cervix is closed down and there is fetal distress, and delivery by the vagina is not feasible. It is also indicated in transverse lie when the shoulder becomes impacted. In the Aberdeen series for 1951–1983 there were only six occasions when twin II was delivered by caesarean section after vaginal delivery of twin I.

The type of delivery for the total population of Aberdeen City District between 1951 and 1983 twin and singleton pregnancies are shown in Table

Table 8.7. Breech delivery rate (%) in Aberdeen City District (1951–1983) in twin and singleton pregnancies by time

Years	Twin I		Twin II		Singletons	
	%	No.	%	No.	%	No.
1951–55	18.72	44	32.77	77	1.66	269
1956–60	12.32	26	30.33	64	1.57	273
1961–65	18.57	39	27.14	78	1.41	244
1966–70	19.89	35	35.80	63	1.78	278
1971–75	20.45	27	30.30	40	2.05	271
1976–80	12.71	15	28.81	34	2.08	238
1981–83	13.24	9	26.47	18	1.61	120

8.6. As expected there are fewer spontaneous deliveries of twins, particularly of twin II, and both forceps and assisted breech deliveries are increased, most markedly assisted breech delivery of twin II.

The breech delivery rate in Aberdeen City District in singletons has shown little change between 1951 and 1983 (Table 8.7). On the other hand, breech delivery for both twin I and twin II remained relatively constant until 1975, but there has been a decline in recent years as caesarean rates increased (Table 8.8). A similar caesarean section rate (27.3%) was found in the 1983 Scottish Twin Survey (Patel et al., 1984).

Table 8.9 examines the incidence of caesarean section in relation to gestation length and presentation of the twins. The highest rates are found for all types of presentation between 34 and 36 weeks. There is also a high rate of caesarean section when twin I is a breech presentation regardless of gestation, the respective rates for twin I as breech or cephalic presentation being 12.5%

Table 8.8. Caesarean section rate (%) in Aberdeen City District (1951–1983) in twin and singleton pregnancies by time

Years	Twin I		Twin II		Singletons	
	%	No.	%	No.	%	No.
1951–55	3.4	8	2.98	7	3.03	489
1956–60	4.74	10	4.74	10	4.27	742
1961–65	8.10	17	8.57	18	5.18	895
1966–70	1.70	3	2.27	4	5.93	927
1971–75	6.06	8	5.82	9	7.4	979
1976–80	17.80	21	18.64	22	8.83	1 010
1981–83	22.06	15	26.47	18	10.75	793

Table 8.9. Caesarean section (CS) rate (%) in Aberdeen City District twin pregnancies (1967–1983) by presentation and gestation at delivery

	34 weeks			34–36 weeks			≥ 37 weeks		
	Twin I % CS	Total no.	Twin II % CS	Twin I % CS	Total no.	Twin II % CS	Twin I % CS	Total no.	Twin II % CS
Cephalic/cephalic	—	21	—	12.7	55	12.7	8.3	144	9.7
Cephalic/breech	11.1	18	11.1	8.3	24	8.3	4.5	67	7.5
Cephalic/other	50.0	2	50.0	—	1	—	—	2	—
Breech/cephalic	—	7	—	11.1	9	22.2	220.7	29	24.1
Breech/Breech	12.5	8	12.5	25.0	12	25.0	14.8	27	14.8
Breech/other	100.0	1	100.0	—	1	100.0	—	—	—
Other/other	50.0	2	50.0	100.0	1	100.0	—	—	—
Total	10.2	59	10.2	13.6	103	15.5	9.3	269	11.2

Table 8.10. Type of delivery in twin pregnancies in Aberdeen City District (1969–1983) by zygosity and placentation

Type of delivery	MZ MC	MZ DC	MZ (NS)	DZ DC	Not known	Total
(A) Twin I						
Spontaneous vaginal	50.0 (34)	33.8 (25)	66.7 (4)	42.2 (84)	35.1 (13)	41.7 (160)
Caesarean section	11.8 (8)	14.9 (11)		12.1 (24)	10.8 (4)	12.2 (47)
Forceps + vacuum extraction	27.9 (19)	13.1 (23)	33.0 (2)	26.6 (53)	24.3 (9)	27.6 (106)
Assisted breech	8.8 (6)	17.6 (13)		18.1 (36)	29.7 (11)	17.2 (66)
Not known	1.5 (1)	2.7 (2)		1.0 (2)		1.3 (5)
Total	100 (68)	100.1 (74)	100 (6)	100 (199)	99.9 (37)	100 (384)
(B) Twin II						
Spontaneous vaginal	30.9 (21)	27.0 (20)	16.7 (1)	35.2 (70)	18.9 (7)	31.0 (119)
Caesarean section	11.8 (8)	14.9 (11)		14.6 (29)	13.5 (5)	13.8 (53)
Forceps + vacuum	25.0 (17)	29.7 (22)	50.0 (3)	19.6 (39)	24.3 (9)	23.4 (90)
Assisted breech	30.9 (21)	27.0 (20)	16.7 (1)	29.2 (58)	43.2 (16)	30.2 (116)
Not known	1.5 (1)	1.4 (1)	16.7 (1)	1.5 (3)		1.6 (6)
Total	100.1 (68)	100 (74)	100.1 (6)	100.1 (199)	99.9 (37)	100 (384)

Numbers in brackets are total numbers in each group.

vs 7.3% less than 34 weeks, 18.2% *vs* 11.3% between 34 and 36 weeks, and 17.9% *vs* 7.0% over 37 weeks. In six cases, caesarean section was performed for twin II, the presentation of twin II was cephalic on three occasions, breech on two, and other on one.

The type of delivery for twin I or twin II is not influenced by zygosity or placentation (Table 8.10).

The Third Stage

It is usual for the placenta or placentae to be delivered after the birth of both babies, but occasionally the first placenta is delivered before the second twin. This does not usually cause any problem. Rarely there may be heavy vaginal bleeding in which case the second twin has to be delivered as expeditiously as possible so that the uterus can be made to contract, thus controlling the bleeding. There is no greater risk of primary postpartum haemorrhage following a twin delivery than a singleton if oxytocics are given and controlled cord traction is employed (Wood and Pinkerton, 1966). In the Aberdeen City District series (1951–1983) the incidence of manual removal of the placenta was 3.0% in twins compared with 1.2% in singletons (Table 8.11). However, there have been no cases of twin pregnancies requiring manual removal in more recent years since there has been routine active management of the third stage. Secondary postpartum haemorrhage, however, was found to be significantly more common after twin deliveries (Table 8.12).

Table 8.11. Manual removal of placenta (% rate) in Aberdeen City District (1951–1983) in twin and singleton pregnancies

	Twins (1 150)		Singletons (98 565)	
	%	No.	%	No.
1951–55	2.55	6	0.16	26
1956–60	3.79	8	0.75	130
1961–65	1.43	3	1.49	258
1966–70	6.82	12	1.90	297
1971–80	4.55	6	1.96	260
1981–83	—	0	1.28	146
	—	0	0.82	61
Total	3.04	35	1.20	1 178

Table 8.12. Incidence of secondary postpartum haemorrhage (% rate) in
Aberdeen City District (1956–1983) in twin and singleton pregnancies

Year	Twins			Singletons		
	No.	Total	%	No.	Total	%
1956–60	2	211	0.95	11	17 394	0.06
1961–65	0	210	—	32	17 275	0.19
1966–70	3	176	1.70	39	15 623	0.25
1971–75	2	132	1.52	63	13 237	0.48
1976–80	2	118	1.69	130	11 436	1.13
1981–83	0	68	—	43	7 443	0.58
Total	9	915	0.98	318	82 408	0.39

Unusual Labour Problems

(a) Obstructed Labour

This is more liable to happen in areas where antenatal care is poor or absent,
for example, in many parts of Africa. Obstructed labour is usually due to
transverse lie of the first twin and only rarely occurs due to twin locking.
Rupture of the uterus is common in such situations in multiparae, but it is
extremely uncommon in primiparae as labour tends to stop. Conversely,
pressure necrosis is more often seen in the primiparous woman. There is
usually a delay in the rate of cervical dilatation in the primipara before the
labour becomes obstructed and this is a reliable early warning sign. Obstruction in multiparous women can occur without any preceding change in the
normal pattern of cervical dilatation, making it more difficult to detect and it
may only be recognised by the slow or arrested rate of descent of the
presenting part. Unless the woman in obstructed labour can be admitted to
hospital quickly, she may die or arrive exhausted and dehydrated with
possible bowel distension. The uterus may already have ruptured or the low
uterine segment may be found to be tender and Bandl's ring may be present.
In such circumstances the fetuses are unlikely to survive.

Caesarean section for obstructed labour in the presence of a transverse lie
can be hazardous to the mother, particularly if a transverse lower uterine
segment incision is made. This is because it may not be possible to deliver the
babies easily even after the use of anaesthetic or other drugs to relax the
uterus, and thus it may be necessary to extend the ends of the tranverse
incision by curving the ends upwards to give more access, but increasing the
likelihood of major haemorrhage. A vertical incision converting the transverse incision into a T-shaped incision should be avoided because it gives rise

to a weak uterine scar. A classical or De Lee incision is preferable in such cases.

As there is a great risk of intrauterine infection, extraperitoneal caesarean section has been recommended by Crichton (1973) for such cases. On the other hand, Phillpott (1980) recommends destructive operative procedures as an alternative to an unnecessary and hazardous caesarean section.

(b) Failure to Diagnose Twins prior to Delivery

Even if an oxytocic has not been given at the delivery of the first twin, there is a danger to the second twin when it has not been diagnosed as there may be undue delay in delivery and birth asphyxia may result. In cases where twin pregnancy is not suspected it is possible that fetal distress may develop in one twin during labour, and be undetected as the other fetal heart is satisfactory. In labour, as soon as twins are suspected the appropriate management should be initiated.

There is a grave risk to twin II from anoxia if an oxytocic agent has been given with the delivery of twin I, and it must be delivered as quickly as possible by the most appropriate method. If the baby is lying transversely and thus cannot be corrected by external version, particularly if the membranes have ruptured, general anaesthetic will be required to cause relaxation of the uterus to allow internal version and breech extraction. It may, in some such cases, be necessary to perform a caesarean section if the cervix has closed down. If twin II has died, time can be allowed for the cervix to dilate again when the effect of the oxytocic drug wears off. Fortunately, in developed countries the vast majority of twin pregnancies are diagnosed antenatally, e.g. in the 1983 Scottish Twin Survey (Patel et al., 1984) over 95%.

(c) Locked Twins

This is an extremely rare complication occurring in about one in a thousand twin deliveries (Nissen, 1958). He described four forms of twin entanglement, collision, impaction, compaction and interlocking.

The classical twin locking is the chin-to-chin type when the first presentation is by the breech and the second by the vertex and is the most difficult to deal with.

The diagnosis of interlocking cannot be made before labour, but when two fetal poles are palpable, either partially or fully, in the pelvis the condition can be suspected and caesarean section performed. Ultrasound scanning will usually reveal the true state of affairs. Chin-to-chin locking, however, is not usually diagnosed until part of the first baby is born and strenuous efforts have been made to deliver it by traction. A general anaesthetic is usually required to determine the extent of the locking and whether it will be possible to disengage the heads. For delivery of chin-to-chin locked babies, forceps are applied to the second twin and traction and hyperextension are applied to the first twin (Kimball and Rand, 1950). The head of the second twin is delivered by flexion. If the first twin is dead, then decapitation is carried out and the second twin is born as quickly as possible. Caesarean section is unfortunately not always of value when there is chin-to-chin locking and the first baby is partially born. The Kimball and Rand procedure is dangerous for both the mother and the baby and is only likely to succeed when the babies are small. For other types of locking or entanglement, caesarean section should be performed.

Fetal mortality is high, variably reported as 31% by Khunda (1972) and 84% by Nissen (1958).

(d) Conjoined Twins

This is also a very rare occurrence. Tan and co-workers (1971) reported an incidence of one in 546 twin deliveries (see Chapter 11). The imperfect division of the embryo after formation of the two embryonic areas can result in various forms of conjoined twins. The possibility of survival of one or both twins will depend on the site and degree of union and sharing of vital organs. Before the advent of ultrasonic scanning the diagnosis was rarely made until labour had become obstructed. Conjoined twins can be suspected on ultrasonic scanning if they are facing one another and the fetal heads are at the same plane, or if the babies tend to move in unison. When the diagnosis is made antenatally the delivery should be by caesarean section. Several cases are now on record of successful surgical separation of conjoined twins, even when the union has been quite extensive.

Delivery of Higher Multiples

Abnormal presentations commonly occur in at least one of higher multiples, so that it is not surprising that some obstetricians advocate caesarean section for most, if not all, of these cases. This is certainly so with quadruplets or higher multiples, unless labour commences at a very early gestation. It is interesting, however, that in a review of seventeen viable higher multiple deliveries resulting from ovulation induction, Schenker et al., (1981) found that some higher multiples have been delivered vaginally (Table 8.13). They concluded that the preferred mode of delivery for higher multiples was caesarean section.

There have been several recent reviews of triplet deliveries (Table 8.14) which show that many triplets are delivered vaginally. However, the perinatal mortality rate ranged from 123 per 1000 births to as high as 444 per 1000 births for vaginal deliveries, and was much lower when caesarean section was the choice for delivery.

Table 8.13. Outcome of multiple gestations following induction of ovulation (from Schenker et al., 1981)

Delivery Number	Quadruplets		Quintuplets		Sextuplets		Septuplets		Nontuplets	
	Vaginal	CS	Vaginal	CS	Vaginal	CS	Vaginal	CS	Vaginal	CS
	2	2	2	6	—	4	1	—	1	—
Outcome	Survived	2 died	Survived	3 died		Survived	2 died (anencephalics)		All died (29 weeks)	

CS = caesarean section.

TWINNING AND TWINS

Table 8.14. Outcome of triplet pregnancies

Authors	Numbers	Deliveries		Stillbirths and neonatal deaths (per 1000 births)	
		Vaginal	CS	Vaginal	CS
Loucopoulos and Jewelewicz (1982)	6	4	2	148	0
Micklewitz et al. (1981)	14	13	1	143	0
Itzkowic (1979)	59	50	9	273	0
Ron-El et al. (1981)	19	13	6	123	62
Holczberg et al. (1982)	31	21	10	444	33
Daw (1978)	14	12	2	361	0

CS = caesarean section.

The risk to subsequent babies after the delivery of the first increases progressively. The mortality rose from 18% in the first triplet to 36% in the third for three delivered vaginally (Itzkowic, 1979), whereas in the series of Micklewitz et al. (1981) the mortality increased from 28.5% for the first baby to 50% in the third baby.

Vaginal delivery of triplets should only be undertaken when the presentations of the babies are not abnormal and there are no other obstetric complications, and the obstetrician is confident and competent to undertake the deliveries.

Twinning and Twins
Edited by I MacGillivray, D. M. Campbell and B. Thompson
© 1988 John Wiley & Sons Ltd

CHAPTER 9

Birthweight standards for twins

DORIS M. CAMPBELL

*Department of Obstetrics and Gynaecology, University of Aberdeen,
Aberdeen, UK*

and

MIKE SAMPHIER

*Medical Research Council Medical Sociology Unit, University of
Glasgow, Glasgow, UK*

Carr-Hill and Pritchard (1985) following their review of the factors affecting birthweight made recommendations for the derivation of birthweight standards for singleton births. They recognised that although the numbers of multiple births are relatively small, nevertheless they contribute disproportionately to perinatal deaths and present special problems in consideration of birthweight.

There were three large studies of fetal growth in multiple pregnancy in the 1950s. McKeown and Record (1952) suggested that mean fetal weight was independent of litter size until about 27 weeks of gestation, the rate of growth of each fetus in a multiple pregnancy being slower than that of a singleton fetus from a stage of gestation varying with the number of fetuses present. They attributed such retardation of fetal growth partly to crowding in the uterus. They also considered that there might be some limitation of fetal growth by placental size. They found the mean birthweight of twins was 5.27 lb with a mean gestation of 261.6 days, and that the rate of growth of twin fetuses slowed from approximately 30 weeks gestation. In addition, sex of the fetuses and birth order were thought to be important factors.

Karn (1952 and 1953) showed that mean birthweight was higher in unlike-sex twins than in like-sex twins. She found that maternal age and parity had approximately the same association with birthweight of twins as of singletons. In contrast, Fraccaro (1957), in an Italian study, showed that like-sex twins had a higher mean birthweight and longer length of gestation than unlike-sex twins at low maternal age and parity. Both Karn and Fraccaro examined the correlation between the birthweights of co-twins. This was higher in unlike-sex twins than in like-sex twins.

More recently, Bleker *et al.* (1977) compared the effects of parity and fetal sex on birthweight and placental weight. They concluded that parity was more important in twin than in singleton pregnancy, but fetal sex had less influence. They suggested that multiparae, possibly due to a uterine vascular system altered as a result of a previous pregnancy, had a uterine environment more favourable for the development of the placenta and this was associated with better fetal development. Bleker *et al.* (1979) showed that twins had a lower placental index (placental weight : birthweight) up to 37–38 weeks, then a higher one compared with singletons. However, McKeown and Record (1953) and Gruenwald (1970) had found higher placental indices at all gestations in twin pregnancies. Thus, there is debate as to the importance of the placenta in limiting fetal growth in twin pregnancy.

Daw and Walker (1975a) have pointed out that, while crowding in the uterus may affect the individual growth of each twin, the combined weight of twins continues to increase to term with no obvious sign of restriction. In a further publication (Daw and Walker, 1975b) they commented on the weight differences between twins. Although the maximum intrapair difference in weight (1600–1700 g) was similar for monozygotic and dizygotic twins, there were more monozygotic twin pairs with a difference of more than 440 g. Bulmer (1970) suggested that the earlier onset of birth in higher multiples was due to uterine distension caused by greater total fetal weight: although mean birthweight of individuals decreased directly according to whether the baby was a twin, triplet or quadruplet, the total fetal weight of multiples at birth increased and was approximately 10, 12 and 12 lb respectively compared with 7 lb for singletons.

Fliegner and Eggers (1984) examined fetal growth for 563 pairs of twins collected over a 10 year period. They concluded that twin growth was similar to singletons up to 32 weeks, but thereafter fetal growth for both twin I and twin II was retarded with no difference between twin I and twin II apparent until after 39 weeks. Although they also claimed that zygosity affected twin birthweight, they classified zygosity by the type of placentation, and this is not valid for dichorionic placentation.

Corney *et al.* (1972) showed that dizygotic twins were heavier than monozygotic twins even when taking into account sex of the baby, placentation, gestation length, maternal age and parity.

If twin birthweights are referred to singleton standards, e.g. those of Thomson *et al.* (1968), all individual twins are identified as growth retarded or light for dates. Although, for certain factors which affect fetal growth, it may be most appropriate to consider the weights of the twins individually, e.g. sex of the baby, for others the difference between weights of co-twins or their combined weights may be relevant. For example, Campbell and MacGillivray (1984) have shown that the expansion of maternal plasma volume in twin pregnancy is correlated with the combined birthweight of the twins rather than with their individual weights.

Earlier work from Aberdeen demonstrated consistent relationships between zygosity and birth order and the corresponding singleton standards controlling for baby sex and parity (Samphier, 1982). At that time the singleton standards used were those of Thomson et al. (1968) modified by Altman and Coles (1980) to produce a standard deviation score for birthweight. This provided a continuous scale rather than the essentially nominal scale derived from centile birthweight tables. The standards are dependent on the distribution being a statistically normal curve. Thus, the standard is the average weight for a given gestation taking account of certain other factors. But this approach is open to criticism.

Carr-Hill and Pritchard (1985) pointed out that it would be unlikely for there to be sufficient numbers of multiple births in any one place in a few years to enable the derivation of clinically useful standards for twin pregnancies. Pooling data for several similar populations might be a possibility.

Aberdeen New Analysis

The Aberdeen Maternity and Neonatal Data Bank (Samphier and Thompson, 1981) provides a unique source of consistently high quality data for a defined geographical population. It had been anticipated that this source would also provide sufficient data for the derivation of twin standards corresponding to those derived for singleton birthweights.

Although there are probably enough observations, they have been accumulated over a 35 year period and this casts doubt on their suitability for use in deriving a standard. Recent work on the Aberdeen data (Carr-Hill and Pritchard, 1983) highlighted a clear trend in birthweight over the period 1951–1980 which could not be attributed to changes in the measurement of birthweight or differences in coding. They showed that there was a decline in mean birthweight for gestation despite progressive improvements in the social environment and in maternity care. This phenomenon has also been reported for Scottish data (Forbes and Small, 1983). It, therefore, seemed prudent to examine the data on twin birthweights for evidence of a similar or related trend.

Data have been extracted from the records of twin deliveries from the Aberdeen City District population for the period 1951 to 1985. Deliveries of uncertain gestation (Hall et al., 1985) have been excluded as have both stillbirths and perinatal deaths due to congenital anomalies. When measures of birthweight are derived by combining or comparing twin pairs, then only those pairs have been included where both infants were born alive and neither suffered from a congenital deformity incompatable with life or leading to death within the first week. Table 9.1. gives details of the numbers of twins by 5 year periods and shows the exclusions. The following analysis, therefore, refers to 963 twin deliveries (Table 9.1). Analysis of variance has been carried out relating various maternal and fetal factors to birthweight.

Table 9.1. Outcome of twin deliveries for Aberdeen City District, 1951–1985

	1951–55	1956–60	1961–65	1966–70	1971–75	1976–80	1981–85	Total
All twin deliveries	235	211	210	176	132	118	116	1198
Twin deliveries of uncertain gestation	27	37	34	25	26	12	3	164
Both twins stillborn[a]	1	2	2	4	3	1	1	14
First twin stillborn	4	2	10	7	3	2	3	31
Second twin stillborn	12	7	11	10	6	3	5	52
Both twins with fetal deformity[a]	0	0	1	0	0	3	0	4
First twin with fetal deformity[a]	1	0	1	0	1	4	1	8
Second twin with fetal deformity	4	1	3	1	2	3	0	14
Deliveries with one or both weights not stated	2	2	4	2	1	1	0	12
Total deliveries excluded	46	41	51	36	31	18	12	235
Total used for analysis	189	170	159	140	101	100	104	963

[a]Important note: The figures for 'both twins' include those given in the subsequent rows for the individual twins—thus in the 1951–55 period there were 16 stillborn twins of which one pair were stillborn.

Table 9.2. Characteristics of twin deliveries usual in analysis; percentage in time period

	1951–55 (189)	1956–60 (170)	1961–65 (159)	1966–70 (140)	1971–75 (101)	1976–80 (100)	1981–85 (104)	Total (963)
Sex combination M/M	37	35	33	33	36	47	44	37
M/F	18	16	16	19	22	8	19	17
F/M	14	18	16	12	16	13	6	14
F/F	31	31	34	36	27	32	31	32
Preterm delivery	44	33	38	39	44	41	40	39
Induction of labour	22	19	30	36	48	43	50	33
Primiparae	26	31	28	29	36	48	41	33
Pre-eclampsia—proteinuric	15	16	14	19	17	19	21	17
mild	17	22	21	19	28	41	31	24
Smoking—not stated	97	47	36	16	28	0	0	38
non-smoker	0.5	29	34	44	36	52	58	33
smoker	2.5	24	30	40	37	48	42	29

Numbers in brackets are total numbers for each time period.

Table 9.2 lists the characteristics of those factors namely, parity, the sex combination, preterm delivery (<37 weeks), induction of labour, pre-eclampsia and smoking, which have been used in the subsequent analyses. Maternal height has been included as a covariant. The distribution of sex pairings of the twin babies is slightly different from expected, there being 37% male/male, giving an overall sex ratio at birth of 1.12, which is slightly higher than the average figure of 1.06 for the Aberdeen population previously reported both in twin (MacGillivray *et al.*, 1982) and singleton birth (Campbell *et al.*, 1983). Thirty-nine per cent of twins delivered preterm. In this population 33% were primigravidae, 17% of the women developed proteinuric pre-eclampsia and a further 24% had mild pre-eclampsia; also 33% of the mothers had labour

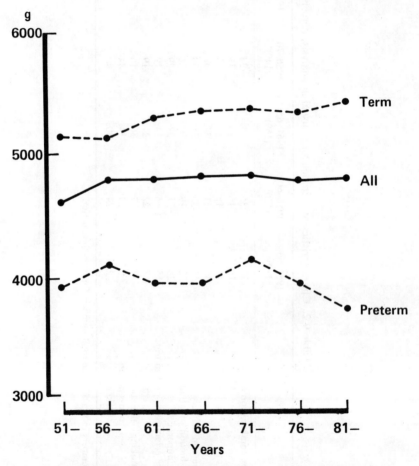

Figure 9.1. Aberdeen City District 1951–1985: combined birthweight twins.

induced. Smoking data are incomplete as details of smoking habits were not recorded routinely in the early years when fewer women smoked. However, in the last decade for which information is complete, 45% of women who delivered twins were smokers.

Figure 9.1 displays the mean combined birthweight for each quinquennium for all twins and also subdivided into term and preterm deliveries. Over the whole period an average increase of 180 g for all twins occurred, but this was almost entirely in the early 1950s. In term deliveries there was an average increase of 280 g and the increase was particularly marked in the late 1950s and the most recent years. Preterm deliveries showed a different pattern. In the early years the average combined birthweight fluctuated, but over the past 15–20 years it progressively declined. This is most likely to be attributable to the earlier detection and management of antenatal problems coupled with the

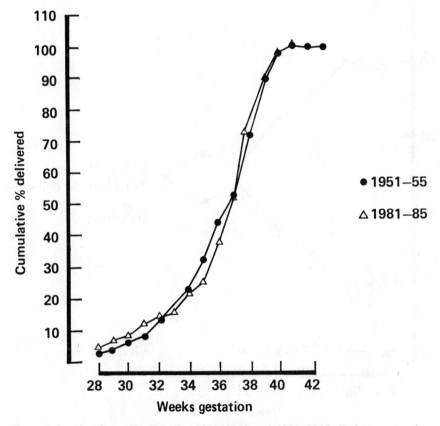

Figure 9.2. Aberdeen City District 1951–1955 and 1981–1985: Twin pregnancies—cumulative distribution of gestation at delivery.

increasing viability of very small preterm infants. It will be noted from Table 9.2. that there has not been any noticeable change in the proportion of deliveries occurring preterm in each 5 year period.

Figure 9.2 shows the cumulative distribution of gestation at delivery for the two extreme time periods studied. There is a difference in the pattern of preterm delivery between 1951–1955 and 1981–1985, in that in the later period there were more early (i.e. 28–32 weeks gestation), and fewer later (i.e. 33–37 weeks) preterm deliveries. This also might account for some of the decline in preterm combined birthweight of twins (Figure 9.1). In the 1981– 1985 period fewer twin pregnancies proceeded beyond 38 weeks gestation. Changes in gestation must, however, be considered in relationship to induction of labour. Figure 9.3 illustrates the progressive increase in elective

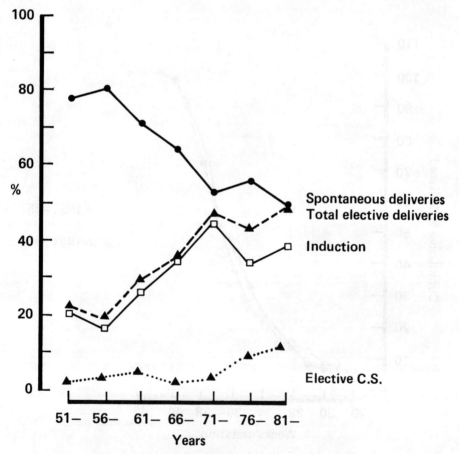

Figure 9.3. Aberdeen City District 1951–1985: Twin pregnancies—induction and elective caesarean section.

intervention in the induction of labour between 1951 and 1985; over the last 10 years, there has been a marked rise in elective caesarean sections. Only 50% of twin pregnancies in the most recent period ended in a spontaneous delivery.

Another factor which affects birthweight is maternal height and for mothers of twins this increased by approximately 2.5 cm on average between the first and last quinquennia studied. Maternal smoking also affects birthweights and although the height of both smokers and non-smokers increased over time, Figure 9.4 shows that in all quinquennia smokers were considerably shorter than non-smokers by an average ranging from 1.2 to 2.2 cm, 1.5 cm overall.

Any tendency for the increasing rate of induction to result in a fall in the mean combined birthweight of twins is in part offset by the fact that women in whom labour was induced were consistently taller than those who delivered spontaneously (Figure 9.5).

Changes in parity distribution discussed in Chapter 5 would also tend to reduce the mean combined birthweight as over the years an increasing proportion of twin pregnancies occur in primigravidae. Higher parity was also associated with short stature and these factors are known to act in opposite directions with respect to singleton birthweights (Carr-Hill and Pritchard, 1985).

In relation to the combined birthweights of twins, sex and birth order have to be considered. Although the number of twin births has declined throughout the period studied, the sex combination remained very similar until the 1970s (Figure 9.6). In the past decade, however, there has been a marked

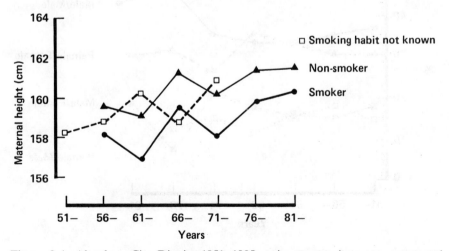

Figure 9.4. Aberdeen City District 1951–1985: twin pregnancies—mean maternal height by smoking.

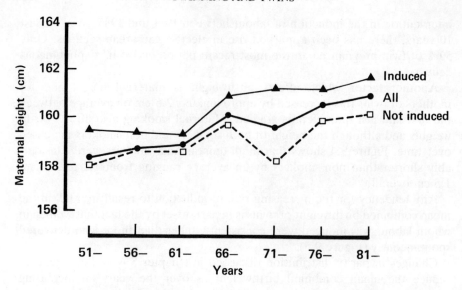

Figure 9.5. Aberdeen City District 1951–1985: twin pregnancies—mean maternal height by induction of labour.

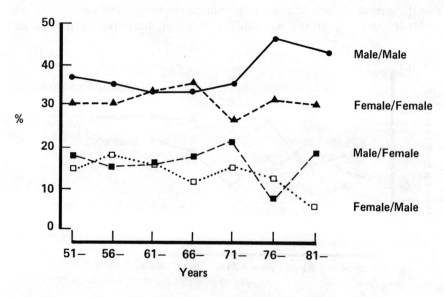

Figure 9.6. Aberdeen City District 1951–1985: twin pregnancies—distribution by sex and birth order.

increase in male : male twins and a fall in unlike-sex pairs. This may be related to the relative increase in the monozygotic twinning rate (see Chapter 4). Given the male birthweight advantage, such a trend should also contribute to increasing the mean combined birthweight.

In an attempt to assess the order of importance of these factors, an analysis of variance (SPSS-X) was performed. Time period, gestation at delivery, parity, sex combination, smoking habit, whether labour was inducud or not, and pre-eclampsia were entered as categorical independent variables. Maternal height and the difference in weights of co-twins as a percentage of their combined birthweights were added as covariants. The adjustments to the mean for changes in these variables are given in Table 9.3 for both the combined and separate birthweights of the twins. Caution should be exercised in interpreting these results since there are too few observations to investigate all potential interactions. Table 9.3 lists only those adjustments for the independent variables which are statistically significant ($p \leqslant 0.05$).

Combined Birthweight

It will be seen from Table 9.3, column 1 that with respect to the combined birthweight of twins, all the independent variables, except the presence or absence of pre-eclampsia have a significant effect. As expected, gestation at delivery taken at 2 week intervals accounts for 50% of the variance in combined birthweight. Despite the missing information on smoking habits, this is the second most important factor in terms of explaining the variation in combined birthweight accounting for 1.7%. Parity and sex combination each account for about 1%, time period for 0.5% and whether the labour was induced or spontaneous 0.4%. These results are similar to what might be expected from our knowledge of birthweights in singleton pregnancies, e.g. the birthweights of babies born to primiparous women are generally accepted to be less than those of multiparae, and smokers are known to have lighter babies than non-smokers. Carr-Hill and Pritchard (1985), however, noted that birthweight for gestation was less in women who had labour induced, particularly marked in those who delivered preterm. This is the opposite to what we have found with respect to the combined weight of twins when in those women whose labour was induced, the babies were heavier than when the onset of labour was spontaneous.

Twin I and Twin II

Previous studies have considered mean birthweight of individual twins rather than the combined birthweight of twins. A similar analysis was, therefore, made to determine the relevance of the same factors for twin I and twin II separately (Table 9.3, columns 2 and 3). Figure 9.7 depicts the change over

Table 9.3. Mean birthweight analysis of variance results for twins combined and separately

	Column 1 Combined birthweight of twins (g)	Column 2 Birthweight (g) Twin I	Column 3 Birthweight (g) Twin II
(A) Grand mean	4 767	2 461	2 307
(B) Adjusted deviations for each factor and the beta value (in brackets)			
1. Time period (years)			
1951–55	−133	12	64
1956–60	−58	12	−77
1961–65	40	64	−7
1966–70	67	10	36
1971–75	70	−53	86
1976–80	55	−50	51
1981–85	62	−72	74
	(0.07)	(0.08)	(0.10)
2. Gestation (weeks)			
<28	−2 721	−1 359	−1 355
28–29	−2 234	−1 150	−1 074
30–31	−1 857	−911	−956
32–33	−1 041	−541	−555
34–35	−394	−237	−165
36–37	97	57	50
38–39	498	257	252
≥40	628	336	280
	(0.71)	(0.69)	(0.64)
3. Parity			
0	−176	−80	−72
1+	84	38	34
	(0.11)	(0.10)	(0.08)
4. Sex combination			
M/M	99	50	43
M/F	84	63	22
F/M	−16	−50	38
F/F	−156	−71	−80
	(0.10)	(0.10)	(0.09)
5. Maternal smoking habit			
Not stated	56	9	20
Non-smoker	118	54	63
Smoker	−208	−73	−97
	(0.13)	(0.09)	(0.11)
6. Onset of labour			
Spontaneous	−43	−27	—
Induced	88	55	—
	(0.06)	(0.07)	
7. Pre-eclampsia			
None	—	—	2
Mild	—	—	26
Proteinuric	—	—	−42
			(0.04)
(C) Regression coefficients of covariants			
1. Maternal height	17.4	11.5	6.7
2. Differences in birthweight as %	—	—	−29.6

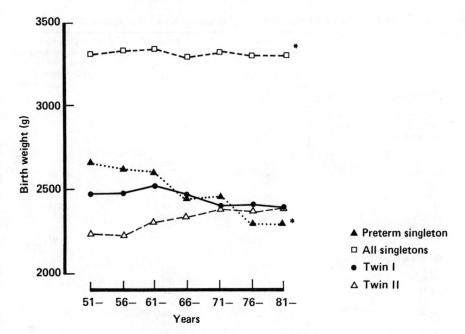

Figure 9.7 Aberdeen City District 1951–1985: mean birthweight of twins and single-tons. * Data available for 1981/83.

the period 1951–1985 in mean birthweight in twins and singletons. The singleton data are taken from Carr-Hill and Pritchard (1985). There is a very slight decline in the average singleton birthweight with a marked fall in singleton preterm birthweights over the period under review. The mean birthweight of twin I shows a slight fall, whereas that of twin II shows a marked increase until in the most recent years there is no difference between the mean birthweights of twin I and twin II. The analysis of variance also points to other interesting findings affecting the birthweight of first and second born twins (Table 9.3). The effect of parity is slightly less for twin II. Sex combination and birth order effects are markedly different—there is a much greater difference between second born females in comparison with first born in like- and unlike-sexed pairs (102 and 21 g respectively). Maternal smoking has a marked effect but is more detrimental to twin II. Whether the labour was spontaneous or induced has a marginal effect on twin I, but twin II is unaffected. Proteinuric pre-eclampsia does not affect twin I, but has a negative effect on the birthweight of twin II, similar to that expected in singletons. The regression coefficient for maternal height in the determina-tion of birthweight is almost halved for a second born twin.

Table 9.4. Differences in birthweights and analysis of variance results

	Column 1 Relative difference in birthweight (Twin I − twin II)	Column 2 Absolute difference (g) between twin I and twin II	Column 3 Absolute difference in birthweight as % total birthweight
(A) Grand mean	155	357	7.8
(B) Adjusted deviations for each factor and the beta value (in brackets)			
1. Time period (years)			
1951–55	156	104	2.6
1956–60	104	2	0.2
1961–65	88	24	0.7
1966–70	−50	−19	−0.7
1971–75	−180	−55	−1.4
1976–80	−155	−68	−1.6
1981–85	−201	−85	−2.1
	(0.31)	(0.21)	(0.23)
2. Gestation (weeks)			
<28	—	−192	—
28–29	—	−169	—
30–31	—	−142	—
32–33	—	−134	—
34–35	—	−30	—
36–37	—	24	—
38–39	—	45	—
⩾40	—	26 (0.22)	—
3. Parity			
0	—	—	0.7
1+	—	—	−0.3
			(0.07)
4. Sex combination			
M/M	—	—	—
M/F	—	—	—
F/M	—	—	—
F/F	—	—	—
5. Maternal smoking habit			
Not stated	−41	−30	−0.8
Non-smoker	−10	4	−0.1
Smoker	65	36	1.1
	(0.19)	(0.09)	(0.11)
6. Onset of labour			
Spontaneous	—	—	—
Induced	—	—	—
7. Pre-eclampsia			
None	−24	—	—
Mild	8	—	—
Proteinuric	71	—	—
	(0.08)		
(C) Regression coefficients of covariants			
1. Maternal height	5.8	—	—
2. Differences in birthweight as %	—	—	—

Intrapair Differences

Analysis of the difference in birthweights within pairs is also intriguing (Table 9.4). Considering first the relative differences in subtracting the weight of twin II from that of twin I, the analysis reveals (Table 9.4, column 1) a significant effect of time period, maternal smoking habit, proteinuric pre-eclampsia and maternal height. The model explains only approximately 11% of the variance of the differences in birthweights and this is accounted for almost entirely by the effect of one variable, time period. At the beginning, in the early 1950s, the mean positive advantage of twin I over twin II was 311 g, whereas from 1971 to date, this has virtually vanished. Both maternal smoking and the presence of proteinuric pre-eclampsia exaggerate the relative difference (Table 9.4, column 1). The relative difference is increased by 65 g if the mother smoked and by 71 g if she had proteinuric pre-eclampsia. Interestingly, the regression coefficient for correction by maternal height for the relative difference between twin birthweights is almost as large as that in the model used to predict the weight of twin II.

In contrast, the analysis of the absolute difference in intrapair weights of twins suggests only three significant factors: time period, gestation, and maternal smoking (Table 9.4, column 2). There is a progressive increase in the absolute differences in birthweights of co-twins with increasing gestational age reaching a peak of some 400 g at 38–39 weeks. Conversely the model shows a decrease of about 200 g over the period of study. Again, maternal smoking widens the intrapair differential, and the model explains only 10% of the variance in the absolute difference in birthweight.

Perhaps, as might have been expected, parity has no effect on either measure of the difference between pairs. It is rather surprising, however, that there is no effect of the different sex combinations and birth order.

Both maternal smoking and the development of proteinuric pre-eclampsia might exert their effect on birthweight in singleton and twin pregnancies by vasoconstriction of uteroplacental blood vessels. It is possible that some alteration in the relative blood supplies to the twins as a result of the disease process in pre-eclampsia or of the mother smoking might lead to a redistribution of blood supply. Figure 9.8 shows the effect of maternal smoking on the intrapair differences in birthweight for the cohort of twins delivered between 1976 and 1985, and indicates a greater difference in birthweights when the mother smoked. It may be noted that this effect of smoking was present during the time period when the difference in birthweight between twin I and twin II diminished.

An alternative approach in considering within pair weight differential is to express the absolute difference as a percentage of the combined birthweight. This has then been used in the analysis of variance (Table 9.4, column 3). The only significant factors in this model which explains only a small proportion of

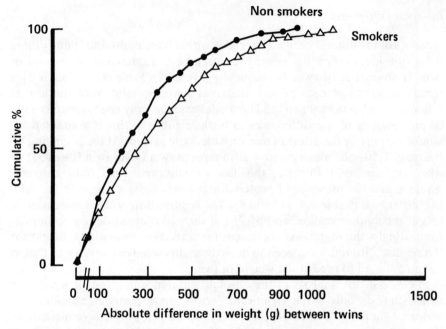

Figure 9.8. Aberdeen City District 1976–1985: twin pregnancies—cumulative distribution of absolute difference in birthweight between twins by smoking.

the variance, namely 4%, are time period, parity and smoking. When the difference in birthweights is expressed in this manner those twins born to primiparae have a greater difference in birthweight than do those resulting from second and subsequent pregnancies. Smoking, as one would expect, exaggerates the difference. Rather surprisingly, maternal height has no effect.

Figure 9.9 depicts the intrapair birthweight difference as a percentage of the total combined weight of twins, and this has decreased for term infants from 10.4% to 5.7%, while that for preterm deliveries shows a similar but less marked overall trend from 8.6% to 7%. Further analysis also suggests that there may be a tendency for the rate of decline to be steeper in unlike-sexed pairs.

Conclusions

With the suggestion from earlier studies (Bulmer, 1970; Daw and Walker, 1975a; 1975b) of a degree of dependency of twin II on twin I, we attempted to account for the possibility that twin birthweights might to some extent be affected by the presence of the second fetus in utero. Several experimental

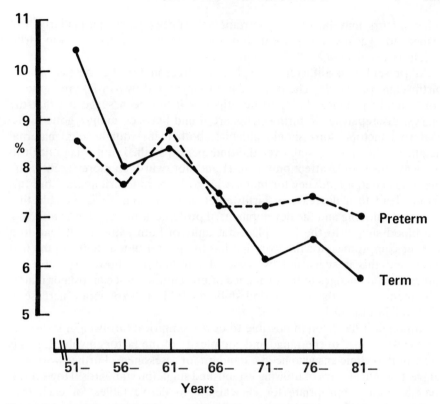

Figure 9.9. Aberdeen City District 1951–1985: twin pregnancies—birthweight difference as % of total combined weight.

indices were added to the models in analyses of variance. The results
indicated that the most useful of these factors in terms of independence and
effect was the difference in twin birthweights expressed as a proportion of the
combined weight which, when entered as a covariant, accounted for some
10% of the variance in the birthweight of twin II, but had no significant effect
on the birthweight of twin I, perhaps indicating a greater vulnerability of
twin II.

It has proved impossible to define birthweight standards for twins as
originally planned because of the secular trend in the birthweight and the
multiplicity of factors involved. Our analyses of variance have shown that
various ways of manipulating and expressing twin birthweights implicate
different factors which might be significant in the determination of birthweight. It is difficult to know which of these factors should be considered
when deriving empirical birthweight standards for twins. In addition, as the
models only explain a portion of the variation in birthweight, it is clear that

other factors may be more important and further work, particularly with respect to zygosity and placentation known to have effects on twin birthweight (Corney *et al.*, 1972) is required.

At present it is difficult to explain the reason for the increase in the birthweight of twin II. The increase in proportion of twins who are monozygotic should produce the opposite effect as it has been suggested that the biggest discrepancies in birthweights are found between monozygotic twins. Maternal factors alone should influence both twins equally, e.g. maternal height has been increasing over the time period studied, but it is difficult to see why this should affect only twin II and not twin I. In more recent years there has been a tendency for more twins to be born to primiparae, but this should lead to a decrease in birthweight in both twins. It is possible that maternal smoking and the development of proteinuric pre-eclampsia affecting the blood supply to the fetal placental units of both twins might lead to a greater compromise for the twin that has the poorer blood supply in the first place and this is suggested by some of our findings; however, Table 9.2 indicates that changes in the incidence of proteinuric pre-eclampsia or maternal smoking over the time period studied could not explain an increase in birthweight of twin II.

Although it has been impossible to devise empirical birthweight standards for twins because of the range and complexity of the factors involved, this is unhelpful to clinicians who need a standard for assessment. Further work may suggest practical ways of utilising established singleton standards. However, it may be more appropriate for clinical use to derive tables for each twin separately and for both twins together, correcting only for gestation at delivery and ignoring all the other factors which contribute much less to the variations found in birthweight. Such tables would have the advantage of being relatively simple to apply and could readily be adapted to take account of secular changes.

Twinning and Twins
Edited by I. MacGillivray, D. M. Campbell and B. Thompson
© 1988 John Wiley & Sons Ltd

CHAPTER 10

Outcome of twin pregnancies

DORIS M. CAMPBELL and IAN MACGILLIVRAY
*Department of Obstetrics and Gynaecology, University of Aberdeen,
Aberdeen, UK*

The perinatal death rate is much higher in twins than in singletons and is even greater for higher multiples. This was so thirty years ago (Beacham and Beacham, 1950; Miettinen, 1954; Kurtz *et al.*, 1958) and is still true (see Chapter 8, section on delivery of higher multiples). Although sextuplets have been delivered successfully and survived (Giovannucci-Uzielli *et al.*, 1981) there is no doubt that the perinatal mortality rises with increasing numbers of multiples.

Recent figures show that there is still a marked difference in the survival rate of twins compared with singletons in various parts of the world. For example, in a multiple hospital study in the USA the perinatal mortality rate for twins was three times greater than in singletons (Ellis *et al.*, 1979). In Nigeria it was four times greater (Nylander, 1979b). In Scotland it was 5.8 times greater, the perinatal mortality rate of multiple births being 55.9 per 1000 compared with 9.7 per 1000 in singletons (Registrar General for Scotland Annual Report, 1983). In our total Aberdeen series between 1951 and 1983, the perinatal mortality rate in twins was also four to five times greater than in singletons, 90.4 compared with 21.2 per 1000 births. Over this period, the perinatal mortality rate in Aberdeen in singleton pregnancies showed a steady decline (Table 10.1) falling to about one-third between 1951 and 1983. Over the same time period, the twin perinatal death rates were more variable, but showed a similar fall. Although overall the perinatal mortality rate for twin I was significantly less than that for twin II ($z = 3.34$, $p < 0.01$) the difference has been steadily decreasing particularly so in recent years. The only significant difference in perinatal mortality rates for twin I and twin II was in the first quinquennium studied ($z = 2.27$, $p < 0.05$).

It is not surprising that the perinatal death rate in multiple pregnancies is higher than in singletons in view of the increased incidence of complications of pregnancy, early delivery, and relatively low birthweight. In addition, there are many other factors which affect the prognosis for the babies.

Table 10.1. Perinatal death rate (per 1000 births) in twin and singleton pregnancies for Aberdeen City District 1951–1983

	Twin I	Twin II	All twins	Singletons
1951–55	72.3	136.2	104.3	29.2
1956–60	47.4	94.8	71.1	28.5
1961–65	95.2	128.6	111.9	23.6
1966–70	85.2	142.1	113.6	18.7
1971–75	83.3	83.3	83.3	16.8
1976–80	50.9	76.3	63.6	11.2
1981–83	29.4	44.1	36.8	9.8
Total	70.4	110.4	90.4	21.2

For numbers of twin and singleton pregnancies in each quinquennium see Chapter 7.

Maternal Factors

Age

The incidence of twinning increases with increasing maternal age up to about 35–40 years (see Chapter 5). However, the effect of age on twin mortality is disputed. Karn (1953) found that when one, or especially both babies died, the mothers were much younger than the mothers of twins who survived. The 1958 British Perinatal Mortality Survey (Butler and Alberman, 1969) also found that twin babies were at greatest risk when the mothers were under 20 years of age. On the other hand, Barr and Stevenson (1961) found no relationship between maternal age and fetal death of twin pregnancies as did Parsons (1964) in a study limited to unlike-sex pairs.

More recently, Nylander (1979b) in Ibadan showed that the perinatal death rate was slightly higher in teenagers, then fell to its lowest in mothers aged 20–24 years, but rose consistently with age to a maximum in those over 40 years of age.

Parity

Earlier studies (Farrell, 1964; Klein, 1964; Parsons, 1964; Law, 1967) showed that perinatal mortality was two to three times higher in twins born to primigravidae than to multigravidae. However, Farrell (1964) found that there was no consistent association between individual parities and mortalities after the first. There was a slight increase in perinatal loss in higher parities, but it did not reach the levels found in primigravidae (Parsons, 1964; Butler and Alberman, 1969).

Table 10.2. Perinatal mortality rate (per 1000 births) in twin pregnancies by age and parity for Aberdeen City District 1951–1983 (gestation >24 weeks)

Age	Parity					
	0	1	2	3	4+	All
(A) Twin I						
≤14	0 (5)	100 (10)	0 (6)	0 (7)	0 (4)	31.3 (32)
15–19	37.7 (55)	142.9 (7)	— (0)	— (0)	— (0)	48.4 (62)
20–24	94.6 (148)	80.4 (112)	96.8 (31)	0 (11)	0 (3)	85.2 (305)
25–29	111.1 (99)	58.4 (154)	0 (66)	117.6 (34)	0 (16)	65.0 (369)
30–34	83.3 (48)	29.4 (68)	83.3 (60)	31.3 (32)	90.9 (33)	62.2 (241)
35–39	62.5 (16)	105.3 (19)	35.7 (28)	0 (14)	105.3 (19)	62.5 (96)
≥40	250.0 (4)	0 (2)	0 (5)	0 (3)	0 (4)	55.6 (18)
Total	88 (375)	64.5 (372)	45.9 (196)	49.5 (101)	63.3 (79)	67.68 (1123)
(B) Twin II						
≤14	200 (5)	200 (10)	0 (6)	285.7 (7)	0 (4)	156.3 (322)
15–19	54.5 (55)	142.9 (7)	— (0)	— (0)	— (0)	64.5 (62)
20–24	148.6 (148)	151.8 (112)	161.3 (31)	0 (11)	0 (3)	144.3 (305)
25–29	70.7 (99)	64.9 (154)	136.4 (66)	176.5 (34)	0 (16)	86.7 (369)
30–34	41.7 (48)	102.9 (68)	116.7 (60)	93.8 (32)	90.9 (33)	91.3 (241)
35–39	125 (16)	263.2 (19)	0 (28)	0 (14)	105.3 (19)	93.3 (96)
≥40	250 (4)	0 (2)	0 (5)	333.3 (3)	0 (4)	111.1 (18)
Total	101.3 (375)	112.9 (372)	107.1 (196)	118.8 (101)	63.3 (79)	105.1 (1123)

Numbers in brackets are the total births in each group.

Nylander (1979b) from Ibadan showed a perinatal mortality rate of 60 per 1000 births in primiparae which fell to 52 in women of parity 1, but rose thereafter to 61 in parity 2, 64 in parities 3 and 4, and to 92 in women of higher parity. Medearis *et al.* (1979) on the other hand, examining risk ratios for perinatal death in twin pregnancy, found an increased risk in women of low gravidity.

Puissant and Leroy (1982) showed lower perinatal mortality rates in primiparae up to 37–38 weeks gestation, then higher rates thereafter. However, when they looked at the confounding effect of birthweight the difference disappeared.

It seems appropriate in view of the earlier documented changes in twinning rates by age and parity together, to examine perinatal outcome also in this manner and to do this for twin I and twin II separately. Table 10.2 shows the outcome of twin pregnancies for Aberdeen City District cases from 1951 to 1983 when the gestation at delivery was greater than 24 weeks. At all parities and ages, the perinatal mortality of twin II was greater than for twin I. Perinatal mortality rates were lowest for twin I in parities 2 and 3 with no effect of maternal age in any parity, while for twin II (part B, Table 10.2) the rates were lowest in parities 0 and 4 with again no effect of maternal age.

Height

Twin perinatal mortality in Aberdeen was found to be greater in short than in tall women when the birthweight was between 1.4 and 2.3 kg (Anderson, 1956), but this did not apply for other birthweights. A similar high perinatal mortality is found in short women in singleton pregnancies, and is associated with a smaller size of babies due either to growth retardation or to preterm labour. More recently analysis of Aberdeen data (Table 10.3) shows different patterns of perinatal mortality rates for twin I and twin II. With respect to twin I, perinatal deaths are commonest in tall women and for twin II perinatal loss is greatest in short women, but the differences are small and not statistically significant. Thus, for all twins together, there is no significant gradient of decreasing perinatal mortality with increasing maternal height.

Social Class

Reports on the outcome of twin pregnancies with changing socioeconomic status are very limited. Alm (1953) in a hospital study of selected male infants only, found that when the mothers were of lower social class, the outcome at follow-up of low birthweight twins was worse than that of singletons of the same weight or of heavier control infants. Medearis *et al.* (1979) suggested a greater risk of perinatal loss in twin pregnancies when the mother had less education.

Table 10.3. Perinatal death (PND) rate (per 1 000 births) maternal height for twin I and twin II and singleton births—Aberdeen City District 1951–1983 (gestation > 24 weeks)

Maternal height (cm)	Twin I			Twin II			All Twins			Singletons		
	PND	Total	PND rate	PND	Total	PND rate	PND	Total	PND rate	PND	Total	PND rate
<154	16	254	63.0	33	254	129.9	49	508	96.5	647	25 036	25.8
155–163	40	597	67.0	59	597	98.8	99	1 194	82.9	1 039	52 143	19.9
≥164	18	246	73.1	24	246	97.6	42	492	85.4	284	18 893	15.0
Not stated	2	26	76.9	2	26	76.9	4	52	76.9	58	1 833	31.6
Total	76	1 123	67.7	118	1 123	105.1	194	2 246	86.4	2 028	97 905	20.7

Table 10.4. Perinatal death (PND) rate (per 1 000 births) by social class of the mother in twin and singleton pregnancy—Aberdeen City District 1951–1983

Social class	Twin I			Twin II			All Twins			Singletons		
	PND	Total	PND rate	PND	Total	PND rate	PND	Total	PND rate	PND	Total	PND rate
I, II, IIIa	20	261	76.6	18	261	69.0	38	522	72.8	495	28 692	17.3
IIb, IIIc	24	425	56.5	43	425	101.2	67	850	78.8	890	40 572	21.9
IV, V	25	325	76.9	46	325	141.5	71	650	109.2	694	27 069	25.6
Widowed, single	3	32	93.8	6	32	187.5	9	64	140.6	83	3 444	24.1
Not stated	4	80	50	5	80	62.5	9	160	56.3	58	3 039	19.1
Total	76	1123	67.7	118	1123	105.1	194	2 246	86.4	2 220	102 816	21.6

Table 10.5. Birthweight (g) (mean ± SD) (gestation > 24/52): Aberdeen City District 1951–1983

Social class	Twin I	Twin II	Singletons
I, II, IIIa	2484.6 ± 621.0	2335.2 ± 616.0	3353.1 ± 519.9
IIIb, IIIc	2431.3 ± 583.2	2260.1 ± 588.0	3291.1 ± 542.1
IV, V	2363.5 ± 606.8	2140.7 ± 675.7	3237.1 ± 565.0
Widowed, single	2415.2 ± 658.6	2141.8 ± 626.1	3146.1 ± 548.6
Not stated	2486.2 ± 591.5	2249.1 ± 607.2	3204.7 ± 578.6

Numbers in each group are given in Table 10.4.

Table 10.4 shows that the perinatal mortality rate in Aberdeen singletons increased with declining social status; that for the widowed and unmarried was similar to that for the wives of semi-skilled and unskilled manual workers although their babies weighed marginally less (Table 10.4, 10.5). Overall the perinatal mortality of twins was similar to that of singletons, but the highest rate, almost double those of the wives of non-manual workers, was in the widowed and unmarried group. There is, however, a difference in the pattern between twin I and II. Although in each social class, the mean birthweight of twin I was higher than that of twin II (Table 10.5) birthweight was always highest in the non-manual group and lowest, albeit marginally, in social classes IV and V. Perinatal mortality for twin II followed the overall pattern for twins, but it was accentuated. Exceptionally, however, the perinatal mortality of twin I in the non-manual group was higher than that of the co-twins, and similar to that of social class IV and V first born.

Smoking

There is a well-known increase in perinatal death rate in singleton babies when the mother smokes, and this is confirmed from the Aberdeen data (Table 10.6). However, smoking did not affect the perinatal mortality of either twin I or twin II.

Although the fetal mortality in twin pregnancies is higher than in singletons, maternal factors do not seem to be exerting a major influence on the outcome of twin pregnancies, whereas the effects of maternal height, social class and smoking on fetal loss, while interrelated, are marked in singleton pregnancies. Factors other than these may be more important in twin pregnancies, for example the onset of preterm labour masking a minor effect of maternal characteristics on perinatal loss.

Table 10.6. Perinatal death rate (per 1000 births) for singletons/twins 1969–1983 in Aberdeen City District by smoking

	Twin I	Twin II	All twins	Singletons (38 179)
Non-smokers (173)	52.02	75.14	63.6	11.53
Smokers (179)	50.28	67.04	58.7	16.05
Smoking not known (32)	125.00	62.05	93.8	8.34
Total (384)	57.29	70.31	63.8	14.12

Numbers in brackets are numbers of twin pregnancies in each category.

Fetal Factors affecting Perinatal Mortality

Sex of the Baby (either as Individual Twins or as Pairs of the Same Sex)

Previous studies have shown that unlike-sex pair twins have a better chance of survival than like-sex pairs (Potter, 1963; Klein, 1964; Dunn, 1965) and that boys are at greater risk than girls (Barr and Stevenson, 1961; Spurway, 1962; Potter, 1963). The highest mortality in twins in the British Perinatal Mortality Survey of 1958 (Butler and Alberman, 1969) was found in like-sex twin boys, when nearly one in ten pregnancies ended in the death of both babies in contrast to like-sex female pairs, when the death of both babies was less common than in any other group. Boys have a better chance of survival if the co-twin is a girl rather than a boy (Potter, 1963) and the lowest death rates in girls occurred in those of unlike-sex pairs (Barr and Stevenson, 1961).

In a recent study of perinatal mortality in a total population of 820 twins pairs born in the north-east of Scotland between 1968 and 1982 (Thompson *et al.*, 1983) the perinatal mortality rate was 61.6 per 1000 in males compared with the 48.8 per 1000 in females (statistically significant $p < 0.05$).

In the 1969–1983 Aberdeen series, however, no difference was found in the perinatal death rate for males compared with females (Table 10.7).

Birth Order

It is generally agreed that the second twin and the succeeding babies in higher multiple pregnancies have a worse prognosis (Beacham and Beacham, 1950; Guttmacher and Kohl, 1958; Kurtz *et al.*, 1958; Little and Friedman, 1958;

Table 10.7. Perinatal death rates (per 1000 births) in twin pregnancies in Aberdeen City District (1969–1983) by sex and birth order

	Total	Rate
Twin I–male	228	52.6
Twin I–female	156	64.1
Twin II–male	204	83.3
Twin II–female	179	55.9
All twin I	384	57.3
All twin II	383	70.5
All twins–male	432	67.1
All twins–female	335	59.7
Total twins	767	63.8

Note: one twin II stillbirth has sex of infant not coded.

Potter, 1963; Wyshak and White, 1963; Klein, 1964; Ferguson, 1964; Law, 1967; Butler and Alberman, 1969; Patten, 1970; Ellis *et al.*, 1979) although in the last named study, the differences are not statistically significant. On the other hand, some authors found that the second baby did as well as, if not better than, the first (Potter and Fuller, 1949; Bender, 1952; Aaron *et al.*, 1961; Graves *et al.*, 1962; Moir, 1964). Some difficulty may arise in interpretation of such studies on account of the small number of cases and biased selection of women, e.g. primigravidae only.

In the series of Thompson *et al.* (1983) from north-east Scotland, the perinatal death rate was 47.6 per 1000 in first born compared with 64.6 in second born twins (statistically significant $p < 0.01$).

Aberdeen data (Table 10.7) have shown no difference in perinatal mortality rates between first born and second born females and although there was a tendency for the second male twins to have a higher perinatal mortality than first male twins, this did not reach statistical significance.

With respect to the time of death of twins, second twins are more likely to die before delivery than in the neonatal period (Butler and Alberman, 1969; Myrianthopoulous, 1970). The stillbirth rate for twin II however is the same as that of first born twins, although the neonatal death rate is twice as high (Little and Friedman, 1958; Sherman and Lowe, 1970).

Table 10.8. Time of perinatal death in Aberden City District twin and singleton pregnancies (1969–1983) by sex and birth order

Time of death	Twin I: M		Twin I: F		Twin II: M		Twin II: F	
(A) Twin pregnancies	%		%		%		%	
Stillbirth	2.19	(5)	2.56	(4)	1.96	(4)	2.79	(5)
First day	1.32	(3)	2.56	(4)	2.45	(5)	1.68	(3)
First week	1.75	(4)	1.28	(2)	3.92	(8)	1.12	(2)
First month	0.44	(1)		(0)	0.49	(1)	0.56	(1)
Live birth	94.3	(215)	93.59	(146)	91.18	(186)	93.85	(168)
Total	100	(228)	100	(156)	100	(204)	100	(179)

(B) Singleton pregnancies		
	%	
Stillbirth	0.84	(319)
First week	0.58	(220)
First month	0.08	(32)
Late deaths	0.04	(14)
Live births	98.46	(37 594)
Total	100	(38 179)

Note: one twin II stillbirth has sex missing.
Numbers in brackets are total numbers in each group.

In Aberdeen, the tendency for the second male twin to die occurs in the first week of life, with no difference in stillbirths or in first day or first month (neonatal) deaths between twin I and twin II (Table 10.8). The outcome for singletons is shown for comparison.

The recent improvement in outcome from that of earlier studies is probably due to better standards of care at delivery and in the neonatal period. Male babies and the second born, although they may have lesser potential for survival, are now given sufficient care to ensure that they do not die. Follow-up studies to determine long-term morbidity are required.

Zygosity

When zygosity is known, perinatal mortality is reported as higher in the monozygotic twins than in dizygotic (Potter, 1963; Myrianthopoulous, 1970; Nylander, 1979b). For example, Potter (1963) found that in 16.4% of monozygotic pairs, one or both twins died compared with 5.3% in dizygotic pairs.

In the study of north-east Scotland (Thompson et al., 1983) the perinatal death rate in monozygotic twins was 50.0 per 1000 births compared with 31.9 per 1000 births in dizygotic. In 10.4% of babies the zygosity was not known and they accounted for 38% of the perinatal deaths. The perinatal death rate was 3.7 times higher in those twins of unknown zygosity compared with all the twins. Other studies have also had to ignore a sizeable proportion of like-sex pairs for which zygosity was not available. Thompson et al. (1983) examine the likely effect of allocating the pairs for whom zygosity is unknown to either all MZ or all DZ. If all such pairs were DZ, the perinatal mortality rate for DZ twins would not differ from the overall. In contrast if all were MZ the rate would be significantly different. Assuming that all the twins of unknown zygosity who survived the first week were MZ, then 73% of deaths would have to be MZ in order for the perinatal mortality rate to reach statistical significance. They comment that it is difficult on account of differential effects of sex and birthweight in MZ and DZ twins to reach any firm conclusions about the relevance of zygosity in perinatal mortality until a series of twins all of known zygosity for all like-sex pairs is available.

Placentation

The highest death rates have been reported in MZ pairs with monochorionic placentae, while unlike-sex DZ pairs with separate placentae have the lowest mortality. In a Birmingham study the stillbirth rate in monoamniotic monochorionic twins was found to be almost twice that in diamniotic monochorionic twins, with one-third of such twins dying in the perinatal period (Wharton et al., 1968).

Gruenwald (1970) reported that the perinatal death rate was 7.1% in monochorionic pairs, 4.6% in dichorionic pairs of the same sex, and 3.6% in dichorionic pairs of the opposite sex. In Myrianthopoulous's 1970 study the stillbirth rate was highest among monoamniotic monochorionic twins (22.2%) and lowest in diamniotic dichorionic twins (3.9%). Neonatal deaths, however, were highest in the diamniotic monochorionic pairs (13.7%) and lowest in the monoamniotic monochorionic pairs (5.6%). The overall perinatal death rate was 27.8% for those who were monoamniotic monochorionic, 22.5% for those who were diamniotic monochorionic, and 10.9% for the diamniotic dichorionic pairs.

Nylander (1979b) again found the highest perinatal mortality rates in monozygotic monochorionic twin pregnancies. In contrast, Thompson *et al.* (1983) found that there was not a significant difference in perinatal mortality rates between monozygotic twins with monochorionic and dichorionic placenta, although again the rate was highest when the placentation was not determined. This still applied whichever way the cases of unknown placentation were allocated and it was concluded that placentation was not an important factor in perinatal mortality in this series of twins.

In the series of 92 perinatal deaths in 820 pairs (Thompson *et al.*, 1983) 48 were accounted for by 24 pairs. There were 10 male, 7 female pairs, and 7 of unlike sex. Stillbirths accounted for 3 pairs. In 13 pairs both twins died in the first week, while in the remaining 8 pairs, one twin was stillborn and the other died within a few days. Zygosity was not stated for the majority of like sex-twins (10 out of 17). Of the 5 MZ pairs, 2 had a MC placenta.

Table 10.9 attempts to examine perinatal mortality in twin pregnancies by sex, birth order, zygosity and placentation. The numbers in some cells of this total population of twin pregnancies are very small and conclusions are, therefore, impossible. Clearly, there is a need for more work in this area on total populations of twins when zygosity and placentation have both been determined in order to identify the significance of these factors in fetal outcome.

Birthweight

Birthweight of twins is generally less than that of singletons of the same gestation (see Chapter 9). Earlier studies (Karn, 1953; Miettinen, 1954; Klein, 1964) identified birthweight as the most important single factor affecting survival of multiple births. At that time the excess mortality in twin pregnancies was attributed mainly to a high incidence of very low birthweight babies (under 1 kg), whereas the twin mortality with birthweights over 2.5 kg was similar to that of singletons, and for those between 1 kg and 2.5 kg it was twice that of singletons (Potter, 1963). It was also noted earlier that the mean birthweight is lower and the intrapair weight differences are greater when

Table 10.9. Perinatal mortality rates (per 1000 births) in twin pregnancies in Aberdeen City District (1969–1983) by birth order, sex of baby, zygosity and placentation

Zygosity and placentation	Twin I				Twin II*			
	Male		Female		Male		Female	
	Total	Rate	Total	Rate	Total	Rate	Total	Rate
MZ MC	35	57.1	33	90.9	35	0	33	90.9
MZ DC	49	0	25	80.0	48	41.7	26	38.6
MZ –	4	0	2	0	4	0	2	0
DZ DC	115	34.8	84	23.8	92	54.4	106	18.9
Not known	25	240.0	12	250.0	25	400.0	12	333.3
Total	228	52.6	156	64.1	204	83.3	179	55.9

*Excluding 1 stillbirth of uncertain sex.

both twins die than when they both survive (Parsons, 1964). A mean lower birthweight and a high incidence of intrapair inequality occurs in monoamniotic twins and they have a poorer prognosis than other twins (Wharton *et al.*, 1968).

More recently, Medearis *et al.* (1979) considered that low birthweight was still a major factor in the elevated perinatal mortality in twin pregnancies, particularly if there were associated pregnancy complications such as preterm labour, antepartum haemorrhage and early rupture of the membranes. Puissant and Leroy (1982) noted as mentioned earlier, difference in perinatal mortality by parity, but found this disappeared when they looked at birthweight specific mortality.

The 1983 Scottish Twin Study (Patel *et al.*, 1984) showed that when the birthweight specific perinatal mortality rates for twin and singleton babies were compared, the perinatal mortality rate was lower for twins in each 500 g weight group between 1000 and 2500 g.

Although Ellis *et al.* (1979) claimed that second twins had a higher birthweight specific perinatal mortality up to 1500 g, the differences they found do not reach statistical significance.

Table 10.10 compares Aberdeen birthweight specific perinatal mortality rates for twin I, twin II and singleton pregnancies. Below 1000 g, the rates are similar in twins and singletons. Thereafter up to birthweights of 2500 g

Table 10.10. Perinatal death (PND) rate (per 1000 births) in twin and singleton pregnancies by birthweight: Aberdeen City District 1951–1983 (gestation >24 weeks)

Birthweight (g)	Twin I		Twin II		Singletons	
	Total	PND rate	Total	PND rate	Total	PND rate
<750	5	1000	23	652.2	152	651.3
750–	22	818.2	39	692.3	178	825.8
1 000–	29	482.8	19	473.7	296	706.1
1 250–	43	302.3	91	318.7	389	532.1
1 500–	65	61.5	28	214.3	430	351.2
1 750–	85	35.3	170	82.4	766	205.0
2 000–	119	50.4	77	64.9	1 159	115.6
2 250–	187	10.7	254	31.5	2 880	47.9
2 500–	218	22.9	250	20.0	5 368	21.6
2 750–	165	18.2	60	0	11 587	13.9
3 000–	120	8.3	87	0	16 585	8.7
3 250–	47	21.3	15	0	20 287	6.9
3 500–	11	0	7	0	22 342	5.7
3 750–	7	166.7	3	0	8 795	4.9
≥4 000	—	—	—	—	6 691	8.1
Total	1 123	67.7	1 123	105.1	97 905	20.7

the perinatal mortality is higher for singletons. Up to 1250 g, the perinatal mortality rate of twin I is greater than that of twin II, from 1250 to 2500 g the rate of twin II is greater than twin I, from 2500 to 2750 g the rates for twin I and II are almost the same, and from 2750 g upwards the rates for twin I are greater than for twin II. However, the rates of twin I and twin II are only significantly different in the category when birthweight lies between 1500 and 1750g ($z = 2.18$, $p < 0.05$). It is interesting to note that all perinatal deaths in twins over 2750 g occurred in twin I. Prematurity is the term which was used in the past to describe small babies, but this did not differentiate between preterm immature and small-for-dates, growth retarded babies, but simply described the heterogeneous group of low birthweight babies. Both immaturity and retarded growth contribute to the lower birthweight in twins and this in turn is a major contributing factor to the higher perinatal mortality rate than in singletons.

Pregnancy Complications

There is no doubt that much of the obstetric management of twin pregnancies is aimed at minimising the antenatal problems arising, particularly preterm labour and pre-eclampsia (see Chapter 7). As yet no effective treatment has been found to prevent the onset of preterm labour, although advocates of hospitalisation with bedrest claim a decrease in perinatal mortality (see Chapter 7 for discussion of problems of such studies).

Medearis *et al.* (1979), examining twin perinatal deaths by birthweight in association with pregnancy complications (not including preterm labour), found that both low birthweight and fetal death were increased in association with antepartum haemorrhage, both abruptio placentae and bleeding of unknown origin, premature rupture of the membranes and miscellaneous other complications. Rather surprisingly, toxaemia was insignificant, but no definition was given for this condition and cases of mild pre-eclampsia may have been included. It is only when proteinuria is present that fetal deaths increase in this condition (MacGillivray, 1983).

Mode of Delivery

The controversy with respect to the best method of delivering twins, particularly at early gestations and when malpresentation is present, is discussed in Chapter 8. Protagonists of liberal use of caesarean section, e.g. Cetrulo (1986), claim to have decreased perinatal mortality in twin pregnancies to that of singletons for those with other than cephalic : cephalic presentation under 34 weeks gestation, and to have eliminated the differential in mortality between twin I and twin II. Others (Ryhdstrom and Ohrlander, 1985; Mueller-Heubach *et al.*, 1985; Bell *et al.*, 1986) in larger studies have shown no improvement in perinatal outcome with increasing caesarean section rates.

Table 10.11. Perinatal mortality (per 1000 births) by type of delivery and gestation in twin pregnancies in Aberdeen City District 1951–83 (gestation > 24 weeks)

Gestation	SD	LUSCS*	Forceps/vacuum	Assisted breech	NS	Total
(A) Twin I						
<28	800 (15)	—	666.7 (3)	800 (5)		782.6 (23)
28–30	379.3 (29)	0 (1)	500 (8)	461.5 (13)	1000 (1)	423.1 (52)
31–33	112.9 (62)	0 (6)	142.9 (14)	0 (11)	—	96.8 (93)
34–36	21.9 (137)	83.3 (24)	49.2 (61)	119.1 (42)		49.2 (264)
37–39	7.02 (285)	24.3 (41)	20.6 (97)	26.3 (76)	0 (2)	14.0 (501)
≥40	9.62 (104)	9 (11)	64.5 (31)	90.9 (44)	—	36.8 (190)
Total	57.0 (632)	36.14 (83)	70.09 (214)	109.9 (191)	333.3 (3)	67.7 (1123)
(B) Twin II						
<28	857.1 (7)	—	750.0 (4)	777.8 (9)	666.7 (3)	782.6 (23)
28–30	600.0 (20)	0 (2)	1000 (4)	480.0 (25)	1000 (1)	557.7 (52)
31–33	170.7 (41)	0 (6)	214.3 (14)	233.3 (30)	0 (2)	182.8 (93)
34–36	54.6 (110)	83.3 (24)	43.5 (46)	92.1 (76)	250 (8)	72.0 (264)
37–39	61.9 (194)	22.2 (45)	44.9 (89)	43.5 (161)	166.7 (12)	51.9 (501)
≥40	30.3 (66)	0 (12)	68.2 (44)	62.5 (64)	0 (4)	47.4 (190)
Total	102.7 (438)	33.7 (89)	94.5 (201)	120.6 (365)	233.3 (30)	105.1 (1123)

Numbers in brackets are the total births in each group.
*Lower uterine segment caesarean section.

Table 10.11 illustrates from the Aberdeen data part of the problem in determining the relevance of different factors with respect to perinatal deaths. Even with this total population of twin pregnancies, some of the cells are empty or contain few cases.

The experiences of twin I and twin II are obviously different and should be considered separately. Whereas for twin I, the total perinatal mortality for breech delivery is significantly higher than for twin I overall ($z = 2.06$, $p < 0.05$), this does not apply to twin II which has a rate similar to that for twin II delivered spontaneously; this latter rate, however, is nearly twice that for spontaneous first born deliveries. When caesarean section is the mode of delivery, the rates for both twins are all very similar, but the significant difference from overall mortality rates is for twin II ($z = 2.16$, $p < 0.05$) rather than twin I ($z = 1.12$, not significant). For all modes of delivery, for both twin I and twin II, perinatal mortality decreased with increasing gestation at least up to 40 weeks; a longer gestation seemed to be beneficial only to twin II delivered spontaneously. It is concluded that gestation at delivery is more relevant to perinatal mortality than mode of delivery.

Causes of Twin Deaths

In all series of twin deaths immaturity is the commonest cause of perinatal deaths.

Asphyxia and anoxia in utero occur less frequently in twins than in singletons, but account for 8–10% of the antepartum deaths (Barr and Stevenson, 1961; Potter, 1963; Myrianthopoulous, 1970). MZ twins are more liable to anoxia than DZ twins and boys are at greater risk than girls (Myrianthopoulous, 1970). Second born twins are more likely to die from intrapartum causes not associated with birth trauma (Butler and Alberman, 1969). Rausen et al. (1965) estimated that of 130 monochorionic twin pregnancies in their series, 15% had twin-to-twin transfusion syndrome and two-thirds (66%) died. This was a similar mortality to that found by Smith and Benjamin (1968).

Ellis et al. (1979) found immaturity to be the most important cause of death accounting for 75% of deaths of twin I and 58% of deaths of twin II. Unfortunately, they were unable to determine the cause in 16% of all twin deaths.

Using the Aberdeen classification of perinatal death (Baird et al., 1954) it was found in the 1983 Scottish Twin Study (Patel et al., 1984) that prematurity (unexplained low birthweight) accounted for 58 out of the 75 deaths i.e., 77.3%. Table 10.12 lists the breakdown of cause of all baby deaths in twins born in the period 1951–1983 in Aberdeen. Again, prematurity accounts for two-thirds of the deaths for both twin I and twin II, but when both babies die, the percentage rises to nearly 80%.

Table 10.12. Causes of all twin deaths: Aberdeen City District 1951–1983

	Twin I		Twin II	
	No.	%	No.	%
(A) All				
Premature unknown	58	62.4	89	67.4
Deformity	8	8.6	12	9.1
Trauma	5	5.4	6	4.5
Toxaemia	4	4.3	6	4.5
Maternal disease	4	4.3	4	3.0
Antepartum haemorrhage	3	3.2	5	3.8
Infection	4	4.3	1	0.8
Mature unknown	2	2.2	3	2.3
Other and not known	5	5.4	6	4.5
(B) For 33 pairs where both twins died				
Premature unknown	26	78.8		
Toxaemia	2	6.1		
Maternal disease	2	6.1		
Antepartum haemorrhage	1	3.0		
Trauma	1	3.0		
Other	1	3.0		

MacGillivray and Campbell (1981) examined the outcome of all twin pregnancies ($n = 321$) in Aberdeen between 1967 and 1978, looking at the obstetric management of twin pregnancies by cause of death and gestation rather than as before by birthweight. This was done because it was considered that gestation length was virtually always known now with the increased use of ultrasound, whereas birthweight was only known after the event. In 46 of the 54 babies who died prematurity (birthweight less than 2500 g) was given as the cause. The gestation was less than 30 weeks, 30–34 weeks and 35 weeks or over in 21, and 17 and 4 deliveries respectively; it was unknown in 4 cases. There were 15 pairs born before 30 weeks with 25 deaths and at such early gestation no pair of twins survived. Attention was focused on the group born between 30 and 34 weeks, 92 babies of whom 18 died, i.e. 19.6%. It was concluded from consideration of the mode of delivery and outcome (both deaths and those with low Apgar scores) that greater resort to caesarean sections might have been of benefit at such gestations, particularly when twin II was presenting by the breech.

Condition of Twins at Birth

The Apgar score is only an approximate way of expressing the condition of babies at birth and not an accurate measurement. It is, however, convenient and widely used.

When both babies were delivered by the vertex, the second twin was more severely asphyxiated than the first (MacDonald, 1962). There was a higher incidence of fair or poor Apgar scores in the second twin compared with the first, particularly when delivered by total breech extraction or version and extraction in the series of Ware (1971). Berger *et al.* (1981) examined the distribution of Apgar scores at 5 minutes by birthweight and mode of delivery and concluded that the predictive effect of birthweight was clearly more important than mode of delivery. Vaginal breech delivery was noted to be particularly a problem when birthweight was less than 1500 g.

In the Scottish Twin Study of 1983 (Patel *et al.*, 1984) the Apgar score at 5 minutes was available for 607 pairs of babies who were born alive. There were only 9 first twins and 9 second twins who were in a very poor condition with Apgar scores of less than 3 at 5 minutes, whereas 95.5% of first twins and 94.2% of second twins had Apgar scores of 7 or more at 5 minutes.

MacGillivray (1980) with Apgar scores available for 270 Aberdeen babies found an Apgar score of 5 or less at 1 minute, but with more than 5 at 5 minutes in 13 first babies, 30 second babies, and in 8 pairs of twins, a total of 59 babies. In only 4, 1 first twin and 3 second twins, was the Apgar score 5 or less at both 1 and 5 minutes.

Gestation length is, however, important in the determination of the condition of the baby at birth. The group which was of particular interest was that with delivery taking place between 30 and 34 weeks (MacGillivray and Campbell, 1981). The Apgar scores of 33 surviving pairs and of 6 of the 7 survivors of pairs in which one twin died were recorded at 1 minute and at 5 minutes and are shown according to the type of delivery (Table 10.13). Four of the 7 twins with Apgar scores of less than 3 at 1 minute and 8 of the 17 scoring 3–6 had been delivered by assisted breech. At 5 minutes the assisted breech deliveries had more low values (3–6). Breech delivery in those twins born between 30 and 34 weeks is, therefore, more commonly associated with both a higher perinatal mortality and a lower Apgar score than other types of delivery.

In singleton pregnancy breech delivery is considered more hazardous in primigravidae than in multigravidae. The outcome (Apgar score and perinatal deaths) for the 25 assisted breech deliveries occurring between 30 and 34 weeks in twin pregnancies were studied by parity and it was found that delivery of the multigravid twin breech was just as hazardous as for primigravidae.

The effect of the zygosity on the Apgar score at 1 and 5 minutes was studied in the Aberdeen series of 1969–1983 (Tables 10.14 and 10.15). At 1 minute the percentage of twin I babies with Apgar scores less than 5, but greater than 0 is double that of singletons, namely 10.1% and 5.03%. The rate by zygosity is as follows: 6.9% for MZ, 10.2% for DZ and 24.2% when zygosity was not known. For twin II the percentage with the Apgar score at 1 minute of less

Table 10.13. Outcome of 72 surviving twins at 30–34 weeks by type of delivery

| Type of delivery | Apgar score | | | | | |
| | <3 | | 3–6 | | >6 | |
	Twin I	Twin II	Twin I	Twin II	Twin I	Twin II
(A) 1 Minute Apgar score						
Spontaneous cephalic	0	2	3	0	19	10
Forceps cephalic	0	1	2	2	6	4
Assisted breech	2	2	3	5	2	6
Caesarean section	0	0	1	1	0	0
Total	2	5	9	8	27	20
(B) 5 Minute Apgar score						
Spontaneous cephalic	0	0	0	0	22	12
Forceps cephalic	0	0	0	1	8	7
Assisted breech	0	0	2	2	5	11
Caesarean section	0	0	1	0	0	1
Total	0	0	3	3	35	31

Note: one survivor did not have Apgar scores recorded.
From MacGillivray and Campbell (1981).

than 5 and greater than 0, 13.6%, is higher than for twin I or singletons. The rate is not affected by zygosity: 14.3% for MZ, 12.7% for DZ and 16.1% when zygosity is not known.

The Apgar scores at 5 minutes again tended to be lower in twins than in singletons (Table 10.15). The proportion of twin I with a score less than 7 was 5.1%, compared to 2.4% of singletons. There was no difference between MZ and DZ twins, the proportions being 3.5% and 4.1%. However, there were 18.2% of those where zygosity was not determined with low scores at 5 minutes. With respect to twin II, the rate of Apgar score less than 7 was similar to twin I, namely 4.8% overall and 4.1% for MZ, 4.1% for DZ and 12.9% for those with unknown zygosity. Placentation among MZ twins does not alter the proportions with low Apgar scores at 1 or 5 minutes. It can be concluded that zygosity and placentation have little, if any, effect on this measure of outcome and rather surprisingly twin II does not fare worse than twin I.

The percentage of Apgar scores at 1 minute or less than 5 was greater in women with singleton pregnancies who smoked than those who did not (Table 10.16), but rather surprisingly, smoking did not appear to have any adverse effect on either twin I or twin II Apgar scores at 1 minute. This was also true of the 5 minute Apgar scores. This finding conforms with the finding that although the perinatal death rate was higher in singleton mothers who

Table 10.14. Distbution of Apgar scores at 1 minute in twin pregnancy by zygosity and singleton pregnancy: Aberdeen City District 1969–1983

Apgar	MZ MC %	MZ DC %	MZ (NS) %	DZ DC %	Not known %	Total %
(A) Twin I						
1–2	1.47 (1)	1.35 (1)		3.52 (7)	8.11 (3)	3.13 (12)
3–4	2.94 (2)	6.76 (5)	16.67 (1)	6.53 (13)	13.51 (5)	6.77 (26)
5–6	22.06 (15)	12.16 (9)		9.05 (18)	8.11 (3)	11.72 (45)
7–8	27.94 (19)	28.38 (21)	33.33 (2)	26.63 (53)	43.24 (16)	28.91 (111)
9–10	41.18 (28)	43.24 (32)	50.00 (3)	52.26 (104)	16.22 (6)	45.05 (173)
0 (SB)	1.47 (1)	2.7 (2)		1.01 (2)	10.81 (4)	2.34 (9)
Not known	2.94 (2)	5.41 (4)		1.01 (2)		2.08 (8)
Total	100 (68)	100 (74)	100 (6)	100 (199)	100 (37)	100 (384)
(B) Twin II						
1–2	5.88 (4)	5.41 (4)		5.03 (10)	8.11 (3)	5.47 (21)
3–4	10.29 (7)	8.11 (6)		7.54 (15)	5.41 (2)	7.81 (30)
5–6	11.76 (8)	17.57 (13)	16.67 (1)	15.58 (31)	21.62 (8)	15.89 (61)
7–8	26.47 (18)	9.46 (7)	33.33 (2)	29.15 (58)	18.92 (7)	23.96 (92)
9–10	32.35 (22)	35.14 (26)	16.67 (1)	31.66 (63)	13.51 (5)	30.47 (117)
0 (SB)	1.47 (1)			1.01 (2)	16.22 (6)	3.34 (9)
Not known	11.76 (8)	24.32 (18)	33.33 (2)	10.05 (20)	16.22 (6)	14.06 (54)
Total	99.98 (68)	100.01 (74)	100 (6)	100.02 (199)	100.01 (37)	100 (384)
(C) Singletons						
1–2	1.66 (632)					
3–4	3.34 (1274)					
5–6	8.76 (3344)					
7–8	29.78 (11 370)					
9–10	54.61 (20 848)					
0 (SB)	0.84 (319)					
Not known	1.03 (392)					
Total	100.02 (38 179)					

Numbers in brackets are numbers in each category.

Table 10.15. Distribution of Apgar score at 5 minutes in twin pregnancy by zygosity and singleton pregnancy: Aberdeen City District 1969–1983

(A) Twin I

Apgar score	MZ MC %	MZ DC %	MZ (NS) %	DZ DC %	Not known %	Total %
1–2	—	—	—	—	7.7 (1)	0.26 (1)
3–4	—	—	—	1.51 (3)	2.7 (1)	1.04 (4)
5–6	2.94 (2)	2.7 (2)	16.67 (1)	2.51 (5)	10.81 (4)	3.65 (14)
7–8	13.24 (9)	12.16 (9)	—	9.55 (19)	18.92 (7)	11.46 (44)
9–10	77.94 (53)	77.03 (57)	83.33 (5)	84.42 (168)	54.05 (20)	78.91 (303)
0 (SB)	1.47 (1)	2.70 (2)	—	1.07 (2)	10.81 (4)	2.34 (9)
Not known	4.41 (3)	5.41 (4)	—	1.07 (2)	—	2.34 (9)
Total	100 (68)	100 (74)	100 (6)	100 (199)	99.94 (37)	100 (384)

(B) Twin II

Apgar score	MZ MC %	MZ DC %	MZ (NS) %	DZ DC %	Not known %	Total %
1–2	—	—	—	—	5.41 (2)	—
3–4	1.47 (1)	1.35 (1)	—	2.01 (4)	5.41 (2)	2.08 (8)
5–6	1.47 (1)	4.05 (3)	—	2.01 (4)	21.62 (8)	2.6 (10)
7–8	13.24 (9)	9.46 (7)	16.67 (1)	14.57 (29)	35.14 (13)	14.06 (54)
9–10	69.12 (47)	60.81 (45)	50.00 (3)	70.35 (140)	16.22 (6)	64.58 (248)
0 (SB)	1.47 (1)	—	—	1.01 (2)	16.22 (6)	2.34 (9)
Not known	13.24 (9)	24.32 (18)	33.33 (2)	10.05 (20)	—	14.32 (55)
Total	101.01 (68)	99.99 (74)	100 (6)	100 (199)	100.02 (37)	100 (384)

(C) Singletons

Apgar score	%
1–2	0.25 (96)
3–4	0.51 (193)
5–6	1.57 (601)
7–8	6.23 (2378)
9–10	89.51 (34 174)
0 (SB)	0.84 (319)
Not known	1.09 (418)
Total	100 (38 179)

Numbers in brackets are numbers in each category.

Table 10.16. Outcome in singleton and twin pregnancies by smoking habits in Aberdeen City District 1969–1983

	Twin I (375)	Twin II (375)	Singleton (37 860)
(A) % 1 minute Apgar <5 (excluding 0, i.e. stillbirth)			
Non-smokers	11.24	15.12	4.58
Smokers	9.77	13.95	5.51
Smoking not known	6.25	3.23	5.08
(B) % 5 minute Apgar <7 (excluding 0, i.e. stillbirth)			
Non-smokers	4.73	5.23	2.09
Smokers	5.75	4.65	2.59
Smoking not known	3.13	3.23	2.55

smoked compared with those who did not, there was no difference in the perinatal mortality rates of either twin I or twin II of mothers who smoked or did not smoke (Table 10.6).

Other Neonatal Problems

Neonatal complications are more likely to arise with twins. The results of the 1983 Scottish Twin Study (Patel *et al.*, 1984) show that nearly two-thirds of the babies were admitted to special care baby units (Table 10.17). The only significant difference between the first and second babies, however, was that more second babies require intermittent positive pressure ventilation for resuscitation.

Table 10.17. Neonatal complications in infants born alive

	Twin I		Twin II	
	No.	%	No.	%
Required intermittent positive pressure ventilation	106	16.5	146	22.5*
Admitted to special care baby unit	391	62.0	410	61.1
Admited to special care baby units 14 days	175	28.5[a]	171	28.4[a]
Convulsions	13	2.1	14	2.2
Apnoea	36	5.7	42	6.7
Assisted ventilation after 30 minutes	33	5.2	47	7.5
Major deformity	19	3.0	15	2.4
Minor deformity	64	10.1	64	10.2

*significant difference at 0.999 level.
[a]%Excludes first week deaths.

Conclusion

It can be concluded that lower birthweight due to shorter gestation and poor fetal growth is responsible in large measure for the much higher perinatal mortality in twins compared with singletons. Although previously twin II's outcome appeared worse than twin I, males poorer than females, MZ worse than DZ, this did not take into account the interrelationship between all the factors affecting the outcome.

Small size of baby appears more important than other problems such as antepartum haemorrhage, pre-eclampsia, infections and maternal disease, but fetal malformation, although not a major cause, is nevertheless more common in twins than in singletons (see Chapter 11).

Higher maternal age and parity, lower social class, short stature and smoking, however, do not have the significant influence on perinatal mortality or Apgar scores as they do in singletons and other unknown factors which cause poor growth and preterm delivery are mainly responsible.

Clearly there is a need for further study to determine the importance of factors affecting perinatal mortality and morbidity in twins, having first taken into account the major effect of early delivery of a low birthweight baby. This requires co-operation between centres as numbers of twin pregnancies in a total defined population are limited and changes in obstetric practice coupled with secular trends, e.g. in birthweight, make it difficult to draw conclusions from long-term series of limited numbers.

Outcome of twin pregnancies: the effect of death of a twin

with ELIZABETH BRYAN

So far this chapter has considered some factors which affect perinatal mortality of twins, in order to increase knowledge and understanding of the process at work which may help to identify possible recommendations for future management of pregnancy and delivery. However, for the parents and family it is a question of facing the tragedy of bereavement. Although individuals react very differently to such loss, there is increasing evidence that the problems of coming to terms with losing a baby have been under-estimated. In the case of twins there are special difficulties if one survives (Lewis, 1983).

There is no bigger anticlimax than the birth of a dead baby. Society shuns it and tries to forget that the baby ever existed (Bourne, 1968). Parents who lose one twin face particular problems. Because they still have a baby they find relatives, friends and often medical staff tend to ignore a very real bereavement. Their reality avoidance is accomplished with even greater ease than with a single baby (Bryan, 1986).

Consciously or not, society forgets the dead baby. All attention is focused on the surviving child. By concentrating on the live baby it is quite possible, once out of the delivery room, never to mention the lost one. Some mothers have found that midwives who they have known well during their pregnancy did not – perhaps could not – even refer to the baby who died.

A pregnancy following too soon after a stillbirth is known to inhibit mourning (Lewis, 1979) and a mother who has not adequately mourned her dead baby may have serious misidentifications of the new child with the dead sibling (Lewis and Page, 1978). Twins are an extreme example of this. The mother experiences the joy of new life and the tragedy of death simultaneously. She is likely to suppress her grief especially as others will encourage her to do so.

It is important that a mother is able clearly to distinguish the two babies in her mind otherwise she may think of the surviving baby, as one mother put it, as 'only half a baby'. Those who have some substantive memories of the dead

one are less likely to feel this confusion, or to fear that the baby was not real –
a 'fantasy' baby.

Most mothers – and often fathers too – need to grieve their dead baby
before they can relate properly to the survivor. They want to talk about the
dead baby; to ask questions about how and why the death happened; to vent
anger; to attribute blame; just to share their feelings, whether rational or not,
about the baby they have lost.

Naming the baby can be particularly important in twins. Not only does it
become easier for the parents to distinguish the babies in their mind and when
they talk about them, but for the suvivor it is obviously easier if he can refer
to his sibling by name. For many parents it is also important to have a
memorable funeral service and an individual grave or memorial to their baby.

Likewise, blood samples should always be taken for zygosity determination. Even if one baby dies, parents usually want to know whether or not their
twins were 'identical'. The zygosity may also be important for reliable genetic
counselling, particularly if either of the babies is malformed. Furthermore,
those with DZ twins may like to know that they have a greatly increased risk
of conceiving twins again.

Similar considerations are relevant when both babies are born alive, but
one is likely to die soon due, for example, to gross congenital abnormalities or
to severe birth asphyxia.

The increased risk of handicap to one or both twins not only poses
problems for the twins, but also for the parents and siblings. The guilt feelings
of parents and siblings may be even stronger in cases of handicap. The
families as well as the handicapped twins require special counselling, guid-
ance and support. The risk of mental illness particularly to the mother of a
handicapped child is increased (Romans-Clarkson et al., 1986). The risks to
the siblings and particularly to the non-handicapped co-twin of feelings of
guilt and of added responsibility are also increased and the chances of mental
illness are almost certainly greater.

Most, if not all, mothers continue to think of their surviving child as a twin
even if the other baby was stillborn (Bryan, 1986).

The price of being the single survivor may be very high. There seems no
doubt that psychiatric morbidity is higher in single surviving twins than in
either the general population or in twins where the co-twin is alive (Reveley et
al., 1981). To be the twin of a stillborn baby may be the worst fate of all.
Many survivors appear to carry a burden concerning their twin's death right
into adulthood. Even those twins who appear psychologically and socially
unscathed may suffer profoundly from their bereavement (Woodward, 1986).

All single surviving twins should hear about their dead twins from the start
and be encouraged to ask questions and express their feelings rational or not.
Many feel angry; angry with the twin for deserting them, for making them feel
guilty; for causing such unhappiness in the family; angry with their parents for

'allowing' their twin to die. Expert counselling services and support groups are now available to help parents not only through their own bereavement, but later as they cope with the often complex feelings of a child deprived of its partner.

Twinning and Twins
Edited by I. MacGillivray, D. M. Campbell and B. Thompson
© 1988 John Wiley & Sons Ltd

CHAPTER 11

Congenital anomalies

JULIAN LITTLE

*Department of Community Medicine and Epidemiology, University of
Nottingham, Nottingham, UK*
and

ELIZABETH M. BRYAN

Queen Charlotte's Maternity and Hammersmith Hospitals, London, UK

Introduction

Congenital anomalies in multiple births present a wider range of problems than those in singleton births. Parents, if more than one of the infants is affected, have to care for more than one handicapped child. If, as is more common, only one child is affected, the parents have to cope with balancing attention between children of the same age, but with different mental and physical needs. The healthy child or children may receive less attention than the affected child and may develop feelings of jealousy and guilt (Bryan, 1983).

The paediatrician may encounter some anomalies unique to the process of multiple conception which may be outside his usual range of experience. Recent advances in prenatal diagnosis and management have created new opportunities, but also new dilemmas. Not only will the obstetrician, together with the paediatrician, make antenatal plans for treatment, but the possibility of selective birth provides a new and difficult choice for parents who will need expert counselling.

In this chapter the subject of congenital anomalies in twins both in general and of specific types is reviewed.

A universally agreed definition of congenital anomalies has yet to be reached (Vowles *et al.*, 1975).

There are at least two reasons for this ambiguity. Firstly, some of the conditions generally accepted as congenital anomalies, such as some heart defects, are not readily detectable at birth. That structural cardiac malformations are of prenatal aetiology is undisputed, but observations of changes in manifestation during early postnatal development raise questions about the exclusion of other conditions, e.g. certain functional and metabolic disorders, from the range of congenital anomalies. Secondly, some anomalous embryos and fetuses abort so that newborn infants with anomalies are a biased sample of affected conceptuses (Carr, 1971; Boue *et al.*, 1975; Roberts and Lowe, 1975; Stein *et al.*, 1975; Lauritsen, 1976; Alberman and Creasy, 1977; Porter and Hook, 1980). Morphological studies of spontaneously aborted embryos and fetuses are difficult so the full range of consequences of prenatal disturbances is unlikely to have been documented fully.

Incidence of Anomalies

The incidence rate of an anomaly is the number affected expressed as a proportion of the total viable during the appropriate period of development. Because estimation of the true incidence of an anomaly is hampered by such factors as undetected or unexamined abortuses, by tissue regeneration concealing damage in earlier fetal development and by delayed manifestation of the anomaly, it is probably more appropriate to consider prevalence at various stages of development rather than incidence.

Prevalence of Fetal Anomalies

Data from series of pregnancies scanned by ultrasound show that the number of twin pregnancies is higher than that of twin births (Landy *et al.*, 1982). It has been found that the frequency of twins amongst spontaneous abortuses is of the order of three times the frequency in live births (Livingston and Poland, 1980; Uchida *et al.*, 1983b).

In their study of spontaneously aborted embryos and fetuses, Livingston and Poland (1980) found 52 twin embryos and 54 twin fetuses. Some 46 (88%) of the twin embryos were abnormal, the majority exhibiting growth disorganisation. Eleven (21%) of the twin fetuses were abnormal, many with cardiac anomalies. These abnormality rates were similar to those observed amongst all abortuses in the study. Uchida *et al.* (1983b) found that five out of 29 (17%) of twin abortions had chromosomal anomalies, approximately a third of the rate in singletons. This suggests that there are other conditions unique to, or increased in, twins that may be the cause of some of the twin abortions. Furthermore, an abnormal fetus may sometimes be maintained by the normal twin by means, for instance, of their shared circulation.

It has been suggested that the dizygotic twinning rate may be affected by changes in the overall incidence of fetal anomalies and that this could have accounted for the decline in the rate of DZ twin births in certain countries between the late 1950s and mid 1970s (Lazar, 1976; Lazar *et al.*, 1978). The phenomenon of the 'vanishing twin' (Landy *et al.*, 1982) suggests that substantial changes in the prevalence of twinning at birth could occur as a result of changes in the rates of early fetal loss. However, there is no clear evidence of a secular increase in spontaneous abortion rates (Elwood, 1985) although the decline in the prevalence of neural tube defects at birth may be suggestive of this (Leck, 1983; Al-Awadi et al., 1984; Carstairs and Cole, 1984; Kirke and Elwood, 1984). Moreover, other evidence suggests that rates of spontaneous abortion of fetuses with anomalies decrease with increasing maternal age (Stein et al., 1975; 1986).

So far as we are aware, there is only one study of embryonic/fetal abnormality and twins amongst products of conception examined following induced abortion (Tanimura and Tanaka, 1977). Amongst 78 pairs of twin embryos obtained following induced abortion for 'socioeconomic' reasons in Japan, two pairs were discordant for polydactyly and two pairs were double monsters. Because of the small numbers involved, it is difficult to compare these data with the results of the systematic study of induced abortions in Japan (Shiota, 1984) which show that the rates of specific anomalies in the early intrauterine population are several times higher than at birth. An additional difficulty is that twin conceptuses may be mistaken as singletons if one or both members of the pair is damaged as a result of the procedure used to terminate the pregnancy. This would explain the lower frequency of twin pairs amongst embryos obtained following induced abortion (0.38%–78/20 417) than that following spontaneous abortion (1.6%–7/448) or ectopic pregnancy (1.8%–4/220).

Prevalence of Anomalies at Birth

The remainder of this paper concentrates on anomalies in infants, which are thus only a small, and unrepresentative proportion of the anomalies occurring in conceptuses as a whole.

A summary comparison of the prevalence at birth of congenital anomalies in twins and singletons is presented in Table 11.1. In most studies, malformations have been found to be commoner in twins than in singletons. In general it is in the smaller studies that the rates of anomalies in twins are lower than those in singletons. Notable exceptions are the series from Norway (Windham and Bjerkedal, 1984), Bombay and Czechoslovakia (Stevenson et al., 1966) but in these the differences in rates are not statistically significant. There are several other possible explanations for this inconsistency, for example:

1. The gestational period used for defining a stillbirth may vary.
2. The differences in the range of specific anomalies included in studies could affect the ratio of the rate in twins to that in singletons.
3. Opportunities for the timing and thoroughness of examination or recording may vary (McIntosh et al., 1954; Neel, 1958; McKeown and Record, 1960; Nevin et al., 1978).

Table 11.1. Comparison of prevalence at birth (live and still) of congenita

Study population	Period of study	Population (P) or hospital (H) series	Method of ascertainment[a]	Singletons Number with anomalies	Rate (%)	RR[b] T:S
Australia, Melbourne				210	1.8	1.1
Brazil, Sao Paulo				222	1.6	1.3
Chile, Santiago	1961–64	H	N	219	0.9	1.1
Colombia, Medellin				218	1.1	2.6
Czechoslovakia				344	1.7	0.7
Czechoslovakia, Prague[d]	1929–62	H	M	67	1.3	2.0
Egypt, Alexandria				106	1.2	0.5
Hong Kong	1961–64	H	N	112	1.2	0.7
India, Bombay				335	0.9	0.6
India, Bombay	1982–83	H	?	280	1.6	1.7
India, Calcutta				58	0.3	0.7
Malaysia, Kuala Lumpur				161	1.0	1.6
Malaysia, Singapore	1961–64	H	N	336	0.9	1.2
Mexico City				353	1.5	1.3
Netherlands, Dordrecht	1981–83	H	?	29	1.2	3.5
Nigeria, Zaria	1976–79	H	N	247	1.1	2.0
Norway[e]	1967–79	P	B	23 424	3.0	0.9
Panama City				324	2.1	0.8
Philippines, Manila				246	0.8	2.1
S. Africa, Cape Town				26	0.9	0.0
S. Africa, Johannesburg	1961–64	H	N	241	2.2	2.0
S. Africa, Pretoria				125	1.3	0.8
Spain, Madrid				257	1.3	1.1
Taiwan, Taipei	1965–68	H	N	338	1.3	1.8
UK, Belfast	1957–63	H	N	545	1.9	1.3
UK, Birmingham	1950–52	P	N, HV, 5	1 204	2.2	1.2
UK, Northern Ireland[f]	1974–79	P	M	6 340	4.0	1.3
USA, Atlanta[g]	1969–76	P	M, 1	6 767	3.3	1.5
USA, Cleveland	1955–63	H	N	?	3.3	3.2
USA, New York	1950–56	H	?	3 698	4.0	1.7
Yugoslavia, Ljubljana	1961–64			163	1.9	1.3
Yugoslavia, Zagreb		H	N	106	1.3	0.5
USA, multicentre	1959–65	H	P, 7	8 288	15.6	1.2
Belgium, Ghent	1964–67	H	?	—	—	—
UK, Birmingham	1963–67	H	?	—	—	—
UK, North-east Scotland	1968–79	H	N	—	—	—

[a]Method of ascertainment: B = review of birth notification records; M = review of routine records from multiple sources, N = neonatal examination; P = physical examination; HV = health visitor.
Number following letter denotes age in year to which infants followed up e.g., 1 to first year.
[b]Ratio of prevalence rate at birth of anomalies in twins to rate in singletons.
[c]Ratio of prevalence rate at birth of anomalies in twins of like sex (LS) to rate in twins of unlike sex (US).

Total		Twins like sex		Unlike sex			
Number with anomalies	Rate (%)	Number with anomalies	Rate (%)	Number with anomalies	Rate (%)	RRᶜ LS : US	Reference
6	1.9	4	1.9	2	1.7	1.1	
9	2.1	8	3.1	1	0.6	5.2	
5	1.0	5	1.5	0	0.0	∞	Stevenson et al. (1966)
11	2.9	8	3.1	3	2.3	1.3	
4	1.2	3	1.4	1	0.8	1.8	
132	2.6	—	—	—	—	—	Onyskowova et al. (1971)
5	0.6	5	1.1	0	0.0	∞	
2	0.8	1	0.5	0	0.0	∞	Stevenson et al. (1966)
5	0.5	5	0.7	0	0.0	∞	
8	2.7	5	2.4	3	3.4	0.7	Shah and Patel (1984)
1	0.2	0	0.0	1	0.5	0.0	
6	1.6	5	1.7	1	1.2	1.4	Stevenson et al. (1966)
7	1.1	6	1.2	1	0.8	1.5	
11	1.9	5	1.3	6	2.9	0.4	
5	4.2	4	9.3	1	1.4	6.6	Ceelie, 1985
35	2.3	—	—	—	—	—	Harrison et al. (1985)
426	2.8	306	2.9	123	2.5	1.2	Windham and Bjerkedal (1984)
5	1.7	3	1.5	2	2.1	0.7	
6	1.7	6	2.2	0	0.0	∞	
0	0.0	0	0.0	0	0.0	∞	Stevenson et al. (1966)
11	4.4	10	5.4	1	1.6	3.4	
4	1.0	3	1.3	1	0.6	2.2	
7	1.4	4	1.1	3	2.0	0.6	
12	2.3	—	—	—	—	—	Emanuel et al. (1972)
27	2.5	21	3.1	6	1.4	2.2	Stevenson et al. (1966)
41	2.6	26	2.8	15	2.4	1.2	McKeown and Record (1960)
172	5.2	115	5.2	51	4.8	1.1	Little and Nevin (1988)
181	4.9	115	4.9	28	2.5	2.0	Layde et al. (1980)
80	10.6	—	—	—	—	—	Hendricks (1966)
182	6.9	—	—	—	—	—	Guttmacher and Kohl (1958)
8	2.5	5	3.7	3	3.3	1.1	Stevenson et al. (1966)
1	0.6	1	1.0	0	0.0	∞	
		MZ		DZ		RR	
		Number with anomalies	Rate (%)	Number with anomalies	Rate (%)	MZ : DZ	
219	18.3	90	24.1	91	14.8	1.6	Myrianthopoulos (1978)
17	2.4	9	3.1	8	1.9	1.6	Cameron et al. (1983)
66	3.1	24	4.0	42	2.7	1.5	
57	4.3	20	5.3	26	3.7	1.4	Corney et al. (1983)

[d]Only a sample of singletons was examined.
[e]Rates are adjusted for maternal age and parity.
[f]Follow-up of variable length to a maximum of 5 years according to year of child's birth and type of anomaly; bias of ascertainment as between singletons and twins throughout to be unlikely.
[g]Live births only.

4. Pregnancies with either twins or suspected congenital anomalies are more likely to be delivered in a hospital.
5. Being a twin infant in itself may affect the detection rate of anomalies, firstly because twins in general stay in hospital longer, and secondly because the detection of an anomaly in one twin should lead to an assiduous search for problems in the co-twin.
6. Age and parity of mothers in the study population, as both dizygotic twinning (Bulmer, 1970) and the risk of malformation in general (Milham and Gittelsohn, 1965; Hay and Barbano, 1972) increase with maternal age. In the only study in which rates are adjusted for maternal age and parity (Windham and Bjerkedal, 1984), there was no excess risk in twins.
7. The rate of malformations in twins is likely to vary according to the proportion of twins of unlike sex as malformations are more common in twins of like than of unlike sex (see Table 11.1).

These factors discussed are all likely to contribute to the observed variation in relative risk but our conclusion is that congenital anomalies are almost certainly more common amongst twins than singletons.

Zygosity

Indirect evidence for the increased prevalence of anomalies in twins being confined to MZ pairs has been provided by many studies where the incidence of anomalies amongst like-sex twins has been higher than amongst those of unlike sex. Small numbers is the likely explanation for the few exceptions to this finding (Stevenson *et al.*, 1966; Shah and Patel, 1984). More recently this appears to have been confirmed in the few studies of twin series in which zygosity has been determined by a direct method (Myrianthopoulos and Chung, 1974; Myrianthopoulos, 1978; Melnick and Myrianthopoulos, 1979; Cameron *et al.*, 1983; Corney *et al.*, 1983 and see Table 11.1). However, in these studies, the numbers of affected twins have been small, and therefore chance is one explanation. In addition there have been substantial numbers of twins of unknown zygosity but in the National Collaborative Perinatal Project (NCPP) study (Melnick and Myrianthopoulos, 1979) and the study from north-east Scotland (Corney *et al.*, 1983), the rate of malformation in twins of unknown zygosity lies midway between the rates in MZ and DZ twins.

Doubts about the validity of the Weinberg rule (see Chapter 2) raise doubts also as to whether an excess rate of malformation in like-sex twins can be taken as evidence of an excess rate in MZ twins. In particular Boklage (1985; 1986) has argued that the assumption that problem frequencies are equal amongst DZ pairs of like and unlike sex is untenable (for further discussion, see p. 232).

Placentation

Monochorial placentation may provide a less favourable environment for the developing fetus and it has been suggested that this could be the explanation for the increased frequency of anomalies in MZ twins (Bulmer, 1970). However, in the two studies on anomalies in general in which this hypothesis has been tested, neither showed any significant difference in the rate of malformations between monochorionic and dichorionic MZ twins (Melnick and Myrianthopoulos, 1979; Corney *et al.*, 1983) nor did studies of dermatoglyphics (Reed *et al.*, 1978). Monochorial placentation may, however, be involved in the aetiology of some specific anomalies, e.g., acardia and congenital heart disease (Cameron *et al.*, 1983).

Concordance and Discordance

The literature on concordance for congenital anomalies relates, in the main, to specific anomalies. A summary of reports of concordance in twins for anomalies of any type is presented in Table 11.2. Some of the discrepancy in concordance rates for MZ twins reported by Myrianthopoulos (1978) and Cameron *et al.* (1983) is likely to be due to differing methods of assembling the twin series and of case ascertainment, but further work is needed. In general, however, discordance is the rule, both for anomalies in general (Table 11.2) and of specific types. This imposes difficult decisions on many parents when termination is being considered.

Specific Anomalies

There have been few studies of specific anomalies in twins in which comparisons have been made between twins of different types as well as singletons (Hay and Wehrung, 1970). Some reviews have been based on data pooled from several studies with the risk of biases and others from case series from undefined populations with no control data.

Anomalies Unique to Multiple Conception

Anomalies unique to the twinning process include conjoined twinning, fetus-in-fetu, acardia and fetus papyraceus.

Conjoined Twins

Conjoined twins are thought to be derived from a single ovum, i.e. to be monozygotic. However, at least one set of twins of unlike sex has been reported, possibly due to pseudohermaphroditism in one twin (Milham,

Table 11.2. Summary of reports of concordance in twins for anomalies

Total pairs (one or both twins with anomalies)	Concordant for anomalies of any type		Concordant for specific anomalies only		Reference
	No.	Rate (%)	No.	Rate (%)	
(a) All twins					
126	12	9.5	6	4.8	Stevenson et al. (1966)
154[a]	29	18.8	21[b]	13.6	Myrianthopoulos (1975)
132	21	15.9	16	12.1	Layde et al. (1980)
55	2	3.6	—	—	Corney et al. (1983)
366	57	15.6	45[c]	12.3	Windham and Bjerkedal (1984)
(b) Dizygotic twins					
85	6	7.1	6	7.1	Myrianthopoulos, (1975)
(c) Monozygotic twins					
69	23	33.3	16[b]	23.2	Myrianthopoulos (1975)
446	—	—	6	1.3	Cameron et al. (1983)

[a] Excludes pairs of unknown zygosity.
[b] One pair of conjoined thoracopagus twins with fused hearts, livers, common umbilical cord and single placenta included.
[c] Pairs concordant for categories of malformation, rather than specific malformations.

1966). It is generally accepted that the anomaly results from imperfect division of the embryo after the formation of two embryonic discs prior to the end of the third week, the 'fission' hypothesis (Zimmerman, 1967; Potter and Craig, 1976). However, it has been suggested that secondary, partial fusion of the blastocysts may occur, the 'fusion' hypothesis (Aird, 1959).

In view of the rarity of the condition it is not surprising to find that reports on the prevalence at birth of conjoined twins vary (Table 11.3). Much of this variation depends on whether the studies were hospital or population based (Hanson, 1975; Edmonds and Layde, 1982). Bulmer (1970) estimated an incidence of one in 100 000 maternities but twice this frequency, about one in 200 monozygotic twin maternities, now seems more likely (Hanson, 1975). Conjoined pairs occur with unexpected frequency in triplet sets (Schinzel et al., 1979).

There is general agreement that the sex ratio in conjoined twins is low (Benirschke and Kim, 1973; Zake, 1984) although there is at least one exception (Metneki et al., 1983). Of 22 cases in Milham's series 20 were female (Milham, 1966). Female conceptions may be at higher risk of late splitting of the zygote or female conjoined conceptuses may be less likely to be aborted spontaneously than male conceptuses. The latter seems the more likely as male fetuses with anomalies tend to be lost more commonly than female (Stein et al., 1975). Another possible explanation is that the overall sex ratio in monoamniotic twins is low (Derom et al., 1987).

There are no known predisposing factors to conjoined twinning but occasional geographical (Bhettay et al., 1975; Viljoen et al., 1983; Zake, 1984) temporal (Kaplan and Eidelman, 1983; Viljoen et al., 1983; Harrison and Rossiter, 1985) and seasonal (Milham, 1966) clusterings have been reported. However, these may well be due either to chance or to a bias in reporting clusters rather than isolated cases. Jaschevatzky et al. (1980) noted that all four cases of conjoined twins born in Tel Aviv during a 15 year period were delivered to Arab mothers, yet Arab women comprised only 13% of the total of women who gave birth during the period.

Maternal factors may be of importance in the aetiology of conjoined twins. Milham (1966) found evidence of poor obstetric histories in a high proportion of cases. Seven out of 33 previous pregnancies had ended in the delivery of a stillborn infant.

As would be expected with monozygotic twins there is little evidence of genetic predisposition to conjoined twinning, nor does maternal age appear to influence the incidence (Rudolph et al., 1967; Edmonds and Layde, 1982; Viljoen et al., 1983). There has been only one report of a second set of conjoined twins in a family (Hamon and Dinno, 1978) and a family history of twins in general is not particularly common.

The site and extent of attachment is highly variable. Thoracopagus is the commonest form and accounts for about 70% of cases (Rudolph et al., 1967;

Table 11.3. Summary of selected reports of prevalence at birth of conjoined twins

Location	Period of study	Population (P) or hospital (H) series	Method of ascertainment	Total number of births	Conjoined pairs		Reference
					Number	Case rate	
Australia	1936-66	H	Hospital records	158 940	4	1/40 000	Beischer and Fortune (1968a)
England and Wales	1961-66	P	Stillbirth registrations	5 180 400	50	1/100 000	Rogers (1969)
Hungary	1970-77	P	Register of congenital malformations	1 364 664	14	1/97 500	Metneki et al. (1983)
India, Madras	1920-28	H	Hospital records	25 000	4	1/6250	Mudaliar (1930)
International	1961-64	H	Neonatal examination	426 932	2	1/200 000	Stevenson et al. (1966)
Israel, Tel Aviv	1963-78	H	Neonatal examination	63 229	4	1/16 000	Jaschevatzky et al. (1980)
Israel (live births)[a]	1970-78	P	?	500 000	6	1/80 000	Ormoy et al. (1980)
Israel	1976-81	P	?	475 000	10	1/47 500	Kaplan and Eidelman (1980)
Nigeria, Zaria[b]	1976-79	P	Neonatal examination	23 467	3	1/7800	Harrison and Rossiter (1985)
Norway	1967-79	P	Birth notification	783 065	2	1/400 000	Windham and Bjerkedal (1984)
Rhodesia	1950-62	H	Hospital records	41 826	3	1/14 000	Bland and Hammer (1962)
Singapore	1960-70	H	Hospital records	406 791	6	1/68 000	Tan et al. (1971)
South Africa, South West[c] Africa and Zimbabwe	1974-82	P	Hospital records and opportunistic notification	8 670 000	31	1/300 000	Vijoen et al. (1983)
Sweden, Lund	1900-33	H	Hospital records	40 000	2	1/20 000	Ryden (1934)
Sweden	1965-74	P	Register of congenital malformations	875 000	10	1/88 000	Kallen and Rybo (1978)
Taiwan, Taipei	1965-68	H	Neonatal examination	25 814	4	1/6500	Emanuel et al. (1972)
Uganda, Mbale	1971-80	H	Neonatal examination	67 872	16	1/4000	Zake (1984)
USA, Cook County Hospital	1905-42	H	Hospital records	85 000	3	1/28 000	Mortimer and Kirschbaum (1942)
USA, Chicago	1931-68	H	Hospital records	over 100 000	2	1/50 000	Potter and Craig (1976)
USA, New York State	1945-65	P	Birth notification	3 645 622	22	1/166 000	Milham (1966)
USA, Los Angeles	1949-69	H	Hospital records	ca. 250 000	5	1/50 000	Compton (1971)
USA, all states[d]	1962-65	H	Birth notification	?	43	1/200 000	Bender (1967)
USA, multicentre	1959-65	H	Physical examinations to age 7	56 249	1	1/56 000	Myrianthopoulos (1978)
USA, Atlanta	1968-78	P	Hospital records	300 000	10	1/30 000	Center for Disease Control (1982)
USA, all states	1970-77	H	Neonatal hospital discharge records	7 903 000	81	1/98 000	Edmonds and Layde (1982)

[a] Investigators aware of a further set among fetuses terminated following prenatal diagnosis of a neural tube defect, and of a further 200 sets amongst 800 spontaneous abortions and stillbirths.
[b] One set of conjoined twins in 15 391 births to booked women, two sets in 8076 births to women who had emergency admissions.
[c] Estimated.
[d] Live born—further 92 sets estimated as stillborn; rate estimated from total of observed and estimated numbers.

Table 11.4. Types of conjoined twins

Inferior conjunction
Diprosopus—two faces with one head and body
Dicephalus—two heads and one body
Ischiopagus—inferior sacrococcygeal fusion
Pygopagus—posterolateral sacrococcygeal fusion

Superior conjunction
Dipygus—two pelves and four legs
Syncephalus—facial + thoracic fusion
Craniopagus—cranial fusion

Mid conjunction
Thoracopagus—thoracic fusion
Omphalopagus—fusion from umbilicus to xiphoid cartilage
Rachipagus—vertebral fusion above sacrum

Edmonds and Layde, 1982). The full range as defined by Guttmacher and Nichols (1967) is shown in Table 11.4.

There is a high incidence of congenital heart disease in thoracopagus twins which seems related to the degree of union, and the anomalies are similar to the defects described in Ivemark's syndrome including anomalous pulmonary venous return, common atrium, single ventricle, conotruncal abnormalities and endocardial cushion defects (Noonan, 1978). Nichols *et al.* (1967) found that 90% of such twins shared a common pericardium and 75% had conjoined hearts.

Edmonds and Layde (1982), noted that 40 of their 81 sets of conjoined twins had malformations which were not obviously associated with the site of junction. Some of the malformations, e.g. imperforate anus and diaphragmatic hernia, could be explained on a mechanical basis. Others seemed to be associated with a more fundamental disturbance of embryogenesis.

Primary discordance, different malformations in non-joined organs, is rare but cases discordant for meningomyelocele, anencephaly and cleft lip have been reported (Ornoy *et al.*, 1980). Cases of differing sex are probably due to pseudohermaphroditism (Szendi, 1939; Khanna *et al.*, 1969; Milham, 1966). However, secondary discordance, different defects of parts of joined organs belonging to each of the twins, is a common finding.

Many physiological responses of a conjoined pair may be autonomous. Heart rhythms may differ and change independently in response to external stimuli. If one of a pair becomes pregnant the other may continue to menstruate. Obviously, prognosis depends on the extent of union and the nature of additional anomalies.

Fetus-in-fetu

The frequency of fetus-in-fetu is unknown. Lord (1956) found 31 published reports of the condition before 1900 (some of which may have been retroperitoneal teratoma) and eleven since then. Grant and Pearn (1969) suggest that the frequency is about one in 20 conjoined twins, but it is not clear how this estimate was derived. The parasitic fetus is most commonly attached near the origin of the superior mesenteric vessels, and usually in the upper retroperitoneal space. However, other sites of attachment have been noted, one of the most striking reported being a cerebral tumour containing five fetuses (Kimmel *et al.*, 1950).

Acardia

Acardia, or chorioangiopagus parasiticus, varies in manifestation from a mass of amorphous tissues to an incomplete but otherwise well-formed fetus weighing up to 3.5 kg. It has been estimated to occur in about one in 30 000–35 000 deliveries (Gillim and Hendricks, 1953; Napolitani and Schreiber, 1960) or in approximately one in every 100 MZ twin pregnancies. It appears to occur more often in triplet pregnancies (Schinzel *et al.*, 1979), as the expected proportion of acardiacs occurring within triplets should be about one in 30 but three times this incidence has been reported (Frutiger, 1969; James, 1978). It is possible that there has been preferential reporting of acardiac fetuses in triplet pregnancies, but this is unlikely to explain a threefold increase.

Acardia occurs almost exclusively in monochorionic, and therefore MZ, pregnancies as survival of the fetus is dependent on a shared circulation with the (usually normal) co-twin. However, in one reported instance, a triploid twin acardiac with a 70, XXX, + 15 karyotype was delivered with a co-twin with a normal male karyotype and a monochorionic placenta (Bieber *et al.*, 1981).

James (1978) has collated reports on 340 acardiac cases. Of the cases where the sex was recorded the sex ratio was 156 : 173, a lower proportion of males than in twins in general.

Frutiger (1969) found that in acardiac pregnancies, the mean maternal age was high, which is consistent with the finding that some acardiacs are trisomic (Kerr and Rashad, 1966; Scott and Ferguson-Smith, 1973).

Reports on placentation are often inadequate but there is some evidence that the risk of acardia is considerably higher in monoamniotic pregnancies (James, 1978). Acardia seems to be associated only with artery-to-artery and vein-to-vein connections, rather than arteriovenus, and it may be that this type of connection is more common between monoamniotic than diamniotic pairs.

There are two theories as to the mechanism by which acardia develops:

1. Primary failure of cardiac development.
2. The heart was present but atrophied as a result of passive perfusion and reversal of circulation.

Evidence as to mechanism is derived from case reports, and may be biased.

Some findings suggest that a general disturbance of morphogenesis may be the cause of acardia. For example, other specific abnormalities have been reported in acardiac twins and not uncommonly the co-twin has anomalies of the same type. Schinzel *et al.* (1979) found that in 10% of 85 cases the co-twin had a similar congenital anomaly. Acardia has been reported in one member of conjoined twins (Geeves, 1928) as have conjoined acardiac monsters associated with a normal infant (Amatuzio and Gorlin, 1981) and a case of acardiac fetus-in-fetu (Junqueira and Pinto 1951).

It has been suggested that acardia is one manifestation of a chromosomal anomaly, but the available evidence does not appear to support this. Another possible mechanism suggested by protagonists of the hypothesis of primary failure of development is that acardia is a consequence of failure of the paired cardiac tubes to fuse (Severn and Holyoke, 1973).

According to the hypothesis of primary agenesis of the heart, it would be expected that singleton acardiac embryos would be conceived but survive only briefly in utero. Whereas, when such embryos are conceived in a twin pregnancy with monochorionic placentation, they are able to survive due to their shared circulation with the co-twin (Potter and Craig, 1976). It is difficult to reject this hypothesis as singleton acardiac embryos, if they exist, would be virtually impossible to detect!

The second hypothesis is that acardia results from an imbalance in the interfetal circulation leading to atrophy of the heart and often resulting in a preferential development of the lower part of the body which tends to be the better developed – the organs most commonly absent or deficient include the head, heart, limbs, lungs, liver, pancreas, kidneys and upper intestine (Schinzel *et al.*, 1979; Van Allen *et al.*, 1983). This hypothetical mechanism first proposed by Campbell and Shepherd (1905) has been named the twin reversed arterial perfusion (TRAP) sequence (Van Allen *et al.*, 1983). There is indirect supporting evidence from studies of embryos in which the developing heart has been manipulated mechanically (Gessner, 1966).

Relatively little attention has been paid to the pump twin. These potentially normal infants have a high mortality rate usually due to the combination of intrauterine cardiac failure and prematurity (Van Allen *et al.*, 1983). The perinatal management of these infants should be greatly improved now that the problems can be foreseen by routine ultrasonic examination.

Fetus Papyraceus

Occasionally the remains of a fetus compressed and embedded in the placenta of a single baby may be noticed at delivery. This fetus is known as a fetus papyraceus and the mother is often unaware that she ever had a twin pregnancy. On other occasions the multiple pregnancy and subsequent fetal death is detected by ultrasound scanning. Most of these embryos or fetuses have died after the eighth week of gestation and before the end of the second trimester. Earlier in pregnancy a dead fetus is usually reabsorbed whereas the fetus that dies in the third trimester presents as a macerated rather than as a compressed fetus. Mummification of the fetus indicates that the death occurred at least 10 weeks before delivery (Saier *et al.*, 1975).

Fetus papyraceus is a rare condition and has been estimated to occur with a frequency of 1 in 1200 live births (Saier *et al.*, 1975) or 1 in 200 twin pregnancies (Baker and Doering, 1982). It has also been reported in higher multiple pregnancies (Aiken, 1969; Skelly *et al.*, 1982).

In a study of 113 cases of aplasia cutis, Mannino *et al.* (1977) found that as many as fifteen had a MZ fetus papyraceus twin. Cerebral abnormalities have been reported in several surviving twins of a fetus papyraceus (Yoshioka *et al.*, 1979; Choulet *et al.*, 1982). Cardiac malformations have also been reported in the co-twin of a fetus papyraceus (Baker and Doering, 1982; Daw, 1983).

The fetofetal transfusion syndrome and entanglement of the umbilical cords in monoamniotic twins account for the deaths of some but many papyraceus fetuses are dichorionic (Kindred, 1944) so other explanations such as separation of the placenta, blood group incompatibility or entanglement of the cords around parts of the fetus must then be considered. A velamentous insertion of the cord appears to increase the risk of fetal death (Daw, 1983).

Anomalies not Unique to Multiple Conception

These anomalies will be reviewed by system.

Neural Tube Defects (NTDs)

It is not clear as to whether the rate of neural tube defects in twins is higher than in singletons. In most studies, the frequency of twin births among series of cases with neural tube defect is considered rather than the prevalence at birth amongst twins. In a comprehensive review of the literature, Elwood and Elwood (1980) found that the total number of twins in series of cases of neural tube defect was slightly lower than expected. In addition, these authors found no consistent positive association between twinning rates and the prevalence at birth of neural tube defects in terms of geographical distribution, of secular and seasonal trends, or in maternal age effects, family history or social class.

Table 11.5. Summary of selected reports on anencephalus (with or without associated spina bifida) in twins and singletons

Population	Period of study	Singleton births			Twin births			Reference
		Total number	Number affected	Rate per 1000	Total number	Number affected	Rate per 1000	
(i) Total number of twin births known								
Canada, British Columbia	1952–70	672 200	457	0.68	14 126	9	0.64	McBride (1979)
Japan, Hiroshima, Nagasaki and Kure	1948–54	63 796	40	0.63	773	1	1.29	Neel (1958)
Norway	1967–79	775 405	344	0.44	15 320	10	0.65	Windham and Bjerkedal, (1984); Windham et al. (1982)
UK, Belfast	1964–68	41 351	171	4.24	1027	4	3.89	Elwood and Nevin (1973)
USA, Atlanta — Blacks	1969–76	63 544	21	0.33	1670	2	1.20 }	Layde et al. (1980)
whites		140 665	128	0.91	2820	6	2.13 }	
USA, Los Angeles	1966–72	848 139	432	0.51	16 880	15	0.89	Windham and Sever (1982)
USA, NCPP	1959–65	53 257	33	0.62	1195	2	1.67	Myrianthopoulos (1975)
Total		2 658 357	1626	0.61	53 811	49	0.91	
(ii) Total number of twin births not known, and inferred as 2% of all births								
France, selected hospitals	1945–55	731 351	395	0.54	14 925	7	0.47	Frezal et al. (1964)
Romania, Bucharest	1977–80	76 467	26	0.34	1560	3	1.92	Christodorescu et al., (1981)
UK, Liverpool and Bootle	1960–62	53 882	179	3.32	1100	1	0.91	Smithells and Franklin (1964)
Oxford	1965–72	116 301	170	1.46	2374	7	2.95	Fedrick, (1976)
Southampton	1958–62	11 669	27	2.31	238	2	8.40	Williamson (1965)
South Wales	1956–62	100 730	241	2.39	2056	6	2.92	Carter et al. (1968)
USA, Alabama	1961–66	435 438	361	0.83	8887	6	0.68	Cassady, (1969)
Central Virginia	1961–69	22 913	22	0.96	468	1	2.14	Solowy and Shepard (1971)
Total		1 548 751	1421	0.92	31 608	33	1.04	

Table 11.6. Summary of selected reports on spina bifida in twins and singletons

Population	Period of study	Singleton births			Twin births			Reference
		Total number	Number affected	Rate per 1000	Total number	Number affected	Rate per 1000	
(i) Total number of twin births known								
Canada, British Columbia	1952–70	672 200	590	0.88	14 126	7	0.50	McBride (1979)
Japan, Hiroshima, Nagasaki and Kure	1948–54	63 796	13	0.21	773	0	0.00	Neel (1958)
Norway	1967–79	775 405	380	0.49	15 320	12	0.78	Windham and Bjerkedal, (1984); Windham et al. (1982)
UK, Belfast	1964–68	41 351	184	4.56	1 027	1	0.97	Elwood and Nevin (1973)
USA, Atlanta — Blacks	1969–76	63 544	40	0.64	1 670	1	0.60 ⎫	Layde et al. (1980)
whites		140 665	199	1.42	2 820	1	0.36 ⎬	
USA, Los Angeles	1966–72	848 139	436	0.51	16 880	6	0.35	Windham and Sever (1982)
USA, NCPP	1959–65	53 257	33	0.62	1 195	0	0.00	Myrianthopoulos (1975)
Total		2 658 357	1 875	0.71	53 811	28	0.53	
(ii) Total number of twin births not known, and inferred as 2% of all births								
Romania, Bucharest	1977–80	76 467	64	0.84	1 560	0	0.00	Christodorescu et al. (1981)
UK, Liverpool and Bootle	1960–63	71 513	257	3.59	1 459	1	0.69	Smithells and Franklin (1964)
Southampton	1958–62	11 669	48	4.11	238	0	0.00	Williamson (1965)
South Wales	1956–62	100 730	271	2.69	2 056	7	3.40	Carter et al. (1968)
Total		260 379	640	2.46	5 313	8	1.51	

Windham *et al.* (1982) suggest that there is a consistent excess of twins among NTD cases in studies in low risk areas, whereas there is no consistent pattern in areas of high risk. Accordingly, results of studies in which the population at risk has been enumerated, or can be indirectly, and the total numbers of twins and singletons with NTDs are known, are summarised for anencephalus (Table 11.5), spina bifida (Table 11.6) and encephalocele (Table 11.7). In Tables 11.5 and 11.6, studies have been included in which the precise number of twin births was not known – this has been estimated as 2% of total births; no account has been taken of secular trends, geographical variation, maternal age or parity. The numbers of affected twin births are too small to permit analysis by overall rate in the population. Accordingly, as there is no reason to suppose that biases of ascertainment of anomalies so obvious externally vary as between twins and singletons, the data have been pooled. The prevalance at birth of anencephalus and of encephalocele in twins is higher than in singletons, but the converse applies for spina bifida. The relative risks (ratio of rate in twin, to that in singletons) are shown in Table 11.8. From this survey, it may be concluded that there is an increased frequency of encephalocele in twins, and there is a suggestion of a slight increase in the frequency of anencephalus.

Not surprisingly, few data are available on rates of neural tube defects in twins by zygosity or sex type. One review suggests that the prevalence rate at birth of anencephalus is highest in twin pairs of like sex (James, 1976) but no such excess was found for anencephalus and spina bifida in a wider review of the literature (Elwood and Elwood, 1980).

As was the case for anomalies in general, neural tube defects generally present in one twin while the co-twin is clinically normal. Elwood and Elwood (1980), using data pooled from the literature, found a concordance rate for anencephalus of 4.1% and for spina bifida of 5.1%. The highest reported concordance rate in the literature on NTDs is 8.3%, for anencephalus (Imaizumi, 1978). The concordance rates for both anomalies were higher for like-sex pairs than for pairs of unlike sex, but the sex could not be determined, or was not reported, in a large number of cases.

While the evidence that rates of neural tube defects differ as between twins and singletons is equivocal, that in favour of a raised twinning rate in first degree relatives of affected births is rather stronger. Elwood and Elwood (1980) estimated a crude rate (i.e. unadjusted for maternal age and parity) of twinning in siblings of propositi with anencephalus or spina bifida in pooled data from the UK of 18.5 per 1000 (95% confidence interval, 13.7–23.1/1000), significantly higher than the twinning rate of 11.5 per 1000 found in the general population. This finding suggests that some women may be predisposed to delivering both twins and infants with NTDs (Janerich, 1975). As some of the available data on the epidemiology of DZ twinning and of NTDs suggest just the opposite (Spiers, 1973), further work is needed on this issue.

Table 11.7. Summary of selected reports on encephalocele in twins and singletons

Population	Period of study	Singleton births			Twin births			Reference
		Total number	Number affected	Rate per 1000	Total number	Number affected	Rate per 1000	
Norway	1967–79	775 405	47	0.06	15 320	0	0.00	Windham and Bjerkedal, (1984); Windham et al. (1982)
USA, Atlanta — Blacks	1969–76	63 544	55	0.87	1 670	0	0.00 }	Layde et al. (1980)
whites		140 665	26	0.18	2 820	2	0.71 }	
USA, Los Angeles	1966–72	848 139	65	0.08	16 880	7[a]	0.41	Windham and Sever (1982)
USA, NCPP	1959–65	53 257	9	0.17	1 195	2	1.67	Myrianthopoulos (1975)
Total		1 881 010	202	0.11	37 885	11	0.29	

[a] 3 spina bifida.

Table 11.8. Risk of neural tube defects in twins as compared to singletons
(based on data in Tables 11.5–11.7)

	Number of twin births known?	Relative risk	
		Point estimate	95% confidence interval
Anencephalus	yes	1.49	1.12–1.98
	no	1.21	0.87–1.19
Spina bifida	yes	0.74	0.51–1.08
	no	0.92	0.52–1.63
Encephalocele	yes	2.70	1.47–4.95

In Norway, the siblings of twins with malformations of any type were found to have a rate of central nervous systems malformations twice as high as those in singletons and similar to the rate in twins (Windham and Bjerkedal, 1984). There are also reports of an excess of twins amongst the parents of infants with spina bifida (Le Marec et al., 1978; Nance, 1981).

Hydrocephalus

There are a few reports of a threefold increase in the risk of isolated hydrocephalus in twins as compared to singletons (Edwards, 1968; Layde et al., 1980; McKeown and Record, 1960; Myrianthopoulos, 1975). Two reports suggest that the increase is confined to twins of the same sex (Hay and Wehrung, 1970; McKeown and Record, 1960), but there is one report of an excess amongst pairs of opposite sex (Layde et al., 1980). Definitive conclusions are difficult to reach because congenital hydrocephalus is often not recognised at birth and because many cases of hydrocephalus in infancy result from neonatal intraventricular haemorrhage or meningitis. It is difficult to exclude the possibility that the apparent excess in twins is due to the inclusion of such cases which are likely to occur more commonly in twins due to their high incidence of prematurity.

Lorber (1984) reports a higher than expected frequency of twins amongst siblings born before index cases with isolated hydrocephalus. As risks of hydrocephalus are raised after having a baby with a NTD, and vice versa, this may be evidence of a close causal connection between twinning, NTDs and hydrocephalus.

Congenital Heart Disease

Comparison of rates of congenital heart disease (CHD) between singletons and twins is particularly difficult to interpret because of the difficulties of diagnosis. Diagnostic criteria are not always included (Burn and Corney, 1984). In addition, the majority of reports are based on data collected in the perinatal period, leading to the erroneous inclusion of innocent murmurs and to the exclusion of some CHD which does not become apparent until later in life (Hardy *et al.*, 1979).

For these reasons, it seems inappropriate to pool the data of Stevenson *et al.* (1966) based on a number of hospital series in different countries. Amongst the reports reviewed (Table 11.9), rates of CHD are, predictably enough, highest in the studies in which a specific protocol of clinical examination was maintained and in which the cohort of births was followed up for a year or more (Mitchell *et al.*, 1971a, 1971b; Richards *et al.*, 1955). The excess of CHD in twins is also more substantial in these studies. Before concluding that these higher rates of CHD in twins are real, three alternative explanations have to be considered. Firstly, diagnosis of CHD in one twin may lead to a more detailed examination of the apparently normal co-twin. Secondly, studies may include less severe congenital heart disease, and this less severe disease may be more common in twins than in singletons. A later report on the NCPP study described by Mitchell *et al.* (1971a, 1971b), for example, revealed that several cases of cardiac enlargement had been included (Myrianthopoulos, 1975) and this is often found in the recipient of fetofetal transfusion syndrome (Burn and Corney, 1984). This explanation does not account for the excess of CHD found by Richards *et al.* (1955). Thirdly, unless certain types of complications of multiple pregnancy are excluded, an excess of CHD in twins would be expected without invoking a particular association between CHD in general and twinning. For instance, cardiac malformation is common in conjoined twins and is thought to be due to secondary internal mechanical factors consequent upon the site and extent of fusion (Noonan, 1978). In addition, as twins are more likely to be born preterm, an excess of patent ductus arteriosus (PDA) is to be expected. Most studies do not allow for this. Furthermore, in most reports from population series, data on the specific type of cardiovascular anomalies are not presented.

The data on specific cardiac anomalies are difficult to interpret because of the problems of ascertainment already mentioned, because of differences in classification, particularly of multiple cardiac anomalies, and because of small numbers.

The findings of the few reports on the prevalence of CHD among twins where sex or zygosity was considered, have not been consistent. An increase of CHD in MZ twins (Kenna *et al.*, 1975; Cameron *et al.*, 1983) and also in those of like sex (McKeown and Record, 1960; Hay and Wehrung, 1970; Layde *et al.*, 1980) has been found by some, but not by others (Burn and Corney, 1984; Windham and Bjerkedal, 1984). Other data pertinent to the issue are based on series of referrals to paediatric cardiology units. Despite

Table 11.9. Comparison of prevalence at birth of congenital heart disease between twins and singletons

Study Population	Period of study	Population (P) or hospital (H) series	Method of ascertainment[a]	Singleton		Twins		RR[b] T:S	Reference
				Number with anomalies	Rate per 1000	Number with anomalies	Rate per 1000		
Norway, all births	1967–79	P	B	1876	2.4	54	3.5	1.5	Windham and Bjerkedal (1984)
UK, Birmingham, all births	1950–54	P	?	?	3.6	?	8.6	2.4	Edwards (1968)
UK, Liverpool, all births	1960–69	P	M	1048	6.6	32	6.5	1.0	Kenna et al. (1975)
USA, New York, all births	1946–53	H	P, 1	47	8.0	3	18.1	2.3	Richards et al. (1955)
USA, 12 centres, all births	1959–65	H	P, 7	437	8.0	20	16.6	2.1	Mitchell et al. (1971a, b)
USA, selected states, live births	1961–66	P	B	5898	0.6	141	0.7	1.2	Hay and Wehrung (1970)

[a]Method of ascertainment: B = birth notification; P = physical examination; M = multiple sources: 1 = to 1 year of age; 7 = to 7 years of age.
[b]Ratio of prevalence rate at birth of anomalies in twins to rate in singletons.

the biases of survival and referral practice inherent in such data, the almost universal finding of an unexpectedly high ratio of like-sex : unlike-sex twins is impressive (Lamy et al., 1957; Uchida and Rowe, 1957; Campbell, 1961; Noonan, 1963; Jorgensen, 1970; Mori, 1975; Anderson, 1977; Burn and Corney, 1984). The only exceptions are reported by Ross (1959) and Nora et al. (1967). Accurate concordance rates are not available for CHD because of differing inclusion criteria and methods of case ascertainment. As for anomalies in general, discordance appears to be the norm (Cameron et al., 1983).

There is one report of a raised frequency of congenital heart disease in the offspring of twins (Kramer et al., 1982).

Orofacial Clefts

There do not appear to be any consistent differences in the frequency of cleft lip and/or cleft palate as between twins and singletons (Edwards, 1968; Hay and Wehrung, 1970; Layde et al., 1980; Myrianthopoulos, 1975; Windham and Bjerkedal, 1984). It seems generally accepted that concordance rates are of the order of 40% for MZ pairs and 8% for DZ pairs (Benirschke and Kim, 1973), but no large unselected series of twins with clefts has been reported within one population and with direct determination of zygosity (Hay and Wehrung, 1970). Again, a raised frequency of oral clefting has been observed in the offspring of Norwegian twins (Kramer et al., 1982).

Oesophageal Atresia with or without Tracheo-Oesophageal Fistula (Tracheo-oesophageal Dysraphism).

Van Staey et al. (1984) have reviewed the literature on familial tracheo-oesophageal dysraphism. Analysis of pooled data from case series shows an excess of twin probands, with just over 5% (70 out of 1365) cases being twins as compared to an expected figure of around 1% (Fraser and Nora, 1975). Virtually all (67 out of 70) of the twin pairs were discordant for the anomaly.

Anomalies of the Urogenital System

Layde et al. (1980) report an excess of urogenital anomalies in twins but this is not confirmed in other reports (Myrianthopoulos, 1975; Windham and Bjerkedal, 1984). Regarding specific anomalies, there have been reports of an excess of twins among cases of hypospadias (De George, 1970b; Roberts and Lloyd, 1973; Neto et al., 1981) of undescended testis (Czeizel et al., 1981) and of clitoral enlargement (De George, 1970b). It is tempting to speculate that endocrine imbalance in twin gestation may be of aetiological importance; there is a lower chorionic gonadotrophin production per fetus in twin gestation (Gaspard and Franchimont, 1974; Roberts and Lloyd, 1973). The relationship, if any, between chorionic gonadotrophin levels and fetal anomalies is yet to be studied.

Chromosomal Anomalies

Most known chromosomal anomalies have been reported in twins (Benirschke and Kim, 1973). These are usually discordant in DZ twins, and surprisingly, also occasionally in MZ. Such MZ twins are known as heterokaryotes. In these cases it is assumed that the maldistribution of chromosomes occurred at about the same time as the twinning process (post-zygotic non-disjunction).

Phenotypically dissimilar twins may have similar chromosome mosaicisms in blood (lymphocyte) cultures, due to the shared fetal circulation in a monochorionic placenta, but show different karyotypes in fibroblast cultures (Potter and Taitz, 1972; Uchida et al., 1983a). As most cytogenetic studies are done on lymphocytes it is likely that some heterokaryote twins will go unrecognised. Extensive studies are required before counselling parents about the phenotypic expression of these genotypes, especially in Turner's syndrome (Paredes et al., 1962; Muller et al., 1970). Whereas MZ twins with Down's or Klinefelter's syndrome are almost always phenotypically and karyotypically concordant, cases of gonadal dysgenesis are often discordant (Karp et al., 1975; Pedersen et al., 1980).

Overall, Down's syndrome is no more common in twins than in singletons (MacGillivray, 1975) and there is some indication that prevalence at birth of Down's syndrome is reduced in twins of like sex (Hay and Wehrung, 1970; Layde et al., 1980; Windham and Bjerkedal, 1984). These findings stand even when allowance is made for maternal age in relation to DZ twinning and Down's syndrome.

There have been rare cases of MZ twins discordant for trisomy 21 (Scott and Ferguson-Smith, 1973; Rogers et al., 1982). Concordance in DZ twins is unusual, not surprisingly. However, several authors have reported a somewhat higher concordance rate in DZ pairs than would be expected even allowing for maternal age (McDonald, 1964; Bulmer, 1970; Avni et al., 1983). There are a number of possible explanations for this, including the operation of an environmental factor or that some women may have a predisposition to the chromosomal anomaly.

Klinefelter's sydrome appears to be more common in twins and in their relatives (Hoefnagel and Benirschke, 1962; Ferguson-Smith, 1966; Soltan, 1968; Nielsen, 1970). The increase appears to be particularly pronounced in sibships of affected DZ twins, but is not explained by an association with maternal age. However, numbers are small and not all investigators agree (Carothers et al., 1984).

There also appears to be an increased incidence of twins amongst people with Turner's syndrome (Lemli and Smith, 1963; Lindsten, 1963; Nance and

Uchida, 1964; Pescia *et al.*, 1975; Carothers *et al.*, 1980) and also amongst their (normal) family members (Nielsen and Dahl, 1976). Carothers *et al.* (1980) suggest that there may be a postzygotic mechanism common to twinning and X chromosome loss.

Single Umbilical Artery (SUA)

Most workers have found that single umbilical arteries are commoner in twins. Heifetz (1984), in his review of the literature, found an incidence of 2.3% in twin infants, between three and four times that found amongst singletons. From the results of thirteen prospective series, the incidence of twins amongst SUA infants was 5.3% – three times that expected (Heifetz, 1984). As in singletons, malformations were more common in the twins with SUA but, apart from acardia, these malformations do not appear to be of a particular type. Indeed, SUA twins have no greater incidence of associated malformations than SUA singletons (Benirschke and Bourne, 1960). In both groups the incidence of malformations was just over 20%. There is some indication that SUA is more common amongst MZ than DZ twins (Strong and Corney, 1967; Boyd and Hamilton, 1970) but the numbers are too small for a definite conclusion to be reached.

It is rare for twins to be concordant for SUA. Concordancy has only been reported in nine cases and in the five cases of known zygosity all were MZ (Heifetz, 1984). Although on this limited evidence more MZ than DZ twin pairs appear to be concordant for the anomaly, the majority remain discordant which suggests that environmental factors are largely responsible for the anomaly.

Greater concordancy amongst MZ twins could indicate that genetic factors were also operating in the genesis of the anomaly but, perhaps more likely, the MZ twinning process itself may have an influence. The type of placentation would also be of interest but unfortunately this is rarely recorded.

SUA tends to occur in the smaller of the two infants; 82.4% of 51 pairs discordant for the anomaly were the lighter of the pair (Heifetz, 1984). This agrees with the finding of a higher incidence of SUA amongst small-for-dates singleton babies (Bryan and Kohler, 1974).

Hydatidiform Mole

The incidence of hydatidiform mole appears to be higher in twin than in singleton pregnancies (Chamberlain, 1963; Beischer and Fortune, 1968b). It has also been suggested that a predisposition to twinning is associated with molar pregnancies. De George (1970a) found that in families where there had been a molar pregnancy there was an unexpectedly high occurrence of twins in both earlier and later pregnancies. Increasing maternal age is also a factor common to both dizygotic twinning and to hydatidiform mole (Bracken et al., 1984).

Hydatidiform mole within a multiple pregnancy should be distinguished from a mole in a single pregnancy with a co-existing fetus – a partial mole. In a single pregnancy the molar tissue only partly replaces the normal placenta leaving sufficient normal placental tissue for the fetus to survive at least for a period. Occasionally the fetus may be delivered as a full term healthy infant. In a twin pregnancy one conceptus is replaced by molar tissue whereas the second may be a normally developing placenta and fetus. Occasionally the otherwise normal placental tissue may have some molar vesicles within it (Beischer and Fortune, 1968b).

Cytogenetic studies have shown that the complete mole in either a single or twin pregnancy is diploid and of androgenetic origin (i.e. derived entirely from the father) whereas partial moles are usually triploid with two androgenetic chromosome components. Furthermore, in the complete mole the two sets of chromosomes are identical, arising from a haploid sperm: in the original mole the chromosomes usually differ suggesting an origin from two sperm.

Analysis of genetic polymorphisms is the most reliable method for distinguishing the partial mole from the dizygotic twin pregnancy (Fisher et al., 1982; Ohama et al., 1985).

Hydatidiform mole has been reported in both MZ and DZ pregnancies. Where karyotyping shows the conceptuses to be of different sex the molar tissue usually has the female karyotype (Beischer and Fortune, 1968b; Fisher et al., 1982). This is consistent with the higher preponderance of female karyotypes in hydatidiform moles in general (Bracken et al., 1984).

Other Anomalies

Many other anomalies have been recorded in twins. In particular, there have been reports of excesses of anomalies of the digestive system (Layde et al., 1980; Myrianthopoulos, 1975), but this was not confirmed in a more recent study (Windham and Bjerkedal, 1984). No other marked excess was observed in the large epidemiological surveys of anomalies of all types in twins and singletons (Stevenson et al., 1966; Edwards, 1968; Hayand Wehrung, 1970; Myrianthopoulos, 1975; Layde et al., 1980; Windham and Bjerkedal, 1984). The remaining evidence is derived from case reports which are particularly subject to ascertainment bias. However, there are reports of higher than expected frequencies of MZ twins amongst cases of amyoplasia (Hall et al., 1983). Finally, increased frequencies of twins in cases of symmelia and exstrophy of the cloaca, both of which are anomalies of midline structures, have been reported (Nance, 1981).

Possible Explanations for Associations between Twinning and Congenital Anomalies

Thus far, the evidence reviewed suggests that, in general, anomalies are more common amongst twins than singletons. The pattern is less clear for specific anomalies other than those unique to twins, and the anomalies unique to twins represent only a small population of cases of congenital malformation in twins. Although it seems widely accepted that most of the excess risk in twins is for monozygotic pairs (Bulmer, 1970), the pattern seems to be consistent only for congenital heart disease, and even in this instance the conclusion can be reached only if it is accepted that Weinberg's rule is valid. Moreover, there are insufficient data relating to specific types of cardiac anomalies. In the main, therefore, the evidence that MZ pairs account for most of the excess risk of anomalies in twins, is derived from studies of congenital anomalies in general (i.e. not classified into specific anomalies) with the zygosity distribution inferred by Weinberg's method. It does, however, seem implausible that there would be uniform associations between anomalies of all types and twinning, sex-pairing and zygosity (Boklage, 1985). This implausibility is demonstrated by considering the evidence as to the aetiology of malformations in twins. Much of this evidence is derived from clinical and pathological case reports.

Proposed explanations for associations between twinning and congenital anomalies fall into two major categories.

1. There is, at least in part, a common aetiology for certain types of anomaly and certain types of twinning. Explanations have included similar predisposition, similar exogenous agents, and the consequences of fission of embryos or of twin embryogenesis.
2. Fetus–fetus interaction. The hypothetical mechanisms include fusion of embryos, the vascular consequences of fetal death and intrauterine constraint.

A common aetiology?

(1) Shared Predispositions?   As already mentioned (see p. 223), reports of raised twinning frequency in siblings of propositi with neural tube defects suggest that some women may be predisposed to delivering both twins and babies with anomalies of this type. Janerich (1975) suggests that there are two causal mechanisms of DZ twinning, one producing high rates of NTD, the other not. One, not associated with NTDs, is the primary overproduction of pituitary gonadotrophin, the other overproduction secondary to defective hormone receptor sites or messenger mechanisms. This hypothesis has not been tested. Elwood and Elwood (1980) suggest that women who are of above average fertility may be predisposed to both conditions. Dizygotic

twinning appears to be more common in illegitimate births, amongst births conceived in the first 3 months of marriage, and women who are delivered of DZ twins have more pregnancies than others (see Chapter 5), but the evidence regarding neural tube defects is more contradictory, with several studies showing a lower risk in illegitimate births and conflicting results about the length of the interval between marriage and birth and between successive births, for mothers of affected infants as compared to other infants (Elwood and Elwood, 1980). One study shows that the sibships of affected invidivuals are larger than comparison sibships; the intervals between births before an affected birth were shorter than in the control group, which suggests that the explanation is a higher fertility state rather than reproductive compensation (Elwood and McBride, 1979). Social influences were not taken into account directly, but the similarity of maternal age at first birth suggests that these are unlikely to have been confounding influences. Attempts should be made to repeat this study in other populations.

Elevated twinning rates in siblings of propositi with Klinefelter's and Turner's syndromes (see p. 229) and in pregnancies ending in birth in women with hydatidiform mole (see p. 230) have also been observed. In the case of Turner's syndrome the association is thought to be with MZ twinning and in that of Klinefelter's syndrome, with DZ twinning (Corney et al., 1981).

Burch (1969, 1981) argues that both DZ twinning and Klinefelter's syndrome are consequences of an autoaggressive process. The high incidence of diabetes mellitus in the parents and close relatives of patients with Klinefelter's syndrome (Nielsen, 1966) is taken as further indirect evidence of this. Burch explains the fall in DZ twinning rates at higher maternal ages, which is at first sight inconsistent with his hypothesis, as a reduction in fertility of mothers of DZ twins, as compared to other women, consequent upon another autoaggressive process. The observation of an earlier age of natural menopause in mothers of twins of unlike sex as compared to mothers of like-sex twins and singletons (Wyshak, 1975, 1978b) is consistent with this. While antibodies to some thyroid, stomach, nuclear and gonadal antigens have been investigated in patients with Klinefelter's syndrome (Vallotton and Forbes, 1967), the key test of the hypothesis – investigation of these antibodies in the mothers of patients with Klinefelter's syndrome – does not appear to have been carried out.

On an intuitive basis, if there are predispositions to certain types of twinning and of congenital anomalies, it would be expected that being a twin oneself might be one predisposition. There is one report that the offspring of twins are at higher risk of congenital heart disease and oral clefting than the general population (Kramer et al., 1982), and some evidence of an excess of twins amongst the parents of propositi with spina bifida (see p. 225). In some other studies, it has been found that women who are themselves twins are more likely to have twin offspring than other women (Weinberg, 1909; Bonnevie and Sverdrup, 1926; Greulich, 1934; Bulmer, 1960b; Wyshak and White, 1965; Propping and Kruger, 1976; Schmidt et al., 1983), but some of these results may have been affected by selection bias in sampling (Eriksson, 1973) and not all authors have found this (Nylander, 1970b). We conclude that further work is necessary to test the hypothesis that being a twin is in itself a predisposing factor to twinning and malformations.

(2) Similar Exogenous Agents?   So far as we are aware, the only exogenous factors which have been hypothesised as linked both with twinning and congenital anomalies are ovulation-stimulating agents. In particular, Elwood (1974) suggested that clomiphene-induced ovulation independently affected the probability of both dizygotic twinning and anencephalus, giving rise to the apparent association between the two events. The major problem in assessing the evidence regarding any association between drug and malformation is whether or not the drug or the underlying disease is the aetiological agent. As ovulation-inducing agents are, almost by definition, used only in cases of subfertility, it is impossible to compare the rates of malformation in the offspring of women exposed to these drugs with those for women not so exposed. One approach has been to compare rates in births to women who later received ovulation-inducing therapy but the circumstances of the pregnancies are not truly comparable. James (1977) employed this approach to examine the relationship between clomiphene and anencephalus, and concluded that any association was due to subfertility – the drug in itself was not teratogenic. Evidence already considered above, however, points more in favour of an association with high fertility states. Most other reports of the association between ovulation induction and malformation have been based on studies of clinical case series. The rates of congenital anomalies have ranged between 2% and 9% in the case of clomiphene, between 5% and 13% in the case of human menopausal gonadotrophin (numbers are small) and between 0.9% and 3.5% in the case of bromocriptine, and are considered not to differ substantially from the background rates of the populations concerned (Scialli, 1986). In one study, the same methods of ascertainment of anomalies have been used in a comparison of pregnancy outcome between women exposed to clomiphene, women exposed to human menopausal gonadotrophin and the general population (Kurachi et al., 1983). The rates of anomalies were similar in all three groups and, in the case of clomiphene therapy, there was no dose–response effect.

(3) Consequences of Fission or Twin Embryogenesis?   A number of anomalies have been interpreted as having the same causation as that giving rise to MZ twinning (Schinzel et al., 1979). These anomalies are thought to include, at least in some instances, sacrococcygeal teratoma (SCT), sirenomelus and

related anomalies thought to be due to maldevelopment of the caudal region, e.g. the VATER association, exstrophy of the cloaca malformation sequence, holoprosencephaly and ancencephaly (Schinzel et al., 1979; Jones and Benir-schke, 1983). The possibility that anomalous embryogenesis is characteristic of all twins, and that unlike sex twinning is protective against its effects cannot be excluded (Boklage, 1985).

It has been suggested that SCT is at one extreme of a spectrum of consequences resulting from abnormal segregation of the blastomere, ranging from SCT through fetus-in-fetu, conjoined twins to uncomplicated MZ twin-ning (Gross and Clatworthy, 1951; Potter, 1962). Other authors reject the notion of any connection between twinning and teratoma (Lewis, 1961; Willis, 1962; Tada et al., 1974). Other hypotheses have related to (1) parthogenetic development of germ cells and (2) origin from totipotent cell rests that have escaped the influence of the primary organiser (Ashley, 1973).

It seems clear that there is an association between SCT and duplication anomalies of the hindgut (Fraumeni et al., 1973; Lemire and Beckwith, 1982). Ashley (1973) argues that extragonadal teratomas which arise at sites in which the attachment of conjoined twins has been observed, can most easily be explained as incomplete conjoined twins if the blastula is incompletely divided so that a proportion of cells insufficient for the development of a complete second individual becomes separated. An excess of twins has been reported in patients with teratoma (Gross et al., 1951; Hickey and Layton, 1954) and in their families (Edmonds and Hawkins, 1941) but these observa-tions have not been confirmed. An association between twinning, SCT and anomalies of the caudal region is not implausible in view of the increased frequencies of twins in cases of symmelia and exstrophy of the cloaca, caused by developmental arrest of the primitive streak (Davies et al., 1971) and by the occurrence of complete and partial twinning following experimental induction of primitive streak lesions (Huxley and DeBeer, 1934). Moreover, there has been at least one case report of an infant with a fetus-in-fetu and a maligant teratoma present within the same intra-abdominal mass (Du Plessis et al., 1974). These authors suggest that the phenomenon is a result of abnormal development of triplets.

James (1976) suggests that MZ twins and anencephalus may be associated because of similar relationships between the times of ovulation and concep-tion. He argues that the increasing rate of anencephalus from dichorionic pairs through monochorionic pairs to conjoined pairs is explained by the interval between the time of cleavage of the zygote and the optimum time of the neural tube closure (James, 1981). In dichorionic pairs, the interval is longest, and in conjoined pairs, least, giving the embryos different intervals to catch up on the developmental delay caused by the twinning event and thereby to form a neural tube according to the developmental clock. There are no definitive data on the relationship between time of fertilisation and

NTDs (Elwood and Elwood, 1980). Flannery and Robinow (1986) suggest that variation in the rate of NTDs, and in concordance rates for these defects, in MZ twins, is due to variation in the timing of fission of the zygote. A similar explanation has been proposed for the occurrence of situs viscerum specularis in MZ twins (Gedda *et al.*, 1984).

Boklage (1986) has noted that NTDs, certain congenital cardiac anomalies, orofacial clefts and gastroschisis are, like twinning, associated with the occurrence of non-righthandedness in families. They have also been observed in families of propositi affected by one of the conditions more than would be expected by chance (Fraser *et al.*, 1982). As already discussed, the evidence that there is an excess of anomalies in twins is less certain.

One of the consequences of twin pregnancy is a lowered chorionic gonado-trophin production per fetus. This may be linked to unconfirmed reports of excesses of urogenital anomalies in twins (see p. 228).

Fetus–Fetus Interaction?

(1) Consequences of fusion? So far as we are aware, the possibility that anomalies may be produced following the fusion of embryos has been suggested only for NTDs and conjoined twinning.

Two mechanisms whereby NTDs arise from fusion of twin conceptuses have been proposed:

1. NTDs in one of twin births arise from fusion of two members of a set of triplets and in singletons from fusion of twin conceptuses (Knox, 1970). This was thought to explain the complete lack of concordance found in the study of Yen and MacMahon (1968) but, since then, some concordant pairs have been identified (Elwood and Elwood, 1980; Windham *et al.*, 1982).
2. MZ twins concordant for NTDs fuse to form conjoined twins, whereas DZ twins fuse to form one survivor, the tissue from the co-twin forming a teratoma or an area of skin with different chromosomal sex (Rogers, 1969; 1976). Only indirect supporting evidence is available such as case reports of anencephalus with incomplete twinning (Riccardi and Bergmann, 1977; Fontaine and Vankemmel, 1978), the association of intraspinal teratoma with spina bifida and the analogous phenomenon of fetus-in-fetu (Du Plessis *et al.*, 1974).

(2) Vascular Consequences of Fetal Death? In monochorionic twins, who share a placental blood circulation, if one fetus dies early in pregnancy, emboli and debris may enter the circulation of the survivor causing ischaemia and disruption to the developing organs.

The types of anomalies reported as being secondary to the death of a

Table 11.10. Anomalies in surviving twin thought to be secondary to the death of a co-twin with a monochorionic placenta in utero

Time of death of co-twin	Anomaly	Reference
Late gestation	Cerebellar necrosis	Melnick (1977); Hoyme et al. (1981)
	Spinal cord transection	Hoyme et al. (1981)
	Congenital renal cortical necrosis	Benirschke (1961b); Hoyme et al. (1981)
		Moore et al. (1969); Reisman and Pathak (1966)
Early gestation	Intestinal atresia	Barnard (1956); Hoyme et al. (1981);
		Louw and Barnard (1955); Louw et al. (1981)
Gestation unspecified	Hydranencephaly	Schinzel et al. (1979); Jung et al. (1984)
	Porencephaly	Durkin et al. (1976); Schinzel et al. (1979);
		Jung et al. (1984)
	Multicystic encephalomalacia	Yoshioka et al. (1979)
	Hydrocephalus	Nejedly (1951)
	Microcephaly	Durkin et al. (1976); Roos et al. (1957);
		Schinzel et al. (1979)
	Horseshoe kidney	Hoyme et al. (1981)
	Hemifacial microsomia	Schinzel et al. (1979)
	Aplasia cutis congenita	Mannino et al. (1977)
	Terminal limb defects	Balfour (1976); Schinzel et al. (1979)

co-twin with a monochorionic or fused dichorionic placenta in utero are presented in Table 11.10. Review of pooled data on 53 cases suggests that disruption of the central nervous system is the most common complication (72%), followed by the gastrointestinal system (19%), kidneys (15%) and lungs (8%) (Szymonowicz et al., 1986). Many of these anomalies have also been described in conjunction with disturbed fetal blood flow unrelated to death of a MZ co-twin (Hoyme et al., 1981). With the exception of en-celphaloplastic brain defects (Jung et al., 1984) and congenital skin defects (Mannino et al., 1977), the lesions reported are isolated cases (Johnson and Driscoll, 1986).

The nature of the anomalies seen in the survivor of a MZ twin pair may depend on the time during gestation at which the co-twin dies (Hoyme et al., 1981), although when correlation with ultrasound evidence of the death was attempted, a spectrum of anomalies in the survivor was found (David, 1985; Szymonowicz et al., 1986). An alternative hypothesis is that the type of anomaly determines the time of death and that the anomaly occurred as a result of disturbance of the laterality of development caused by the process of twinning (Burn and Corney, 1984). However, the lack of published reports of a disseminated intravascular coagulation-like syndrome in the surviving members of dichorionic twin pairs, one of whom has died in utero (Johnson and Driscoll, 1986), makes this seem unlikely.

Although routine antenatal ultrasonic screening has shown that death of one twin in utero is not uncommon (Landy et al., 1982) anomalies occurring secondary to this death appear to be rare (Hanna and Hill, 1984). One recent review of fourteen published reports indicated that 46.2% of the liveborn twins suffered major morbidity or death, but this figure is misleading as the reports were gathered retrospectively on the basis of unfavourable outcome (Enbom, 1985).

(3) Intrauterine Constraint? Twins are more likely to suffer from positional defects due to the intrauterine congestion and relative restriction of move-ment to which they are subjected. Minor foot deformities and skull asym-metry may be more common in twins (Edwards, 1968; Hay and Wehrung, 1970; Schinzel et al., 1979) but this has not been confirmed (Myrianthopoulos, 1975; Layde et al., 1980). They are rarely mentioned in twin studies.

For both talipes and congenital dislocation of the hip, the concordance rate for MZ pairs is ten to fifteen times as high as that for DZ pairs (Vogel and Motulsky, 1979) which argues against a purely mechanical explanation for the aetiology of these defects.

Why is Discordance the Norm?

The 'fusion' hypotheses were proposed to account for the lack of concordance for neural tube defects, but the supporting evidence is inconclusive. Quadruplet conception, or aetiological heterogeneity, have to be invoked to account for the concordant cases. Such a mechanism appears implausible for other congenital anomalies. The intrauterine vascular consequences of fetal death can be of relevance only in a minority of cases. However, the not uncommon finding of placental anastomoses in MZ twin pregnancy may in part be as an explanation for discordance – the common circulation may be the means by which an anomalous fetus is kept alive by its unaffected co-twin (Hay and Wehrung, 1970). Affected singletons, DZ twins and concordant MZ twins would be more likely to die early in gestation, leading to an apparent excess of discordant MZ twins. Many authors cite abnormal splitting of the zygote, i.e. the consequences of MZ twinning itself, as a possible mechanism, but the evidence for the association with MZ twinning only is based on Weinberg's rule and the possibility that abnormal embryogenesis affects all twins, and that opposite sexed co-gestation is protective, cannot be ruled out. Finally, twin embryos may achieve different stages of development at particular gestational ages, the degree of disparity being related to the precise mechanism of twinning (see Chapter 2). The evidence from case reports of twins exposed to known teratogens is of particular relevance in this respect.

Even when twin fetuses have been exposed to known teratogens, discordance for anomalies has been reported. In transplacentally acquired intrauterine infections, occasionally one twin alone suffers the teratological insult (Penrose, 1937; Forrester et al., 1966: Satge et al., 1966; Henriksen et al., 1968; Shearer et al., 1972). However, in at least one of the cases reported it was shown that the other twin had in fact been infected but suffered no lasting damage (Forrester et al., 1966). Perhaps the fetuses were infected at slightly, but critically, different stages of embryological development.

As with infections it appears that there may be intrapair differences in fetal response to drugs (Mellin and Katzenstein, 1962; Lenz, 1966; Loughnan et al., 1973; Schmidt and Salzano, 1980) including alcohol (Christoffel and Salafsky, 1975; Abel, 1982; Chasnoff, 1985). These differences were well demonstrated in a trizygotic triplet pregnancy where the effects of maternal Epanutin were expressed differently in each infant (Bustamante and Stumpff, 1978).

This difference may be due to difference in fetal susceptibility to the teratogenic insult. In MZ twin pregnancy, in which placental anastomoses are not uncommon, the inequality in blood supply would place one embryo at a disadvantage, rendering it more susceptible than the co-twin to teratogens (Hay and Wehrung, 1970). In other instances where the teratogenic effect of the drug is sharply limited, as in the case of thalidomide, the discordance in fetal abnormality could be due to the insult acting at the very beginning or end of the sensitive period (Lenz, 1966). As DZ twins can be conceived several days apart, one embryo may be a few days retarded or accelerated in development and therefore escape unscathed.

Other explanations for discordance in DZ twins include polar body twinning and superfetation, and in MZ twins differences in gene penetrance, cytoplasmic inheritance, and occurrence of postcleavage mutation in only one twin (Gericke, 1986).

Twinning and Twins
Edited by I. MacGillivray, D. M. Campbell and B. Thompson
© 1988 John Wiley & Sons Ltd

CHAPTER 12

The relationship of birthweight to later growth and intelligence in twins

CYNTHIA FRASER

Medical Research Council Medical Sociology Unit, University of Aberdeen, Aberdeen, UK

and

PERCY P. S. NYLANDER

Department of Obstetrics and Gynaecology, University College Hospital, Ibadan, Nigeria

There has been much interest in the effects of variation in intrauterine environment on the subsequent development of the infant. In particular, birthweight is frequently used as an easily measured indication of the quality of this environment. For singletons, low birthweight (LBW) has been shown to be associated with subsequent impairment in both physical and intellectual development although social as well as physiological factors have also been implicated (Illsley and Mitchell, 1984). Indeed, it is the problem of disentangling social, medical and physiological factors associated with LBW which has engendered much research in this area in recent years. While at first sight, it might appear that MZ twins provide ideal 'controlled' pairs to examine the effects of birthweight variation, as they share the same genetic composition and similar postnatal environments, the resulting observations cannot necessarily be made applicable to same sex singletons or even DZ twins, since different factors are implicated in intrapair birthweight differences. The phenomenon of the fetofetal transfusion syndrome in MZ twins, whereby a shared fetal circulation can result in disparity in fetal growth, is the most common cause of large intrapair discrepancies in birthweight in MZ twins. There does not appear to be any agreement as to what order of birthweight difference is implicated since studies investigating the issue have used differing criteria to differentiate twins of 'similar' and 'dissimilar' birthweight. Proponents of hereditary origins of intelligence have argued that estimates of the hereditability of intelligence have been under-estimated because no account of the disparate effects on intelligence test scores (IQ) of the fetofetal transfusion syndrome has been made in correlating the IQs of MZ twins.

Research has attempted to document IQ and birthweight differences between MZ twins and where large discrepancies in birthweight have been associated with substantial IQ difference, the fetofetal transfusion syndrome is said to be implicated. However, to substantiate these claims intrapair birthweight differences in DZ and MZ twins should be compared to determine whether similar degrees of variation in development are found. One might anticipate that IQ differences among DZ twins would be greater since there is evidence that the development of DZ twins diverges as they grow older while MZ twins develop in parallel (Wilson, 1983). However, if the IQ advantage of the heavier MZ twins should exceed that in like-sexed DZ pairs, then it is argued that the cause is fetofetal transfusion (Kamin, 1978). However, from present research, the evidence is inconclusive (James, 1982b).

Of eight studies that have examined the associated outcomes of birthweight differences in MZ twins (Churchill, 1965; Willerman and Churchill, 1967; Kaelber and Pugh, 1969; Scarr, 1969; Babson and Philips, 1973; Fujikura and Froehlich, 1974; Wilson, 1979; Marsh, 1980), all have found the heavier twin to have a higher IQ and (when examined) to be taller; but not all have found the difference to be significant (Kaelber and Pugh, 1969; Fujikura and Froehlich, 1974). The size of the noted IQ difference varies between studies from 1.7 to 9 points. Of course, different tests have been used on subjects at different ages so it is not surprising that variation exists. Kamin (1978), in combining results from six of these studies noted, on average, a 5.44 IQ points difference between heavier and lighter twins which he found to be statistically a highly significant result. Only two studies (Babson and Philips, 1973; Wilson, 1979) looked at intrapair height variation. Babson and Philips found an average intrapair discrepancy of 5.6 cm in favour of the heavier twin, at 9 years of age, while Wilson found only a marginal difference.

Not all the studies have been rigorous in establishing the zygosity of their twins by blood sampling. Those of Scarr (1969), Babson and Philips (1973), Fujikura and Froehlich (1974), and Marsh (1980) did; while those of Churchill (1965), Willerman and Churchill (1967), and Kaelber and Pugh (1969) included twins where some had been blood tested, some identified from a monochorionic placenta and some considered clinically identical from doctor's statements. Willerman and Churchill considered separately those who were confirmed as being MZ. Similarly, Churchill analysed the results of his monochorionic placenta (MC) twins separately from those of his clinically identical twins. From these studies, only the MZ confirmed and MC subsamples have been considered in this discussion. It was, however, impossible to differentiate Kaelber and Pugh's MC and blood tested pairs from those who were considered to be MZ solely from a doctor's statement (27.3% of their sample); thus the results of this study should be viewed with caution.

Most of the studies had highly selected samples: Churchill's (1965) sample were all patients at a psychology clinic while Willerman and Churchill's (1967) sample comprised those from Churchill's study plus others who were from white middle class homes; Marsh (1980) asked for volunteers from an adult group of MZ twins. Babson and Philips (1973) adopted a strict criterion in their sample selection to produce a highly selected group of twins who had at least a 25% difference in birthweight and with the lighter twin also weighing below 2000 g. Over an 8 years period they succeeded in identifying only 20 pairs who fulfilled these criteria. Fujikura and Froehlich (1974), in the only prospectively collected sample, had a high drop-out rate – only 75 out of 176 pairs were tested at 4 years of age. Kaelber and Pugh (1969), due to their testing criterion and difficulty in establishing zygosity, also had a high drop-out rate but were able to show that those included did not differ significantly from the rest on many variables including birthweight, age and parity. Finally Scarr's (1969) sample was selected from a larger longitudinal study which was found to be representative of the total study in basic demographic variables.

These studies disagree as to whether the size of the difference in birthweight between MZ pairs is important in determining the extent of the subsequent IQ difference. The studies themselves vary in their distribution of birthweight differences between pairs. While most have an average birthweight difference of around 300 g with a variety of subsequent differences from 1.7 to 9 points in IQ scores, Marsh (1980) with an average difference of 137 g in his sample noted a 3 points difference and Babson and Philips (1973) with a large average difference of 845 g noted a 6.6 points difference on the Stanford–Binet and 8.7 points on the Weschler Intelligence Score for Children. Bryan (1983) has suggested that the time of intrauterine growth retardation may be important; the earlier the in utero malnutrition the poorer the long-term prognosis.

In their own studies, Churchill (1965), Willerman and Churchill (1967) and Babson and Philips (1973) did not look at this association. Each had very small samples and so such analysis would have been impossible. Marsh (1980) found no association between IQ and birthweight difference but, as already mentioned, his sample tended to have small birthweight differences. Scarr (1969) found the size of birthweight difference to be important while Kaelber and Pugh (1969) and Fujikura and Froehlich (1974) both noted a larger but non-significant difference in their twin pairs who had 'dissimilar' birthweights. These studies have all taken what appear to be arbitrary cut off points to differentiate their 'similar' and 'dissimilar' pairs. Kaelber and Pugh (1969) chose a difference of 300 g, and Fujikura and Froehlich (1974) a 15% difference while Scarr (1969) looked at pairs where both were above 2500 g, both below and those where one was above and one was below this birthweight. Munsinger (1977) attempted to collate these studies to examine the association between birthweight and IQ differences and concluded that 'similar' pairs with a birthweight disparity of less than 300 g had an average of 2.49 IQ points difference while those pairs with more than a 300 g disparity differed, on average, by 7 IQ points. Kamin (1978), however, described many errors in this analysis and corrected these figures to 3.91 and 5.15 IQ points respectively and so concluded that the size of the weight difference is not associated with the size of the IQ difference. To overcome the problem of artificially creating 'similar' and 'dissimilar' groups regression analysis would seem a better technique to examine the nature of any relationship between size of birthweight differences and subsequent IQ differences.

DZ twins, on the other hand, with intrapair genetic variation, might be anticipated to have larger IQ differences than MZ twins with similar magnitude of birthweight differences. Indeed Wilson (1979) has shown that the correlation of IQ scores between DZ twins diverges with age while remaining constant for MZ pairs. In three studies which compared IQ and birthweight differences of MZ and DZ twins the difference in birthweight is larger for DZ pairs though not to any great extent, while the corresponding intrapair IQ differences are similar. Kaelber and Pugh (1969), on a sample where zygosity is not confirmed for some cases had IQ differences for MZ and DZ twins of 2.52 and 0.19 points respectively; Babson and Philips (1973) with a small sample noted a 6.56 and 7.00 points difference while Churchill (1965) found his MC sample to have 1.7 points difference compared with 3.7 points for his DZ sample. Thus, at present it has not been shown that any intrapair birthweight effect on IQ observed within twin pairs is a function of zygosity.

The Present Study

The Sample

The present study overcomes some of the deficiencies of previous research. The sample comprised all twins born in 1952–1954 at Aberdeen Maternity Hospital to Aberdeen residents, i.e. a total geographical population of twin births over 3 years. There were 25 pairs of MZ twins and 46 pairs of like-sex DZ twins as well as 53 pairs of unlike-sex DZ twins. Zygosity for like-sex twins was determined by blood analysis. The children's scores on IQ tests taken routinely at age 7, 9 and 11 years were obtained from the local education authority, as well as their height, as measured at their medical examination on entry to primary school at around 5 years of age. Three pairs of MZ twins were excluded because one twin was physically disabled, blind or deaf and so could not be tested, while a fourth pair had left the area during the period of testing. Similarly for the DZ twins, one pair was excluded because one twin could not be tested due to mental subnormality and two pairs had left the area. Thus details of IQ scores are available for 21 MZ twins

(12 male and 9 female pairs) and 43 like-sex DZ twins (25 male and 18 female pairs). For height 22 MZ pairs and 41 like-sex DZ pairs were measured.

Results

Birthweight   As shown in Table 12.1, like-sex DZ twins tended to be heavier than MZ twins with mean birthweights of 2854.8 g and 2475.6 g respectively for the heavier twin and 2456.2 g and 2150.8 g respectively for the lighter in each pair. Average birthweight difference was also greater for DZ pairs: 398.7 g compared with 324.8 g for MZ pairs. These findings also hold true for male and female pairs considered separately. Average birthweight was very similar for both DZ and MZ first and second twins (Table 12.1). When considering pairs of twins it was noted that the second twin tended to be heavier (57.1% of MZ pairs and 60.5% of DZ pairs).

Intelligence   Table 12.2 shows mean IQ for heavier and lighter twins as well as the mean IQ differences. For both males and females, MZ twins had more disparate scores than DZ twins, with the heavier twin having higher IQ scores. For DZ pairs, however, at 7+ and 9+ tests, the lighter twin tended to score higher. None of the mean IQ differences between heavier and lighter twins show statistical significance even for all MZ and all DZ pairs which had reasonable sample sizes. Thus, it does not appear that heavier twins are substantially better off in terms of subsequent IQ scores, a finding similar to that of Kaelber and Pugh (1969) and Fujikura and Froehlich (1974). On comparing first and second twins, minimal difference was noted in IQ scores.

Height   Table 12.3 shows mean height at approximately 5 years of age for heavier and lighter and for first and second born MZ and DZ twins, and shows minimal differences, on average, between pairs. Again, none of these differences are statistically significant.

It is possible that although averages between heavier and lighter twins are not significantly different some underlying relationship between IQ and birthweight is obscured by looking at the data in this way. Table 12.4 shows the correlation coefficient for the IQ and birthweight for MZ and DZ twins.

There is a significant positive relationship between IQ scores and birthweight particularly for MZ twins. Thus as birthweight increases, IQ increases accordingly. For height, a much weaker association exists, reaching a significant level only for DZ lighter twins. Bivariate regression analysis (Table 12.5) shows that a significant linear relationship exists between birthweight and IQ for both lighter and heavier twins, whether MZ or DZ (with the exception of heavier DZ twins and 9+ scores). Using the regression equation to calculate predicted IQ scores, at any given weight, the lighter twin will

Table 12.1. Mean birthweight (g) by zygosity

(a) Heavier and lighter

	Males			Females			All		
	Heavier	Lighter	Diff.	Heavier	Lighter	Diff.	Heavier	Lighter	Diff.
MZ	2695.7	2347.7	348.0	2182.1	1888.2	293.9	2475.6	2150.8	324.8
DZ	2899.9	2510.3	389.6	2794.9	2384.1	410.8	2854.8	2456.2	398.7

(b) Birth order

	Males			Females			All		
	First	Second	Diff.	First	Second	Diff.	First	Second	Diff.
MZ	2574.0	2469.3	104.7	2049.8	2020.6	29.2	2349.3	2277.0	72.3
DZ	2641.3	2748.1	−106.8	2596.9	2582.1	14.8	2629.5	2678.6	−49.1

Table 12.2. Mean IQ scores by zygosity

(a) Heavier and lighter

	Male			Female			All		
	Heavier	Lighter	Diff.	Heavier	Lighter	Diff.	Heavier	Lighter	Diff.
MZ									
7+	106.9	104.7	2.2	96.6	93.3	3.3	102.5	99.8	2.7
9+	110.3	105.0	5.3	102.9	100.7	2.2	107.1	103.1	4.0
11+	98.7	95.3	3.4	93.1	91.4	1.7	96.3	93.7	2.6
DZ									
7+	101.5	103.1	−1.6	100.3	102.0	−1.7	101.0	102.6	−1.6
9+	103.6	107.7	−4.1	107.2	105.9	1.3	105.1	106.9	−1.8
11+	95.8	95.1	0.7	97.9	95.6	2.3	96.7	95.3	1.4

(b) Birth order

	Male			Female			All		
	First	Second	Diff.	First	Second	Diff.	First	Second	Diff.
MZ									
7+	106.7	104.8	1.9	95.3	96.1	−0.8	101.9	100.4	1.5
9+	108.2	107.1	1.1	99.7	103.9	−4.2	104.6	105.7	−1.1
11+	97.3	96.7	0.6	92.3	92.2	0.1	95.2	94.8	0.4
DZ									
7+	101.8	103.4	−1.6	105.2	97.2	8.0	103.2	100.8	2.4
9+	106.9	105.4	1.5	107.1	106.0	1.1	106.9	105.6	1.3
11+	95.9	95.2	0.7	97.5	96.0	1.5	96.6	95.5	1.1

Table 12.3. Mean height (inches) by zygosity

(a) Heavier and lighter

	Males			Females			All		
	Heavier	Lighter	Diff.	Heavier	Lighter	Diff.	Heavier	Lighter	Diff.
MZ	42.1	41.9	0.2	41.2	41.9	−0.7	41.7	41.9	−0.2
DZ	42.6	42.0	0.6	41.9	41.6	0.3	42.3	41.8	0.5

(b) Birth order

	Males			Females			All		
	First	Second	Diff.	First	Second	Diff.	First	Second	Diff.
MZ	41.9	42.0	−0.1	42.0	41.0	1.0	41.9	41.6	0.3
DZ	42.2	42.4	−0.2	42.1	42.3	−0.2	42.2	42.3	−0.1

Table 12.4. Pearson correlation coefficients: birthweight by IQ at different ages and height by zygosity

		7+	9+	11+	Height
MZ	heavier	0.64****	0.58****	0.59****	0.19
	lighter	0.55**	0.57****	0.44	0.15
	first	0.67****	0.58****	0.60****	0.07
	second	0.49**	0.58****	0.42	0.20
DZ	heavier	0.31	0.28	0.35**	0.15
	lighter	0.44****	0.32**	0.33**	0.38**
	first	0.45****	0.47****	0.51****	0.15
	second	0.20	0.09	0.18	0.15

****$p \leqslant 0.01$.
**$p \leqslant 0.05$.

have a higher IQ than a heavier twin. Figure 12.1 demonstrates the regression lines of birthweight and predicts IQs at 7+ and 11+ tests. While the regression lines for heavier and lighter MZ twins are almost parallel and close together, for DZ twins, the line for the lighter twin is similar to that for MZ twins while for heavier DZ twins the regression line suggests that an increase in birthweight confers a smaller increase in IQ scores.

Table 12.5. Regression of birthweight on IQ at different ages and height by zygosity for heavier and lighter twins

			Regression equation	F values	Predicted values	
					1500 g	3500 g
MZ	7+	H	$y = 61.47 + 0.016x$	13.17****	85.47	117.47
		L	$y = 65.57 + 0.016x$	8.23****	89.57	121.57
	9+	H	$y = 58.59 + 0.019x$	9.52****	87.09	125.09
		L	$y = 70.38 + 0.015x$	9.35****	92.88	132.88
	11+	H	$y = 60.87 + 0.014x$	10.27****	81.87	109.87
		L	$y = 69.64 + 0.011x$	4.68**	86.14	108.14
DZ	7+	H	$y = 75.00 + 0.009x$	4.11**	88.50	106.50
		L	$y = 61.20 + 0.017x$	9.57****	86.70	120.70
	9+	H	$y = 74.61 + 0.010x$	3.49	89.61	109.61
		L	$y = 76.79 + 0.012x$	4.73**	94.80	118.80
	11+	H	$y = 65.69 + 0.010x$	5.43**	80.69	100.69
		L	$y = 68.46 + 0.011x$	4.74**	85.00	107.00
MZ height		H	$y = 39.98 + 0.0007x$	0.74	41.03	42.43
		L	$y = 40.37 + 0.0007x$	0.49	41.42	42.82
DZ height		H	$y = 40.10 + 0.0007x$	0.94	41.15	42.55
		L	$y = 37.74 + 0.002x$	6.48**	40.74	44.74

**$p \leqslant 0.05$.
****$p \leqslant 0.01$.

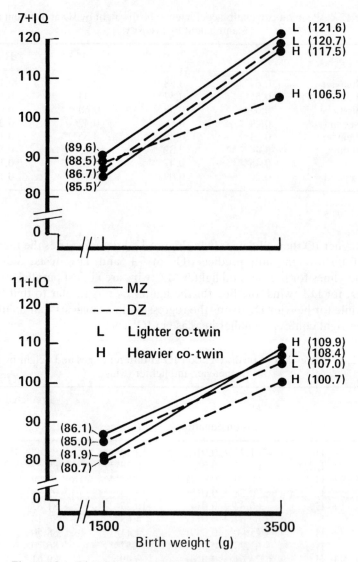

Figure 12.1. Bivariate regression of birthweight on IQ scores at 7+
and 11+ for MZ and DZ twins.

There is little evidence that any linear relationship exists between birth-weight and subsequent height. Only for the lighter DZ twin does the height–birthweight association show any significant relationship.

Looking at the relationship between differences in birthweight between co-twins and differences in outcome (Table 12.6), it appears that differences

Table 12.6. Pearson correlation coefficients: differences in birthweight and outcome by zygosity

	7+	9+	11+	Height
MZ	−0.153	−0.382	−0.195	0.150
DZ	0.337**	0.216	0.190	0.295

**$p \leqslant 0.05$.

in birthweight are not related to differences in IQ or height. The only case in which a significant correlation occurs is for DZ twins and their 7+ scores. The bivariate linear regression analysis is significant (at 5% level) only for this set of data and suggests that approximately 500 g difference is required before the heavier twin would have a larger 7+ score than his lighter co-twin ($y = -7.974 + 0.016x$).

Discussion

Little evidence was found to substantiate the claim that heavier twins will go on to grow taller and have higher IQ scores than their lighter co-twin. Indeed while the heavier twin in an MZ pair tended to have a slight advantage in IQ scores, for DZ twins the lighter twin had a slight advantage. On considering subsequent height, the reverse was true, with the lighter MZ and the heavier DZ being slightly taller than their respective co-twins. None of the differences, however, comparing heavier and lighter twins were of statistical significance.

Birthweight was found to be significantly positively associated with IQ, particularly for MZ twins, and with height only for lighter DZ twins. Furthermore a linear relationship between IQ and birthweight was noted and showed that at a given birthweight, a lighter twin, whether MZ or DZ, will have a higher IQ score than a heavier twin of identical birthweight. Perhaps the birthweight of a twin is not on its own an indication of the quality of the prenatal environment but has to be viewed in relation to that of its co-twin. Thus a twin weighing 1500 g will do better if his/her co-twin is heavier than if he/she is lighter.

There was little evidence for either MZ or DZ pairs that the size of difference in birthweight between pairs was indicative of the size of difference in subsequent IQ score and height between pairs. Where a significant linear relationship was noted (DZ twins and 7+ score) a difference in birthweight of 500 g was required before any difference in IQ scores would be predicted. Few of our twins had such a large difference (3 MZ pairs and 9 DZ pairs).

There was no evidence that the lighter MZ twin was unduly impaired as is suggested by the fetofetal transfusion syndrome. The IQ and birthweight association for the heavier and lighter twins is very similar in nature, with the regression lines being close to parallel (Figure 12.1). Our lighter MZ twins did, on average, score slightly less on the IQ tests but this was not statistically significant. No deficit was observed when considering the height of the twins at 5 years.

Twinning and Twins
Edited by I. MacGillivray, D. M. Campbell and B. Thompson
© 1988 John Wiley & Sons Ltd

CHAPTER 13

Some aspects of first births and the heights of twin sisters of known zygosity

BARBARA THOMPSON and CYNTHIA FRASER

Department of Obstetrics and Gynaecology, and Medical Research Council Medical Sociology Unit, University of Aberdeen, Aberdeen, UK

This chapter considers possible genetic influences in childbearing by comparing the experience of twin sisters of known zygosity. Since MZ twins are genetically identical, in general differences must be due to environmental factors, some of which may already be present in utero, e.g. size difference and birth order. Genetic differences may be obvious in some DZ twins, e.g. unlike sex. Conclusions on genetic effects derived from twin studies must be applicable to the whole population and, therefore, certain assumptions have to be made about the similar environment of twins and singletons. However, twins do differ from singletons in a number of physiological parameters, e.g. birthweight, perinatal mortality or congenital abnormalities as discussed in earlier chapters.

An initial study of 69 pairs of twin sisters, of all parities, demonstrated genetic influences in height and age at menarche, but numbers were inadequate for comparison of obstetric experience because of the complexities of the factors involved (Thompson *et al.*, 1981). Incomplete reproductive histories, complications of pregnancy, twin pregnancy, stillbirth, congenital anomaly and other factors affecting one (or both) twin sisters meant that the pair might have to be excluded, which for certain purposes left very small numbers for analysis. In order to obviate some of these problems, the present study is restricted to primiparae only.

Population and Method

The data refer to residents of Aberdeen City District (total population approximately 200 000) where both twins delivered their first baby in the Aberdeen Maternity Hospital (AMH) between 1951 and 1985. In 1951, 87%

of Aberdeen primigravidae were delived in AMH and since the late 1950s virtually all births have occurred there. Routinely, throughout the years women attending the antenatal clinic were asked if they were a twin and gradually a series of twin sisters was built up manually, and was used in the initial study. However, once the computerised Aberdeen Maternity and Neonatal Data Bank was established (Samphier and Thompson, 1981) twin sisters could be identified using date of birth and maiden name.

The analysis has been limited to 68 pairs of twin sisters for whom zygosity had been determined from blood samples (27 MZ, 41 DZ), who both delivered their first baby in AMH. Seven pairs had to be excluded as one or both of the sisters refused to co-operate and zygosity was unknown for a further pair as blood samples were unsuitable for testing when received at the laboratory.

Zygosity was available from two sources depending on when the twins were born and whether they had been at school in Aberdeen.

1. Initially, twins born before 1950 who could be traced and were available in the late 1960s were asked to give blood samples for zygosity determination at the Galton Laboratories (Corney *et al.*, 1972). Later a similar procedure was adopted for twins born from 1950, but not included in the series below.
2. Twins born in the 1950s and early 1960s who had attended school in Aberdeen had been included in studies carried out by Nylander (1970a) on three 5 year birth cohorts. He obtained blood samples and zygosity was determined locally.

There is a range of methods of analysis available, e.g. construction of broad heritability estimates or of models for estimating genetic variance. For present purposes, as the data were complicated and numbers relatively small, a simple method has been adopted in measuring the proportion of the variance of the difference between DZ twins that can be attributed to genetic variation. Inability to control for environmental factors and, therefore, the assumptions made which pose problems of interpretation are fully discussed by Cavalli-Sforza and Bodmer (1971).

Height

Adult height is largely determined by genetic factors, for example Cavalli-Sforza and Bodmer (1971), Hytten and Leitch (1971), Mittler (1971), Tanner (1978), and the numbers in the present study are adequate to demonstrate this. The correlation coefficient of the height of the twin sisters was higher for MZ than for DZ co-twins, 0.92 and 0.73 respectively and both were highly significant ($p \leq 0.001$). Corey *et al.* (1981) have reported similar findings in adult Norwegian twins.

Table 13.1. Comparison of own actual birthweights and adult heights of twin sisters

Re. co-twin		Birthweight difference between co-twins					
		Under 600 g			600 g and over		
Adult height	Weight at birth	No. of pairs (g)	Range (g)	Mean (g)	No. of pairs	Range (g)	Mean (g)
Taller	Lighter	7 (2)	26–568	303			
Taller	Heavier	6 (1)	29–425	214	6 (2)	633–1134	844
Same		1		511			
Total pairs		14 (3)			6 (2)		

Numbers in brackets are number of MZ twins.

Twenty pairs of the twin sisters (5 MZ, 15 DZ) had been born in AMH and their own birthweights were recorded. The differences in birthweight of the MZ twins ranged from 26–773 g and adult height from 1 to 2.5 cm. The DZ co-twins showed much greater variation from 29 to 1134 g difference in birthweight and from 0 to 10 cm in adult height. In twelve pairs of twins the heavier at birth (mean difference 241 g) was the taller adult (mean difference 5 cm). Seven twins lighter at birth (mean difference 303 g) grew to be taller (mean difference 2.7 cm) than their co-twin. The remaining pair of twin sisters with a birthweight difference of 511 g attained the same adult height. The indications were that there was a threshold at about 600 g difference (Table 13.1) – the heavier twin with at least that difference in birthweight was always the taller adult, whereas some twins lighter by less than this amount grew to be taller than their co-twin. It would have been interesting to compare length at birth with adult height, but this length has only been recorded in recent years.

Age at First Birth

At the birth of their first baby the women were aged from 16 to 37 and on average MZ twin sisters were over a year older than DZ twin sisters (24.4 years MZ, 23.2 years DZ).

The difference in time between co-twins having their first babies varied from one month to over 15 years (Table 13.2). About one quarter of twin sisters of both types delivered their first baby within a year of each other (26% MZ, 24% DZ). The smallest difference was for a DZ pair who had had a double wedding, the only one reported. More MZ sisters' first babies were born at least 5 years apart – 33% compared with 19% for DZ sisters – but the difference is not statistically significant. The maximum difference was over 15

Table 13.2. Age at first birth of twin sisters by zygosity

	MZ	DZ
No. of pairs	27	41
Actual range (years)	17.83–37.83	16.92–33.58
Difference between co-twins		
Range (years)	0.33–15.50	0.08–10.50
5 years or more	33%	19%
Correlation coefficient	0.066	0.419*

*$p \leqslant 0.02$.

years for an MZ pair. The correlation coefficiencies also show that DZ sisters tended to have their first babies closer together ($r = 0.4$; $p \leqslant 0.02$), there being more divergence between births to MZ sisters.

Many factors affect the timing of pregnancy and delay may be voluntary or due to various factors including relative infertility, infrequent coitus and gynaecological problems. More than 5 years had elapsed after marriage before one sister in each of 7 MZ and 4 DZ pairs had a first child, but the difference is not statistically significant. Three MZ sisters married for at least 5 years had had spontaneous abortions. Pregnancy followed infertility investigation in 2 MZ and 3 DZ sisters. Whether less recourse to fertility investigation by MZ twins reflects some fatalistic acceptance of the myth that one of a pair of identical twins is likely to be infertile, is not known.

The reasons for infertility were varied and included vaginal stenosis, scanty periods due to endocrine disorder, very infrequent menstruation coupled with the husband's prolonged absence in the Armed Forces and other menstrual irregularities and dysmenorrhoea, none of which affected the co-twins. One MZ twin with little expectation of ever becoming pregnant had adopted a child.

Infertility did not explain the delay in respect of the fourth DZ twin who was the only divorced woman in the series; an early and brief marriage was childless, but she became pregnant soon after remarriage in her mid-thirties. There was no explanation for the delay of over 8 years in one MZ twin whose sister married about one year earlier, had a baby within 18 months. One twin of 2 MZ and 3 DZ pairs had been unmarried when their first child was born.

About half the first born MZ and DZ twins married before their co-twin – 13 out of 27 MZ and 19 out of 41 DZ; one DZ pair married at the same time. Usually the first married was the first to have a baby, the exceptions (7 MZ, 10 DZ) mainly being accounted for by one twin becoming an unmarried mother, infertility or there being only a few months difference between when the twin sisters married and between when they delivered. Somewhat different results were reported by Corey et al. (1980) who found that the first born

MZ twin tended to marry earlier than her co-twin and that MZ twins tended to be more similar for the interval between marriage and the birth of their first child.

Experience of Pregnancy and Outcome

Table 13.3 gives details of certain features of the twin sisters' experience of pregnancy, first delivery and the outcome.

Previous Pregnancies. One twin in 7 MZ and 9 DZ pairs had had one or two previous pregnancies (Table 13.3), but there was no concordance between co-twins. Three twins (2 MZ, 1 DZ) had had a pregnancy terminated. No twin had had both a termination and a spontaneous abortion. It was noted

Table 13.3. Some factors in reproductive performance and outcome of first births to twin sisters by zygosity (total number of pairs: 27 MZ, 41 DZ)

| | No. of pairs affected | |
	MZ	DZ
Previous pregnancy:		
Abortion(s) only	5	8
Termination only	2	1
Complications of pregnancy:		
Threatened abortion	1	3
Hypertension	7 (4)	3 (1)
Proteinuric PE	4	1
APH	2	3
Complications of delivery:		
Breech/transverse lie	2	2
Cord round neck	2 (1)	2
PPH	2	3
Operative delivery[a]	14 (4)	24 (4)
Outcome:		
Twins	1	—
Stillbirth	3	1
Congenital anomaly	2	—

Numbers in brackets are numbers of twin pairs concordant
[a] See Table 13.4

that all 5 twins (3 MZ, 2 DZ) who had had two spontaneous abortions were
second born twins; this is of doubtful significance unless it implies that the
second twin is more prone to abortion. It is well known that the second twin is
more likely to suffer from certain conditions, e.g. hypoxia at birth (Derom
and Thiery, 1976), and some long-term effect might be implicated.

Complications of Pregnancy.   There was no concordance between co-twins
in threatened abortion (1 MZ, 3 DZ) or for antepartum haemorrhage (APH)
(2 MZ, 3 DZ).

One twin in each of 3 pairs of MZ twins had hydramnios, gestational
diabetes and congestive heart failure respectively.

The classification of pre-eclampsia (PE) used here was established by
Nelson (1955) – see Chapter 7. More MZ than DZ twin pairs were affected by
all degrees of hypertension and PE ($p \leqslant 0.01$). No co-twins suffered from
proteinuric PE, whereas in half the pairs affected by hypertension in pregnancy there was concordance (4 of 7 MZ; 1 of 3 DZ). A familial predisposition to hypertension in pregnancy is well established (Adams and Finlayson,
1961; Chesley *et al.*, 1961) and may be a precursor to essential hypertension in
later life. The lack of MZ twin sister concordance for proteinuric PE, mainly a
disease of primigravidae, is consistent with the view that it has a different
pathological aetiology to mild PE or hypertension. Sutherland *et al.* (1981)
studied mothers and mothers-in-law of women with proteinuric PE and
controls: she assumed that the condition could be a simple recessive trait and
concluded that her findings fully supported a maternal genotype hypothesis
though multifactorial inheritance could not be ruled out.

Weight Gain

Weight gain was considered up to about 30 weeks gestation and as near as
possible comparable for each twin, e.g. if both twins had been weighed at 29
weeks, these weights were taken in preference to weights at 30 and 32 weeks.
Average weekly gain was calculated by dividing the difference between the
woman's weight at about 30 weeks and at her first antenatal clinic attendance
by the number of weeks. Only 21 MZ and 38 DZ pairs have been included in
the analysis. If either twin sister was affected by certain factors likely to
interfere with normal weight gain, e.g. proteinuric PE, carrying twins or a
baby with certain congenital anomalies, or no relevant weights were
recorded, both twins were excluded from the analysis.

The correlation coefficient for the average weekly weight gain of MZ and
DZ co-twins was 0.447 and 0.188 respectively, significant at the 5% level for
MZ twins only. This indicates that MZ co-twins tended to have a more similar
average weekly weight gain in the first 30 weeks of pregnancy than DZ pairs
and suggests a genetic contribution. Sutherland (1980) who studied average

weekly weight gain throughout pregnancy, without exclusions for complications and including estimates in the case of incomplete histories, reported correlation coefficients of 0.374 and 0.367 for MZ and DZ co-twins respectively, both significant at the 5% level. She inferred the existence of a non-genetic contribution towards variations in weight gain, but suggested further studies with unselected women before coming to a definitive conclusion.

At one time it seemed that the pattern, i.e. the time of gain and rate of increase, rather than the actual amount of weight gain might be important. This hypothesis was tested by Sutherland (1980) for a combined Aberdeen and Edinburgh series of twin sisters. However, the results showed that the pattern of weight gain was no more similar for MZ than for DZ twin sisters.

Types of Delivery

The twins were concordant for type of delivery in 56% of MZ and 46% of DZ pairs, not a significant difference. Two pairs of MZ twins were delivered by caesarean section and 2 pairs of DZ twins had forceps deliveries (Table 13.4). Thirteen pairs of MZ and 17 pairs of DZ twins had spontaneous deliveries.

Table 13.4. Type of delivery of twin sisters

Type of delivery	MZ			DZ		
		No.	%		No.	%
Operative — both twins						
Both caesarean section	2			—		
Both forceps	—	4	15	2	4	10
One caesarean section; other forceps	2			2		
Operative — 1 twin only						
One caesarean section, other spontaneous delivery	2			5		
One forceps, other spontaneous delivery	7	10	37	13	20	49
One assisted breech, other spontaneous delivery	1			2		
Spontaneous — both twins		13	48		17	41
Total		27	100		41	100

The sisters experienced different operative procedures – one a caesarean section, the other forceps – in 2 pairs of MZ and DZ pairs respectively. The type of intervention depends to some extent on clinical practice and it may be noted that the reasons for the operation whether concordant or not for caesarean section and forceps were similar for the 4 pairs of MZ sisters, namely: short stature with contracted pelvises (1 caesarean section, the other forceps); large head/fetus and disproportion (both caesarean section); in the remaining 2 pairs (1 both caesarean section; the other caesarean section and forceps) both twins developed increasing hypertension in late pregnancy. In contrast the reasons for operative delivery of DZ pairs were different, e.g. fetal distress and severe proteinuric PE (both forceps); APH and fetal distress (1 forceps, other caesarean section).

Outcome

Most of the twin sisters had normal, liveborn singleton births. With the exception of an unexplained stillbirth to a DZ sister who had threatened to abort in early pregnancy, all the problems were with MZ sisters, but were not concordant between pairs. One MZ twin delivered unlike-sex twins, one of whom had hydrocephalus and died; her sister, also in her early twenties, had a normal pregnancy and outcome. An MZ sister who had suffered from hydramnios delivered a stillborn baby who had multiple abnormalities including anencephaly; her sister developed proteinuric PE, but had a normal liveborn baby – both were in their mid-twenties and had spontaneous deliveries. The central nervous system malformations both occurred in the offspring of second born MZ sisters. Two other MZ sisters, both first born, had stillbirths in association with APH.

Birthweight

In considering birthweight, the two cases of congenital anomaly (both MZ) have been excluded, which automatically excludes the twin pregnancy and one of the stillbirths. In 8 of the remaining 25 pairs of MZ twins, both sisters delivered boys and in 8 both sisters delivered girls; in the remaining 9 pairs the cousins were of different sexes. Thus, the MZ sisters had 25 boys and 25 girls. The DZ twins delivered 37 boys and 45 girls; 6 pairs had boys, 10 pairs had girls, and in 25 pairs one twin had a boy and the other a girl. No exclusions have been made on account of previous pregnancies, partly because of small numbers, but also because most of the women affected had had one abortion and this has been shown to have no effect on subsequent birthweight (Billewicz and Thomson, 1973; Pickering, 1987) and in certain circumstances it may be beneficial (Alberman et al., 1980).

Gestation was recorded in completed weeks and where necessary the best

Table 13.5. Sex and birthweight, crude means (g) of first births to twin sisters by zygosity

			MZ		DZ	
			No. of pairs (25[a])	Crude mean birthweight (g)	No. of pairs (41)	Crude mean birthweight (g)
Cousins:						
Like sex	Male	Male	8	3064.3	6	3198.5
	Female	Female	8	3164.1	10	3115.7
Unlike sex	Male		9	3402.9	25	3343.3
	Female			3377.7		3245.4
All males				3177.3 ± 609.1		3290.3 ± 422.6
All females				3241.0 ± 593.0		3195.1 ± 461.9

[a] Excluding pairs affected by twins or congenital anomalies.

estimate taken, having regard to all the evidence (Hall et al., 1985). Labour had been induced in 2 pairs of DZ sisters and in one sister in 7 MZ and 11 DZ pairs. There was no difference overall between MZ and DZ pairs in the length of gestation or in the difference between co-twins. Most sisters had delivered at 39–41 weeks gestation (82% MZ; 74% DZ) and at the same gestation or 1 week different from their co-twin. The biggest discrepancies of 5 and 6 weeks were associated with the two stillbirths following antepartum haemorrhage.

There was a wide range of birthweights from 1360 to 4394 g and it was greater for offspring of MZ sisters. Table 13.5 shows that overall girls born to MZ twins weighed more than boys, who were particularly disadvantaged if both cousins were boys. It may be noted that the birthweight of the cousins was greater if they were of different sexes. When the babies were of unlike sex, the boys tended to be heavier than the girls.

Cousin pair correlation coefficients for birthweight are shown in Table 13.6. Initially, birthweights were standardised for sex only. DZ twins tended to produce babies of more similar birthweight than MZ twins ($r = 0.300$ and 0.188 respectively), but the strength of the association was weak and not statistically significant. It was thought that these results might be distorted by a few very low birthweights associated with short gestations. The data were, therefore, adjusted for sex and gestation by standardising to male birthweights at 40 weeks gestation (Robson, 1955), using centile tables based on over 52 000 Aberdeen singleton live births delivered in 1948–1954 (Thomson et al., 1968).

Controlling for variation in gestation, the strength of association in birthweight between cousins was reduced for both MZ and DZ twin sisters,

Table 13.6. Correlation coefficient of birthweights of first births to twin sisters by zygosity

	MZ	DZ
No. of pairs	25[a]	41
Birthweights adjusted for:		
Sex only	0.188	0.300
Sex and gestation:		
all pairs	0.046	0.251
excluding pairs affected by:		
stillbirths	−0.036	0.263
stillbirths and proteinuric PE	0.124	0.284

[a] Excluding pairs affected by twins or congenital anomalies.

although again, DZ twins still had babies of more similar birthweight. Excluding pairs where one twin had either delivered a stillborn baby or had proteinuric PE (factors likely to depress birthweight) correlation coefficients still remained low.

Discussion

The 27 MZ and 41 DZ pairs of twin sisters in the study were adequate to demonstrate a genetic influence on height. They also suggest that the rate of weight gain up to 30 weeks may to a small extent be controlled by the maternal genotype. However, this needs to be confirmed.

MZ twin sisters had a greater range of experience than the corresponding DZ twin sisters and they were less efficient in reproduction. They experienced more abortions, complications of pregnancy and labour and more problems with stillbirths and congenital anomalies. However, MZ co-twins were found to be no more similar than DZ twins in their experiences of pregnancy and labour. MZ twins were discordant for threatened abortion, APH, proteinuric PE, hypertension, hydramnios, abnormal lie, cord round neck, twin pregnancy, baby with central nervous system congenital anomaly, stillbirth, sex of offspring and postpartum haemorrhage. Some concordance was found in both MZ and DZ twins for hypertension and both babies to one pair of MZ sisters had the cord round their neck. Larger numbers would be needed to determine whether the first or second born twin is at a disadvantage in reproduction.

The type of intervention in labour partly depends on clinical practice. Although more MZ twin pairs were affected by operative delivery they were usually discordant. However, it may be noted that where both MZ twins had a caesarean section or forceps delivery the reasons were the same, and related to either stature or hypertension. In contrast, the reason for operative delivery in DZ pairs were different.

The analysis of birthweight, even when different exclusions were made and taking into account sex and gestation, shows that birthweight is not under the direct control of the maternal genotype which is in accordance with other studies (Robson, 1955; Sutherland, 1980; Magnus, 1984). Some sophisticated methods of analysis are being developed to assess the contributions of genetic, familial and environmental factors in determining birthweight (e.g. Nance and Corey, 1976; Magnus, 1984).

The problems of assessing length of gestation and the practice adopted in Aberdeen have been discussed by Hall et al. (1985). In this study there was no difference between the MZ and DZ twin pairs in length of gestation. However, Sutherland (1980) suggested that the main genetic contribution to gestation length was likely to come from the male and recommended a study of the wives of twin brothers. As the dates of birth of husbands is not routinely recorded in the maternity records twin brothers as husbands can only be identified by direct questioning of the wives. This has been in progress for about 3 years. As with the twin sisters, at any particular time twin pairs may have to be excluded because one has had no children or births have taken place elsewhere. However, with twin brothers an added complication in building up a series of primiparae is that one or both sisters-in-law may have had their first child by a previous partner.

Since August, 1968, the zygosity of like-sex twins born in AMH has been determined routinely from blood samples and placentation. As over half primigravidae and their husbands have been born and brought up in Aberdeen, zygosity will already be available for the majority of twin sisters and husbands who are twin brothers, who attend AMH in the future.

Twinning and Twins
Edited by I. MacGillivray, D. M. Campbell and B. Thompson
© 1988 John Wiley & Sons Ltd

CHAPTER 14

Summary of main conclusions with implications for research and practice

IAN MACGILLIVRAY and DORIS M. CAMPBELL

Department of Obstetrics and Gynaecology, University of Aberdeen, Aberdeen, UK

and

BARBARA THOMPSON

Medical Research Council Medical Sociology Unit and Department of Obstetrics and Gynaecology, University of Aberdeen, Aberdeen, UK

The increasing interest in twinning manifest in recent years has resulted in a plethora of studies on many different aspects from many parts of the world. Findings, however, have often been contradictory or equivocal and many studies have been of questionable validity. Nevertheless, some pronouncements have been acclaimed and perpetuated without critical assessment and the real state of knowledge on twinning is confused.

In this book we have reviewed reports on certain biological, environmental and clinical aspects of twinning augmented by analysis of data for a total population of a geographical area in north-east Scotland available for up to 35 years. This has enabled us to draw some conclusions with implications for further research and for clinical practice.

Types and Aetiology of Twinning

Two types of twinning have for long been recognised and zygosity determination at birth is often straightforward. Sex difference indicates dizygotic twins (with the rare exception of heterokaryotypic pairs), whereas all twins with a monochorionic placenta are monozygotic. Thus, from simple observations of sex and placentation, the zygosity of about half of all twins can be determined at birth.

Where there are two placentae, either separate or fused, or problems in classification arise and the twins are of the same sex, injection of a contrast medium can demonstrate transplacental circulation which, with rare exceptions, proves monochorionicity.

Vascular anastomosis gives rise to the twin transfusion syndrome, but the pathophysiology of this condition, which on some estimates affects 15% of monochorionic pairs, is not fully understood. Vascular communication in dichorionic placentae is common in animals giving rise to chimerism, but is extremely rare in humans. Like-sex twins with a dichorionic placenta may be dizygotic or monozygotic – the ratio among Europeans seems to be about 3 to 1. The probability of dizygosity can be calculated from analysis of blood group and serum polymorphism. However, new methods of genetic 'finger-printing' based on highly variable DNA markers should reduce the need for these complex calculations in future. Until now many studies have relied on Weinberg's method which estimates the number of DZ twins by doubling the number of unlike-sex pairs. However, small samples and the tendency of DZ twins more often to be of like sex introduce errors. There is evidence that the sex ratio in DZ twins varies markedly with the time between ovulation and insemination.

Although much is known about the factors which influence dizygotic twinning, the causes of monozygotic twinning are more obscure. Until recently the remarkable constancy with which MZ twinning was reported throughout the world at about 3.5 per 1000 deliveries ruled out the likelihood of major environmental factors. Studies of the armadillo which invariably produces monozygotic litters have provided some insight. It is probable that a rare genetic change has become established in the armadillo which affects the interaction of blastomeres so that their developmental separation is precipi-tated. However, in humans, genetic factors may also play a part as a familial tendency to MZ twinning has been described, although it appears to be rare.

It has been proposed that with respect to MZ twinning, developmental separation may be represented by dichorionic, monochorionic, monoamnio-tic, and conjoined twins on a time-span extending over the first 2 weeks of gestation. Studies relating to delayed ovulation, late conception and implantation and sex ratio in twinning have highlighted the importance of the timing of these early events, not only to the time of fertilisation, but also to the timing of follicular maturation. The possibility of a developmental 'clock' coupled with 'unequal X inactivation' is an area for further biological research. Support for the idea that delayed implantation may predispose to MZ twinning results from observations that monozygotic twinning may follow in vitro fertilisation, possibly due either to the use of clomiphene and gonadotrophins causing early division of the embryo, or a weakness of the embryo itself.

Dizygotic twinning results from the development of two ova released from the ovaries which are fertilised simultaneously. Fertilisation at different times in a single menstrual cycle, that is superfecundation, has occasionally been reported. The implantation of a fertilised ovum in an already pregnant uterus, that is superfetation, has not yet been proven to occur in humans.

Pituitary gonadotrphins are responsible for controlling the release of ova, and either an excess of pituitary stimulation or a failure of the inhibiting mechanism which allows only one maturing follicle to be dominant and survive may result in dizygotic twinning. Increasing maternal age is associated with both increasing levels of pituitary gonadotrophin and of dizygotic twinning. Also, Nigerian women who have had twins have higher levels of follicle stimulating hormone than mothers of singletons and Japanese women with low dizygotic twinning rates have low levels of both follicle stimulating and luteinising hormones. It is well known also that stimulation with gonado-trophins in infertile women can produce multiple births. However, it is necessary for studies to be undertaken to determine whether there is a genetic or inherent predisposition to the production of gonadotrophins by mothers of twins, or whether there is some environmental factor involved, such as an item of diet. Such factors as psychological stress, nutrition, or climate might modify hypothalamic–pituitary–ovarian function leading to increased ovula-tion with many follicles being developed, ripened and ruptured.

It has been suggested that oral contraception may influence twinning by affecting the hypothalamic–pituitary–ovarian axis hormones. However, the only known prospective study of a total population in which zygosity was accurately determined showed no association between oral contraceptive use prior to pregnancy and either monozygotic or dizygotic twinning. The type of pill, however, was not considered.

In vitro fertilisation resulting in DZ twinning is increased the greater the number of embryos that are replaced, coupled with the quality of the embryos. Further studies of the phenomenon of 'helping' which accounts for this increase are needed.

Epidemiological Factors

Data on the incidence of twinning and higher multiple conceptions are unsatisfactory because of the problems of studying abortions and the occur-rence of the 'vanishing' twin. Thus, studies of the epidemiology of twinning have to be based on births. In most respects the epidemiology of higher multiple maternities resembles that of twinning, but the pattern has become confused by the use of ovulation-stimulating preparations in the treatment of infertility.

Throughout the world, there are undoubtedly large differences in the incidence of twin births, mainly accounted for by unlike-sex twins and attributed to DZ twinning. There are few large population-based series of twins in which diagnosis of zygosity has been made by direct techniques. The epidemiology of twins of different types has usually been based on Wein-berg's method and, therefore, subject to criticism already mentioned. Know-ledge of geographical variation is best provided from Nigeria, USA and Canada, parts of Europe, Japan, Australia and New Zealand, with frag-mented or incomplete data from other countries or areas. Reported rates of twinning are highest in Nigeria, lowest in Japan and cluster between 8 and 20 per 1000 maternities in most other countries. In Europe and the USA at least, rates appear to increase with latitude. Clustering of twin births has been reported from isolated communities and may be due to factors such as inbreeding, a twin-prone sedentes population or to localised environmental effects.

Evidence suggests that twinning rates are usually modified by migration. For example migrants from West Africa have lower twinning rates than sedentes. However, migrants from Japan tend to keep their low rates. Also differences in twinning rates apparent in Europe are not found in the offspring of migrants to Canada. More detailed analysis of available data, e.g. European migrants to Israel, would be helpful.

Between the end of the 1950s and the late 1960s or early 1970s, unlike-sex twinning rates declined in most Western countries. The picture regarding other countries is unclear in the absence of reliable data over the longer term. Trends in twinning rates in Western countries from the early 1970s are difficult to interpret partly because the use of ovulation-stimulating agents has not yet been quantified specifically in relation to these trends.

Throughout the epidemiological review of twinning, direct comparison of findings reported were bedevilled by a multitude of recurring factors. These included:

1. Differences in the basis of data, e.g. population, area, hospital, selected group, etc.
2. Differences in the detail and standard of recording.
3. Differences in the timing or time period and classification of data, particularly important because of secular changes in childbearing.
4. Differences in the role of abortion legislation and practice.
5. Differences in the incidence of spontaneous abortion.
6. Inadequate information on ovulation stimulation treatment for infertility and in vitro fertilisation.
7. Different methods of zygosity determination, e.g. Weinberg's method, blood samples, appearance, etc.
8. Different methods of statistical analysis.

Factors affecting Twinning

In view of the wide variations in unlike-sex twinning, attention has focused on studies reporting on certain genetic, familial and environmental factors which might help to explain the phenomenon. Problems encountered in making comparisons were similar to those referred to above in relation to epidemiology. Nevertheless, some broad conclusions may be made.

There is general agreement that DZ twinning increases with maternal age to a peak and then declines. Reasons for the different ages at which twinning peaks are uncertain, but the age at which childbearing starts may be a factor. A parity affect is less certain, but may be mediated through age, indicating Milham's gonadotrophin hypothesis. Taller and heavier women are more likely to have twins than short and thin women, but they do not have a higher nutritional intake. Whether such women have overactivity of hypothalamic–pituitary–ovarian axis hormones is unknown. Smoking, which may affect appetite, does not seem to have any effect on twinning. Although there may be no association with nutrition, there is some speculation that a specific item(s) in the diet could sometimes be involved, e.g. yams in Nigeria. This might help to explain definite geographical and ethnic differences and possible seasonal variations, but the findings on seasonal influences are difficult to interpret.

The evidence of a relationship between twinning and social class is contradictory. Classifications of social class are varied and there is evidence of marked secular changes so that the association changes over time. Such major problems make it impossible to come to any conclusion.

There is conclusive evidence of a familial tendency to DZ twinning through the maternal line; transmission through the father is uncertain. The same may rarely apply to MZ twinning, but the findings are more confused.

The fecundability hypothesis is difficult to test. It is based on observations on premarital conceptions, on the rapidity of conception after marriage or following the return of husbands from military service. Interpretation of the data is difficult, however, because of the differential use of efficient contraception and restrictions on family size.

The interrelationship of many of the factors considered is complex and secular trends make comparisons difficult. Until there is adequate comparable population data available it must be recognised that some findings reported may be artefacts.

Antenatal Management

In normal human pregnancy there is considerable maternal physiological adaptation and in women with twin pregnancies the response is exaggerated, triggered by increased production of both steroid and protein hormones from the fetoplacental unit. This exaggerated maternal response is important in ensuring good sized healthy babies, but is also relevant to the practising clinician. Different standards of normality have to be accepted for multiple pregnancies compared with singleton pregnancies and allowance made for more frequent occurrence of abnormalities. In addition, an exaggerated maternal response, for example, excessive weight gain, might lead the clinician to suspect the presence of a multiple pregnancy.

Early diagnosis of multiple pregnancy is important in the interests of both mother and babies. Ultrasonic scanning has revolutionised the situation making it possible much earlier in gestation to confirm the presence of a suspected twin pregnancy. Routine ultrasonic scanning at booking for all pregnant women is unlikely to detect all multiple pregnancies as the gestation of such a scan may not be optimal for the diagnosis to be made; also the ultrasonographer may not be alerted by a clinical suspicion of multiple pregnancy.

While most pregnancy complications are slightly increased in women expecting twins, the major problems with respect to management are preterm delivery and proteinuric pre-eclampsia, both of which are markedly increased in twin pregnancies. Both these complications lead to problems for the babies who are delivered too soon and often with retarded growth. This leads to much increased perinatal mortality in twins compared with singletons.

As the aetiology of preterm labour and proteinuric pre-eclampsia remains unknown, management has to be empirical and aims at minimising the potential ill-effects. The efficacy of bedrest, hotly debated over the years, although still advocated by some obstetricians, would appear to have no major obstetric advantage as it does not improve the outcome with respect to perinatal mortaility or birthweight, or affect the incidence of preterm labour or pre-eclampsia. Trying to identify those women who will deliver preterm or develop proteinuric pre-eclampsia has proved very difficult, even for women expecting twins, despite their more frequent visits to antenatal clinics.

Because of the exaggerated maternal response in twin pregnancy, women expecting twins are important in research into preterm labour and proteinuric pre-eclampsia. They may well provide pointers to the aetiology of these conditions and clues as to predictors with important implications for clinical management.

Management of Labour

Women expecting twins should be delivered under the best conditions where specialist paediatric care is available. Labour in multiple pregnancies carries more risk both to mother and babies because of malpresentations and malposition of the fetuses, coupled with the low birthweight of the babies. Elective caesarean section for malpresentation in preterm labour, particularly advocated in the USA is a highly controversial practice. In Europe a more conservative approach with respect to caesarean section has not resulted in a poorer outcome for twins, although the elective caesarean section rate is still higher than in singleton pregnancy.

Fetal Outcome

With respect to the outcome of twin pregnancy, it has generally been reported that twin II, particularly if a male, was smaller and fared worse with respect to perinatal mortality and morbidity than twin I. Recent studies from Aberdeen, however, have demonstrated secular trends and have shown that this no longer applies. Attempting to derive birthweight standards for twins proved impossible because of the range and complexity of the factors involved coupled with the secular trends in birthweight. As in singletons the birthweight of twin I has decreased over time whereas the birthweight of twin II increased until there is now no difference in the average birthweight of twin I and twin II. Attempts to examine the effects of maternal and fetal factors on birthweight implicate different factors according to whether the combined birthweight or individual birthweights of twins I and II, or the difference in birthweight between the twin pairs, are considered, No maternal or fetal factors at present readily explain the increase in weight of twin II over the time period studied. Further work is needed in this field.

The perinatal death rate has always been much higher in twins than in singletons and this is still true, mainly due to the lower birthweight associated with shorter gestation and poor fetal growth. Although previously with respect to perinatal mortality and morbidity, twin II was found to fare worse than twin I, males poorer than females, monozygotic worse than dizygotic, this is not so now, perhaps because earlier work did not take into account the interrelationship between all factors affecting outcome. Now the small size of the baby appears to be much more important than other factors. It is of particular interest that maternal factors such as age, parity, social class, and smoking do not have a significant influence on perinatal mortality or morbidity as they do in singletons. With respect to the effect of zygosity on perinatal mortality this needs to be studied much more closely with the accurate determination of zygosity for twins, whether the babies die or survive. As indicated earlier problems of interpretation arise when zygosity is inferred from other methods. Even in centres with a special interest in twinning, complete zygosity determination has not yet been possible.

Congenital Anomalies

A fetal anomaly in a multiple pregnancy has many implications that differ from an anomaly in a pregnancy where only one fetus is involved.

For clinicians and parents alike, the key feature of the occurrence of anomalies in twins is discordance. Whereas, until a decade or so, it was unusual for congenital anomalies in twins to be diagnosed antenatally, recent technical innovations have enabled the detection of the fetus with certain anomalies.

The incidence of congenital anomalies in twins is difficult to estimate because of problems not only of studying abortion both spontaneous and induced, but also of ascertainment of anomalies in neonates. The frequency of abortions in twins appears to be three times higher than in singletons and many of the aborted fetuses are abnormal. In most studies anomalies diagnosed at birth have been found to be more prevalent in twins than in singletons. The rates reported have varied due to such factors as small numbers, thoroughness of examination for anomalies, the age and parity of mothers. Evidence available indicates that anomalies are more frequent in like-sex than unlike-sex twins and zygosity studies tend to show that monozygotic twins are more liable to have congenital anomalies than dizygotic. Placentation does not appear to influence the overall prevalence at birth of anomalies, but monochorionic placentation may be involved in the aetiology of some specific anomalies, e.g. acardia and certain structural defects of the heart. Some anomalies such as conjoined twins, fetus-in-fetu, acardia and fetus papyraceus are unique to multiple conception.

The possible explanations for this association between twinning and congenital anomalies have been discussed under two headings. (i) a common aetiology for certain types of anomaly and certain types of twinning, explanations including a similar predisposition, similar exogenous agents, and the consequences of fusion of embryos or twin embryogenesis. (ii) Fetus–fetus interaction, including fusion of embryos, the vascular consequences of fetal death and intrauterine constraint.

The discordance of anomalies may be due to many factors such as the greater likelihood of survival if only one is affected; abnormal splitting of the zygote; or differences between the twins in their stage of development and, therefore, susceptiblity at the time when exposed to an insult, e.g. teratogens.

If one of the twins is abnormal special problems arise, and depending on the condition and when diagnosed, there may be problems in clinical management. However, in all instances, careful and sympathetic counselling is essential to enable the mother and the family to take whatever decisions are necessary and to come to terms with the situation.

Progress in studying the association between twinning and certain congenital anomalies seems to lie in the development of multi-centre registers (Weatherall et al., 1979) which should help to resolve the present inherent problems of bias of ascertainment, zygosity determination and small numbers. However, routine data collected for epidemiological purposes do not permit sufficiently precise information for analytical studies designed to test hypotheses, and more rigorous methods of data collection are essential.

Development of Twins

Findings on the relationship between birthweight, height and intelligence of twins are conflicting. However, most studies have been based on highly selected and usually small samples varying in the age at which children were followed up, in the tests used, in the method of zygosity determination and in the type of analysis.

An Aberdeen population-based prospective study with zygosity of like-sexed twins determined from blood samples found no support for the hypothesis that the heavier twin will grow taller and have a higher IQ score than the lighter co-twin. Furthermore, the lighter MZ twins were not impaired as suggested by the fetofetal transfusion hypothesis. It was also found that birthweight was positively associated with IQ score giving a linear relationship. However, it is suggested that the birthweight of the co-twin should be considered in assessing the quality of the prenatal environment.

Twin Sisters becoming Mothers

Further studies of genetic influences were carried out by an analysis of first births to twin sisters whose zygosity had been accurately determined. These indicated that MZ sisters were less efficient in reproduction compared with corresponding DZ sisters. However, MZ sisters were no more concordant than DZ sisters in their experience of pregnancy and labour. Both MZ and DZ twins were concordant for gestational hypertension, confirming the well-known familial predisposition to the condition. In accordance with other studies birthweight was found not to be under the direct control of the maternal genotype. Limited data on birthweight and adult height suggested a threshold in the difference in birthweight over which the lighter twin never 'caught up' in height with the heavier co-twin.

It was concluded that further studies of adult twins are required into the possibility of maternal weight gain being controlled by maternal genotype; the second born twin being at some disadvantage in reproduction; and that gestation length may be determined paternally.

The Future

The immediate future holds great promise for a better understanding of the biological and physiological aspects of twinning and higher multiples as the more sophisticated techniques associated with DNA probes and in vitro fertilisation are developed and become readily available. With the new techniques it should be possible to define precisely the incidence of MZ and DZ twinning on a scale not previously feasible and also to determine the paternal contribution, if any, to twinning. Frequently in our review the role of hormonal control has been questioned, e.g. regarding twinning and height, fertility; and further work is required to establish the levels of hormone production which may be important.

Clarification of the importance of factors affecting twinning is often obscured by the lack of comparable population data and of knowledge of how changes taking place in society may affect interpretation, e.g. differential changes in secular trends in age, use of contraception. Progress depends on identifying artefacts. With respect to the clinical aspects of twin pregnancies, again there is a deficiency of geographically defined population-based data. At present many conclusions are drawn from individual hospital reports and thus based on highly selected groups making useful comparisons between outcomes very difficult. Properly conducted population studies should in the future give clues as to the aetiology of pregnancy complications, allowing earlier prediction and preventive action where appropriate. The multiplicity of and interaction between factors affecting pregnancy outcome needs a fresh approach.

The different experiences of the first and second twin in utero, in childhood development, and in reproductive experience raise some intriguing questions. This area merits further research in order to assess possible preventive measures which may be taken to help reduce any disadvantage relevant to the birth order of the twins.

As yet there is controversy with respect to the importance of genetic and environmental influences on human reproduction, e.g. birthweight. Studies of twin pregnancies with their exaggerated maternal response, and twins themselves, both together and separately comparing the difference between them, provide useful models for certain types of further research.

The way ahead is a challenge to local, national and international collaborators to utilise existing and elaborate new techniques in pursuing the causation and physiological outcome of twinning, and to study appropriate populations taking advantage of computing facilities and of statistical techniques being developed, thus advancing knowledge on all aspects of twinning and twins.

References

Aaron, J. B., Silverman, S. H. and Halperin, J. (1961). Fetal survival in twin delivery. *American Journal of Obstetrics and Gynecology*, **81**, 331–334.

Abel, E. L. (1982). Consumption of alcohol during pregnancy: a review of effects on growth and development of offspring. *Human Biology*, **54**, 421–453.

Aberg, A., Mitelman, F. and Cantz, M. (1978). Cardiac puncture of fetus with Hurler's disease avoiding abortion of unaffected co-twin. *Lancet*, **ii**, 990–991.

Adams, E. M. and Finlayson, A. (1961). Familial aspects of pre-eclampsia and hypertension in pregnancy. *Lancet*, **ii**, 1375–1378.

Adeleye, J. A. (1972). Retained second twin in Ibadan: its fate and management. *American Journal of Obstetrics and Gynecology*, **114**, 204–207.

Aherne, W., Strong, S. J. and Corney, G. (1968). The structure of the placenta in the twin transfusion syndrome. *Biologia Neonatorum*, **12**, 121–135.

Aiken, R. A. (1969). An account of the Birmingham "sextuplets". *Journal of Obstetrics and Gynaecology of the British Commonwealth*, **76**, 684–691.

Aird, I. (1959). Conjoined twins—further observations. *British Medical Journal*, **ii**, 1313–1315.

Al-Awadi, S. A., Farag, T. I., Teebi, A. S., Naguib, K. K. and El-Khalifa, M. Y. (1984). Anencephaly: disappearing in Kuwait? *Lancet*, **ii**, 701–702.

Alberman, E. D. and Creasy, M. R. (1977). Frequency of chromosomal abnormalities in miscarriages and perinatal deaths. *Journal of Medical Genetics*, **14**, 313–315.

Alberman, E. D., Roman, E., Phoroath, P. O. D. and Chamberlain, G. (1980). Birthweight before and after spontaneous abortion, *British Journal of Obstetrics and Gynaecology*, **87**, 275–280.

Allen, G. (1960). A differential method for estimation of type frequencies in triplets and quadruplets. *American Journal of Human Genetics*, **12**, 210–224.

Allen, G. (1978). The parity effect and fertility in mothers of twins. In: *Twin Research 3, Biology and Epidemiology*, Nance, W. E., Allen, G. and Parisi, P. (eds.), Alan R. Liss, New York, pp. 89–97.

Allen, G. (1981). Errors of Weinberg's difference method. In: *Twin Research 3: Part A, Twin Biology and Multiple Pregnancy*, Gedda, L., Parisi, P. and Nance, W. E. (eds.), Alan R. Liss, New York, pp. 71–74.

Allen, G. (1986). The non-decline in US, twin birth rates 1964–1980. *Acta Geneticae Medicae et Gemellologiae*, **35**, Abstracts, p. 28.

Allen, G. and Schachter, J. (1970). Do conception delays explain some changes in twinning rates? *Acta Geneticae Medicae et Gemellologiae*, **19**, 30–34.

Allen, G. and Schachter, J. (1971). Ease of conception in mothers of twins. *Social Biology*, **18**, 18–27.

Allen, G. and Hrubec, Z. (1986). The MZ twinning rate: how nearly constant? *Acta Geneticae Medicae et Gemellologiae*, **35**, Abstracts, p. 51.

Alm, I. (1953). The longterm prognosis for prematurely born children. *Acta Paediatrica*, **42** (Suppl. 94), 9016.

Altman, D. G. and Coles, E. C. (1980). Assessing birthweight-for-dates on a continuous scale. *Annals of Human Biology*, **7**, 35–44.

Amatuzio, J. C. and Gorlin, R. J. (1981). Conjoined acardiac monsters. *Archives of Pathology and Laboratory Medicine*, **105**, 253–255.

Anderson, R. C. (1977). Congenital cardiac malformations in 109 sets of twins and triplets. *American Journal of Cardiology*, **39**, 1045–1050.

Anderson, W. J. R. (1956). Stillbirth and neonatal mortality in twin pregnancy. *Journal of Obstetrics and Gynaecology of the British Empire*, **63**, 205–215.

Archer, C. R. (1973). Twins in Papua. *Nursing Mirror*, **137**, 34–38.

Arts, N. F. T. and Lohman, A. H. M. (1971). The vascular anatomy of monochorionic diamniotic twin placentas and the transfusion syndrome. *European Journal of Obstetrics and Gynecology*, **3**, 85–93.

Ashley, D. J. B. (1973). Origin of teratomas. *Cancer*, **32**, 390–394.

Avni, A., Amir, J., Wilunsky, E., Katznelson, M. B. M. and Reisner, S. H. (1983). Down's syndrome in twins of unlike sex. *Journal of Medical Genetics*, **20**, 94–96.

Azubuike, J. C. (1982). Multiple births in Igbo women. *British Journal of Obstetrics and Gynaecology*, **89**, 77–79.

Babson, S. G. and Philips, D. S. (1973). Growth and development of twins, dissimilar in size at birth. *New England Journal of Medicine*, **289**, 937–940.

Bailey, D., Flynn, A. M., Kelly, J. and O'Connor, M. (1980). Antepartum fetal heart monitoring in multiple pregnancy. *British Journal of Obstetrics and Gynaecology*, **87**, 561–564.

Baird, D., Walker, J. and Thomson, A. M. (1954). Cause and prevention of stillbirths and first week deaths. *Journal of Obstetrics and Gynaecology of the British Empire*, **61**, 54, 432–448.

Baker, R. J. and Nelder, J. A. (1978). *The GLIM System, Release 3: Generalised Linear Interactive Modelling*, Numerical Algorithms Group, Oxford.

Baker, V. V. and Doering, M. C. (1982). Fetus papyraceus: an unreported congenital anomaly of the surviving infant. *American Journal of Obstetrics and Gynecology*, **142**, 234.

Balard, P. (1924). Twin births. *Journal of the American Medical Association*, **83**, 778.

Balfour, R. P. (1976). Fetus papyraceus. *Obstetrics and Gynecology*, **47**, 507.

Ballantyne, J. W. (1902). *Manual of Antenatal Pathology and Hygiene*, Green, Edinburgh, pp. 470–475.

Bang, J., Nielsen, H. and Philip, J. (1975). Prenatal karyotyping of twins by ultrasonically guided amniocentesis. *American Journal of Obstetrics and Gynecology*, **123**, 695–696.

Barber-Riley, G., Gaetyee, A. E., Richards, T. G. and Thompson, J. Y. (1961). The transfer of bromsulphthalein from the plasma to the bile in man. *Clinical Science*, **20**, 149–159.

Barnard, C. H. (1956). The genesis of intestinal atresia. *Surgical Forum*, **7**, 393–396.

Barr, A. and Stevenson, A. C. (1961). Stillbirths and infant mortality in twins. *Annals of Human Genetics*, **25**, 131–140.

Barter, R. H., Hsui, I., Erkenbeck, R. V. and Pugsley, L. Q. (1965). The prevention of prematurity in multiple pregnancy. *American Journal of Obstetrics and Gynecology*, **91**, 787–796.

Bayani-Sioson, P. S., Cruz, I. T. and Sioson, C. (1967). Twinning characteristics of the contemporary Filipino population. *Acta Medica Philippina*, **4**, 56–63.

Beacham, D. W. and Beacham, W. D. (1950). Triplet gestation and delivery with a report of fifteen cases. *Western Journal of Obstetrics and Gynaecology (Portland)*, **58**, 54–56.

Beazley, J. M. and Tindall, V. R. (1966). Changes in liver function during multiple pregnancy—using a modified bromsulphthalein test. *Journal of Obstetrics and Gynaecology of the British Commonwealth*, **73**, 658–661.

Beck, L., Terinde, R., Rohrborn, G., Claussen, U., Gebauer, H. J. and Rehder, H. (1981). Twin pregnancy, abortion of one fetus with Down's syndrome by sectio parva, the other delivered mature and healthy. *European Journal of Obstetrics, Gynecology and Reproductive Biology*, **12**, 257–259.

Beischer, N. A. and Fortune, D. W. (1968a). Double monsters. *Obstetrics and Gynecology*, **32**, 158–170.

Beischer, N. A. and Fortune, D. W. (1968b). Significance of chromatin patterns in cases of hydatidiform mole with an associated fetus. *American Journal of Obstetrics and Gynecology*, **100**, 276–282.

Beischer, N. A., Brown, J. B. and Smith, M. A. (1968). The significance of high urinary oestriol excretion during pregnancy. *Journal of Obstetrics and Gynaecology of the British Commonwealth*, **75**, 622–628.

Bell, D., Johansson, D., McLean, F. H. and Usher, R. H. (1986). Birth asphyxia, trauma and mortality in twins: Has caesarean section improved outcome? *American Journal of Obstetrics and Gynecology*, **154**, 235–239.

Bender, C. (1967). Studies on symmetrically conjoined twins. *Journal of Pediatrics*, **70**, 1010–1011.

Bender, S. (1952). Twin pregnancy: a review of 472 cases. *Journal of Obstetrics and Gynaecology of the British Empire*, **59**, 510–517.

Benirschke, K. (1961a). Accurate recording of twin placentation. A plea to the obstetrician. *Obstetrics and Gynecology*, **18**, 334–347.

Benirschke, K. (1961b). Twin placenta in perinatal mortality. *New York State Journal of Medicine*, **61**, 1499–1508.

Benirschke, K. (1970). Spontaneous chimerism in mammals: a critical review. *Current Topics in Pathology*, **51**, 1–61.

Benirschke, K. (1981). Lessons from multiple pregnancies in mammals. In: *Twin Research 3, Part A, Twin Biology and Multiple Pregnancy*, Gedda, L., Parisi, P. and Nance, W. E. (eds.). Alan R. Liss, New York, pp. 135–139.

Benirschke, K. (1984). Multiple gestation: incidence, etiology and inheritance. In: *Maternal-Fetal Medicine: Principles and Practice*, Creasy, R. K. and Resnik, R. (eds.) W. B. Saunders, London, pp. 511–526.

Benirschke, K. and Bourne, G. L. (1960). The incidence and prognostic implication of congenital absence of one umbilical artery. *American Journal of Obstetrics and Gynecology*, **79**, 251–254.

Benirschke, K. and Driscoll, S. G. (1967). *The Pathology of the Human Placenta*, Springer-Verlag, New York.

Benirschke, K. and Kim, C. K. (1973). Multiple pregnancy. *New England Journal of Medicine*, **288**, 1276–1284, 1329–1336.

Berger, G. S., Keith, L. G., Ellis, R. and Depp, R. (1981). The Northwestern University Multihospital Twin Study: III Obstetric characteristics and outcome. In: *Twin Research 3, Part A, Twin Biology and Multiple Pregnancy*, Gedda, L., Parisi, P. and Nance, W. E. (eds.), Alan R. Liss, New York, pp. 207–215.

Bernard, R. M. (1952). The size and shape of the female pelvis. *Edinburgh Medical Journal*, **59**, Transactions of the Edinburgh Obstetrical Society, pp. 1–15.

Bertillon, M. (1874). Des combinaisons de sexe dans les grossesses gemellaires (doubles ou triples) de leur cause et de leur caractère ethnique. *Bulletin de la Société d'Anthropologie de Paris*, **9**, 267–290.

Bhettay, E., Nelson, M. M. and Beighton, P. (1975). Epidemic of conjoined twins in Southern Africa? *Lancet*, **ii**, 741–743.

Bieber, F. R., Nance, W. E., Morton, C. C., Brown, J. A., Redwine, F. O., Jordan, R. L. and Mohanakumar, T. (1981). Genetic studies of an acardiac monster: evidence of polar body twinning in man. *Science*, **213**, 775–777.

Bildhaiya, G. S. (1978). A study of twin births. *Indian Pediatrics*, **15**, 931–934.

Billewicz, W. Z. and Thomson, A. M. (1973). Birthweight in consecutive pregnancies. *Journal of Obstetrics and Gynaecology of the British Commonwealth*, **80**, 491–498.

Bland, K. G. and Hammer, B. (1962). Xiphopagus twins. Report of obstetrics and surgical management of a case. *Central African Journal of Medicine*, **8**, 371–375.

Bleker, O. P., Kloosterman, G. J., Huidekoper, B. L. and Breur, W. (1977). Intrauterine growth of twins as estimated from birthweight and the fetal biparietal diameter. *European Journal of Obstetrics, Gynecology and Reproductive Biology*, **7**, 85–90.

Bleker, O. P., Breur, W. and Huidekoper, B. L. (1979). A study of birthweight, placental weight and mortality of twins as compared to singletons. *British Journal of Obstetrics and Gynaecology*, **86**, 111–118.

Boklage, C. E. (1981). On the timing of monozygotic twinning events. In: *Twin Research 3, Part A, Twin Biology and Multiple Pregnancy*, Gedda, L., Parisi, P. and Nance, W. E. (eds.), Alan R. Liss, New York, pp. 155–65.

Boklage, C. E. (1985). Interactions between opposite sex dizygotic fetuses and the assumptions of Weinberg difference method epidemiology. *American Journal of Human Genetics*, **37**, 591–605.

Boklage, C. E. (1986). Twinning, nonrighthandedness and fusion malformations: evidence for heritable causal elements held in common. *Acta Geneticae Medicae et Gemellologiae*, **35**, Abstract, 44.

Boldman, R. and Reed, D. M. (1977). Worldwide variations in low birthweight. In: *The Epidemiology of Prematurity*, Reed, D. M. and Stanley, F. J. (eds.), Urban and Schwarzenburg, Baltimore, pp. 39–52.

Bolognesi, M. and Milani-Comparetti, M. (1970). Twinning and blood groups. I ABO frequencies in twins and controls: immunological considerations. *Acta Geneticae Medicae et Gemellologiae*, **19**, 232–234.

Bomsel-Helmreich, O. and Papiernik-Berkhauer, E. (1976). Delayed ovulation and monozygotic twinning. *Acta Geneticae Medicae et Gemellologiae*, **25**, 73–76.

Bonnevie, K. and Sverdrup, A. (1926). Hereditary predispositions to dizygotic twin births in Norwegian peasant families. *Journal of Genetics*, **16**, 125–188.

Boue, J., Boue, A. and Lazar, P. (1975). Retrospective and prospective epidemiological studies of 1500 karyotyped spontaneous human abortions. *Teratology*, **12**, 11–26.

Bourne, S. (1968). The psychological effects of stillbirths on women and their doctors. *Journal of the Royal College of General Practitioners*, **16**, 103–112.

Boyd, J. D. and Hamilton, W. J. (1970). *The Human Placenta*, Heffer, Cambridge.

Bracken, M. B. (1979). Oral contraception and twinning: an epidemiological study. *American Journal of Obstetrics and Gynecology*, **133**, 432–434.

Bracken, M. B., Brinton, L. A. and Hayashi, K. (1984). Epidemiology of hydatidiform mole and chriocarcinoma. *Epidemiologic Reviews*, **6**, 52–75.

Brackenridge, C. J. (1977). The secular variation of Australian twin births over fifty years. *Annals of Human Biology*, **4**, 559–564.

Brackenridge, C. J. (1978). Aspects of the increasing triplet rate in Australia. *Journal of Biosocial Science*, **10**, 183–188.

Brennan, J. N., Diwan, R. V., Rosen, M. G. and Bellon, E. M. (1982). Fetofetal transfusion syndrome: prenatal ultrasonographic diagnosis. *Radiology*, **143**, 535–536.

Bressers, M., Kostense, P. J. and Eriksson, A. W. (1986). Increasing trend in the MZ twinning rate. *Acta Geneticae Medicae et Gemellologiae*, **35**, Abstracts, 51.

Brown, G. and Daw, E. (1980). Some aspects of triplet pregnancies in England and Wales 1971–1975. *British Journal of Clinical Practice*, **34**(5), 134–135.

Browne, F. J. (1946). *Antenatal and Postnatal Care*, 6th edition, Churchill, London.

Browne, F. J. and Dixon, H. G. (1963). Twin pregnancy. *Journal of Obstetrics and Gynaecology of the British Commonwealth*, **70**, 251–257.

Bruns, P. D. and Cooper, W. E. (1961). Basic factors influencing premature birth. *Clinical Obstetrics and Gynecology*, **4**, 341–351.

Bryan, E. M. (1976). Serum immunoglobulins in twin pregnancy with particular reference to the fetofetal transfusion syndrome. MD Thesis, University of London.

Bryan, E. M. (1977). IgG deficiency with placental oedema. *Early Human Development*, **1**, 133–143.

Bryan, E. M. (1983). *The Nature and Nurture of Twins*, Baillière Tindall, Eastbourne.

Bryan, E. M. (1986). The death of a newborn twin. *Acta Geneticae Medicae et Gemellologiae*, **35**, 115–118.

Bryan, E. M. and Kohler, H. G. (1974). The missing umbilical artery. I. Prospective study based on a maternity unit. *Archives of Disease in Childhood*, **49**, 844–852.

Bryan, E. M. and Slavin, B. (1974). Serum IgG levels in feto-fetal transfusion syndrome. *Archives of Disease in Childhood*, **49**, 908–910.

Bryan, E. M., Slavin, B. and Nicholson, E. (1976). Serum immunoglobulins in multiple pregnancy. *Archives of Disease in Childhood*, **51**, 354–359.

Bulmer, M. G. (1958). The number of human multiple births. *Annals of Human Genetics*, **22**, 158–164.

Bulmer, M. G. (1959a). The effect of parental age, parity and duration of marriage on the twinning rate. *Annals of Human Genetics*, **23**, 454–458.

Bulmer, M. G. (1959b). Twinning rate in Europe during the war. *British Medical Journal*, **i**, 29–30.

Bulmer, M. G. (1960a). The twinning rate in Europe and Africa. *Annals of Human Genetics*, **24**, 121–125.

Bulmer, M. G. (1960b). The familial incidence of twinning. *Annals of Human Genetics*, **24**, 1–3.

Bulmer, M. G. (1970). *The Biology of Twinning in Man*, Clarendon Press, Oxford.

Burch, P. R. J. (1969). Klinefelter's syndrome, dizygotic twinning and diabetes mellitus. *Nature*, **221**, 175–177.

Burch, P. R. J. (1981). The age distribution of dizygotic twinning in humans and cattle: etiologic implications. In: *Twin Research 3, Part A, Twin Biology and Multiple Pregnancy*, Gedda, L., Parisi, P. and Nance, W. E. (eds.), Alan R. Liss, New York, pp. 115–122.

Burn, J. and Corney, G. (1984). Congenital heart defects and twinning. *Acta Geneticae Medicae et Gemellologiae*, **33**: 61–69.

Burn, J., Povey, S., Boyd, Y., Munro, E. A., West, L., Harper, K. and Thomas, D. (1986). Duchenne muscular dystrophy in one of monozygotic twin girls. *Journal of Medical Genetics*, **23**, 494–500

Bustamante, S. A. and Stumpff, L. C. (1978). Fetal hydantoin syndrome in triplets: a unique experiment of nature. *American Journal of Diseases of Children*, **132**, 978–979.

Butler, N. R. and Bonham, D. G. (1963). *British Perinatal Mortality Survey—First Report: Perinatal Mortality*, Livingstone, Edinburgh.

Butler, N. R. and Alberman, E. D. (1969). *British Perinatal Mortality Survey— Second Report: Perinatal Problems*, Livingstone, Edinburgh.

Byrne, J. and Warburton, D. (1987). Male excess among anatomically normal fetuses in spontaneous abortions. *American Journal of Medical Genetics*, **26**, 605–611.

Cameron, A. H. (1968). The Birmingham Twin Survey. *Proceedings of the Royal Society of Medicine*, **61**, 229–234.

Cameron, A. H., Edwards, J. H., Derom, R., Thiery, M. and Boelaert, R. (1983). The value of twin surveys in the study of malformations. *European Journal of Obstetrics, Gynecology and Reproductive Biology*, **14**, 347–356.

Campbell, D. M. and MacGillivray, I. (1972). Comparison of maternal response in first and second pregnancies in relation to baby weight. *Journal of Obstetrics and Gynaecology of the British Commonwealth*, **79**, 684–693.

Campbell, D. M., Campbell, A. J. and MacGillivray, I. (1974). Maternal characteristics of women having twin pregnancies. *Journal of Biosocial Science*, **6**, 463–470.

Campbell, D. M. and MacGillivray, I. (1977). Maternal physiological responses and birthweight in singleton and twin pregnancies by parity. *European Journal of Obstetrics, Gynecology and Reproductive Biology*, **7/1**, 17–24.

Campbell, D. M., MacGillivray, I. and Thompson, B. (1977). Twin zygosity and pre-eclampsia. *Lancet*, **i**, 97.

Campbell, D. M. and MacGillivray, I. (1979). Glucose tolerance in twin pregnancy. *Acta Geneticae Medicae et Gemellologiae*, **28**(4), 283–287.

Campbell, D. M., MacGillivray, I. and Tuttle, S. (1982). Maternal nutrition in twin pregnancy. *Acta Geneticae Medicae et Gemellologiae*, **31**, 221–227.

Campbell, D. M., MacGillivray, I., Carr-Hill, R. and Samphier, M. (1983). Fetal sex and pre-eclampsia in primigravidae. *British Journal of Obstetrics and Gynaecology*, **90**, 26–27.

Campbell, D. M. and MacGillivray, I. (1984). The importance of plasma volume expansion and nutrition in twin pregnancy. *Acta Geneticae Medicae et Gemellologiae*, **33**, 19–24.

Campbell, D. M. and Campbell, A. J. (1985). Arterial blood pressure—the pattern of change in twin pregnancies. *Acta Geneticae Medicae et Gemellologiae*, **34** (3–4), 217–223.

Campbell, D. M., Haites, N., MacLennan, F. and Rawles, J. (1985). Cardiac output in twin pregnancy. *Acta Geneticae Medicae et Gemellologiae*, **34** (3–4), 225–228.

Campbell, D. M., Thompson, B., Pritchard, C. and Samphier, M. (1987). Does the use of oral contraception depress DZ twinning rates? *Acta Geneticae Medicae et Gemellologiae*, **36**, 409–415.

Campbell, M. (1961). Twins and congenital heart disease. *Acta Geneticae Medicae et Gemellologiae*, **10**, 443–455.

Campbell, M. and Shepherd, H. D. (1905). The circulatory and anatomical abnormalities of an acardiac fetus of rare form. *Lancet*, **ii**, 941–944.

Carmelli, D., Hasstedt, S. and Anderson, S. (1981). Demography and genetics of human twinning in the Utah Mormon geneology. In: *Twin Research 3, Part A, Twin Biology and Multiple Pregnancy*, Gedda, L., Parisi, P. and Nance, W. E. (eds.), Alan R. Liss, New York, pp. 81–93.

Carothers, A. D., Prackiewicz, A., deMey, R., Collyer, S., Polani, P. E., Osztoovicas, M., Horvath, K., Dapp, Z. May, H. M. and Ferguson-Smith, M. A. (1980). A collaborative study of the aetiology of Turner syndrome. *Annals of Human Genetics, London*, **43**, 353–368.

Carothers, A. D., Collyer, S., deMey R. and Johnston, I. (1984). An aetiological study of 290 XYY males, with special reference to the role of paternal age. *Human Genetics*, **68**, 248–253.

Carr, D. H. (1971). Chromosomes and abortion. In: *Advances in Human Genetics*, Harris, H. and Hirschhorn, K. (eds.), Plenum Press, New York, London.

Carr-Hill, R. A. and Pritchard, C. W. (1983). Reviewing birthweight standards. *British Journal of Obstetrics and Gynaecology*, **90**, 718–724.

Carr-Hill, R. and Pritchard, C. (1985). *The Development and Exploitation of Empirical Birthweight Standards*, Macmillan Press, London.

Carstairs, V. and Cole, S. (1984). Spina bifida and anencephaly in Scotland. *British Medical Journal*, **289**, 1182–1184.

Carter, C. O., David, P. A., and Laurence, K. M. (1968). A family study of major central nervous system malformations in South Wales. *Journal of Medical Genetics*, **5**, 81–106.

Caspi, E., Ronen, J., Schreyer, P. and Goldberg, M. D. (1976). The outcome of pregnancy after gonadotrophin therapy. *British Journal of Obstetrics and Gynaecology*, **83**, 967–973.

Cassady, G. (1969). Anencephaly: a 6-year study of 367 cases. *American Journal of Obstetrics and Gynecology*, **103**, 1154–1159.

Cavalli-Sforza, L. L. and Bodmer, W. A. (1971). *The Genetics of Human Populations*, W. H. Freeman, San Francisco.

Ceelie, N. (1985). Eenelige tweelinger en congenitale afwijkingen. *Tijdschr Kindergeneeskd*, **53**, 142–145.

Center for Disease Control (1982). Congenital malformations surveillance. Unpublished data, cited by Edmonds, L. D. and Layde, P. M. (1982). *Teratology*, **25**, 301–308.

Cetrulo, C. L. (1986). The controversy of mode of delivery in twins: the intrapartum management of twin gestation (Part I). *Seminars in Perinatology*, **10**, 39–43.

Cetrulo, C. L. and Freeman, R. K. (1976). Ritodrine HCl for the prevention of premature labour in twin pregnancies. *Acta Geneticae Medicae et Gemellologiae*, **25**, 321–324.

Cetrulo, C. L., Ingardia, C. J. and Sbarra, A. J. (1980). Management of multiple gestations. *Clinics in Obstetrics and Gynecology*, **23**, 533–548.

Chamberlain, G. (1963). Hydatidiform mole in twin pregnancy. *American Journal of Obstetrics and Gynecology*, **87**, 140.

Chanarin, I., Rothman, D., Ward, A. and Peng, J. (1968). Folate studies and requirement in pregnancy. *British Medical Journal*, **ii**, 390–394.

Chasnoff, I. J. (1985). Fetal alcohol syndrome in twin pregnancies. *Acta Geneticae Medicae et Gemellologiae*, **34**, 229–232.

Cheng, Y. J., Chen, C. J., Lin, T. M. and Chang, C. (1986). Twinning rates in Taiwan. *Acta Geneticae Medicae et Gemellologiae*, **35**, Abstracts, p. 52.

Chervenak, F. A. (1986). The controversy of mode of delivery in twins: the intrapartum management of twin gestation (Part II). *Seminars in Perinatology*, **10**, 44–49.

Chesley, L. C., Annitto, J. E. and Cosgrove, R. A. (1961). Pregnancy in the sisters and daughters of eclamptic women. *Pathology and Microbiology, Basle*, **24**, 662–666.

Choulet, J. J., Leclerc, M. A., and Saint Martin, J. (1982). Malformation cérébrale et jumeau survivant. *Archives of French Pediatrics*, **39**, 105–107.

Christodorescu, D., Alupului, A., Cristescu, F., Sandu, A. and Urse, M. (1981). Incidence of neural tube malformations in Bucharest over 1977–1980. *Neurologie et Psychiatrie (Bucuresti)*, **19**, 235–246.

Christoffel, K. K. and Salafsky, I. (1975). Fetal alcohol syndrome in dizygotic twins. *Journal of Pediatrics*, **78**, 963–967.

Churchill, J. A. (1965). The relationship between intelligence and birthweight in twins. *Neurology*, **15**, 341–347.

Compton, H. L. (1971). Conjoined twins. *Obstetrics and Gynecology*, **37**, 27–33.

Condie, R. and Campbell, D. M. (1978). Components of the haemostatic mechanisms in twin pregnancy. *British Journal of Obstetrics and Gynaecology*, **85**, 37–39.

Corey, L. A., Golden, W. L., Nance, W. E. and Berg, K. (1980). Analysis of timing similarities in marital and pregnancy history of twins. *American Journal of Human Genetics*, Abstract, 425.

Corey, L. A., Magnus, P., Nance, W. E. and Berg, K. (1981). Determinants of height in adult Norwegian twins and their spouses. *American Journal of Human Genetics*, **33**, Abstract 408.

Corney, G. (1975a). Mythology and customs associated with twins. In: *Human Multiple Reproduction*, MacGillivray, I., Nylander, P. P. S. and Corney, G. (eds.), W. B. Saunders, London, pp. 4–15.

Corney, G. (1975b). Placentation. In: *Human Multiple Reproduction*, MacGillivray, I., Nylander, P. P. S. and Corney, G. (eds.), W. B. Saunders, London, pp. 40–76.

Corney, G. and Aherne, W. (1965). The placental transfusion syndrome in monozygous twins. *Archives of Disease in Childhood*, **40**, 264–270.

Corney, G., Robson, E. B. and Strong, S. J. (1972). The effect of zygosity on the birthweight of twins. *Annals of Human Genetics*, **36**, 45–59.

Corney, G. and Robson, E. B. (1975). Types of twinning and determination of zygosity. In: *Human Multiple Reproduction*, MacGillivray, I., Nylander, P. P. S. and Corney, G. (eds.), W. B. Saunders, London, pp. 16–39.

Corney, G., Thompson, B., Campbell, D. M., MacGillivray, I., Seedburgh, D. and Timlin, D. (1979). The effect of zygosity on the birthweight of twins in Aberdeen and North-East Scotland. *Acta Geneticae Medicae et Gemellologiae*, **28**, 353–360.

Corney, G., Seedburgh, D., Thompson, B., Campbell, D. M., MacGillivray, I. and Timlin, D. (1981). Multiple and singleton pregnancy differences between mother as well as offspring. In: *Twin Research 3, Part A, Twin Biology and Multiple Pregnancy*, Gedda, L., Parisi, P. and Nance, W. E. (eds.), Alan R. Liss, New York, pp. 107–114.

Corney, G., MacGillivray, I., Campbell, D. M., Thompson, B. and Little, J. (1983). Congential anomalies in twins in Aberdeen and North-East Scotland. *Acta Geneticae Medicae et Gemellologiae*, **32**, 31–35.

Cox, M. L. (1963). Incidence and aetiology of multiple births in Nigeria. *Journal of Obstetrics and Gynaecology of the British Empire*, **70**, 878–884.

Coyle, M. G. and Brown, J. B. (1963). Urinary excretion of oestriol during pregnancy. II. Results in normal and abnormal pregnancies. *Journal of Obstetrics and Gynaecology of the British Commonwealth*, **70**, 225–231.

Creasy, M. R., Crolla, J. A. and Alberman, E. D. (1976). A cytogenetic study of human spontaneous abortions using banding techniques. *Human Genetics*, **37**, 777–796.

Crichton, D. (1973). A simple technique of extraperitoneal lower segment caesarean section. *South African Medical Journal*, **47**, 2011–2012.

Cristalli, G. (1924). L'accouchement multiple à Naples de 1914 a 1921. *Revue française Gynécologie*, **19**, 161–183.

Czeizel, A. (1974). Unexplainable demographic phenomena of multiple births in Hungary. *Acta Geneticae Medicae et Gemellologiae*, **22**, 213–218.

Czeizel, A., Pazonyi, I., Metneki, J. and Tomka, M. (1979). The first five years of the Budapest twin register 1970–1974. *Acta Geneticae Medicae et Gemellologiae*, **28**, 73–76.

Czeizel, A., Erodi, E. and Toch, J. (1981). An epidemiological study on undescended testes. *Journal of Urology*, **126**, 524–527.

Dahlberg, G. (1926). *Twin Births and Twins from a Hereditary Point of View*, A. B. Tidens Trycker, Stockholm.

Dahlberg, G. (1952). Die tendenz eu zwillingsgeburton. *Acta Geneticae Medicae et Gemellologiae*, **1**, 80–87

Dallapiccola, B., Stomeo, C., Ferranti, G., DiLecci, A. and Purpura, M. (1985). Discordant sex in one of three monozygotic triplets. *Journal of Medical Genetics*, **22**, 6–11.

D'Alton, M. E. and Dudley, D. K. L. (1986). Ultrasound in the antenatal management of twin gestation. *Seminars in Perinatology*, **10**, 30–38.

Danforth, C. H. (1916). Is twinning hereditary? *Journal of Heredity*, **7**, 195–202.

Danielson, C. (1960). Twin pregnancy and birth. *Acta Obstetricia et Gynecologica Scandinavica*, **39**, 63–87

Davenport, W. C. B. (1930). Litter size and latitude. *Archives fur Rassen und Gesellschaftsbiologie*, **24**, 97–99.

David, T. J. (1985). Vascular basis for malformations in a twin. *Archives of Disease in Childhood*, **60**, 166–167.

Davies, J., Chazen, E. and Nance, W. E. (1971). Symmelia in one of monozygotic twins. *Teratology*, **4**, 367–378.

Davis, B. R. and Fuentes, L. (1984). Co-existing hydatidiform mole with a live fetus. *American Journal of Obstetrics and Gynecology*, **150**, 901–902.

Daw, E. (1983). Fetus papyraceus—11 cases. *Postgraduate Medical Journal*, **59**, 598–600.

Daw, E. (1978). Triplet pregnancy. *British Journal of Obstetrics and Gynaecology*, **85**, 505–509.

Daw, E. and Walker, J. (1975a). Growth differences in twin pregnancy. *British Journal of Clinical Practice*, **29**, 150–152.

Daw, E. and Walker, J. (1975b). Biological aspects of twin pregnancy in Dundee. *British Journal of Obstetrics and Gynaecology*, **82**, 29–34.

Dawood, M. Y., Ratnam, S. S. and Lim, Y. C. (1975). Twin pregnancy in Singapore. *Australian and New Zealand Journal of Obstetrics and Gynaecology*, **15**, 93–98.

De George, F. V. (1970a). Hydatidiform moles in other pregnancies of mothers of twins. *American Journal of Obstetrics and Gynecology*, **108**, 369–371.

De George, F. V. (1970b). Maternal and fetal disorders in pregnancies of mothers of twins. *American Journal of Obstetrics and Gynecology*, **108**, 975–978.

Department of Health and Social Security (1979). Recommended daily amounts of food energy and nutrients for groups of people in the United Kingdom. Report on Health and Social Subjects 15, HMSO, London.

Department of Health and Social Security. (1980). Inequalities in health. Report of a Research Working Group. HMSO, London.

Depp, R., Keith, L. and Sciarri, J. (1986). The mode of delivery in twin pregnancy. Paper given at Fifth Congress of International Society for Twin Studies, Amsterdam (unpublished).

Derom, R. and Thiery, M. (1976). Intrauterine hypoxia—a phenomenon peculiar to the second twin. *Acta Geneticae Medicae et Gemellologiae*, **25**, 314–316.

Derom, C., Derom, R., Vlietnick, R., Van Den Berghe, H. and Thiery, M. (1987). Increased monozygotic twinning rate after ovulation induction. *Lancet*, **i**, 1236.

Dobbie, H. G., Whittle, M. J., Wilson, A. I. and Whitfield, C. R. (1983). Amniotic fluid phospholipid profile in multiple pregnancy and the effect of zygosity. *British Journal of Obstetrics and Gynaecology*, **90**, 1001–1006.

Dor, J., Itzkowic, D. J., Mashiach, S., Luenfeld, B. and Serr, D. (1980). Cumulative conception rates following gonadotrophin therapy. *American Journal of Obstetrics and Gynecology*, **136**, 102–105.

Dor, J., Shaler, J., Mashiach, S., Blankenstein, J. and Serr, D. M. (1982). Elective cervical suture of twin pregnancies diagnosed ultrasonically in the first trimester following induced ovulation. *Gynaecological and Obstetrical Investigation*, **13**, 55–60.

Dudley, D. K. L. and D'Alton, M. E. (1986). Single fetal death in twin gestation. *Seminars in Perinatology*, **10**, 65–72.

Duncan, J. Matthews (1865). On the comparative frequency of twin-bearing in different pregnancies. *Edinburgh Medical Journal*, **10**, 928–929.

Dunn, B. (1961). Bed rest in twin pregnancy. *Journal of Obstetrics and Gynaecology of the British Commonwealth*, **68**, 685–687.

Dunn, P. M. (1965). Some perinatal observations on twins. *Developmental Medicine and Child Neurology*, **7**, 121–134.

Du Plessis, J. P. G., Winship, W. S. and Kirsten, J. D. L. (1974). Fetus in fetu and teratoma. A case report and review. *South African Medical Journal*, **48**, 2119–2122.

Durkin, M. V., Kaveggia, E. G., Pendleton, E., Neuhauser, G. and Opitz, J. M. (1976). Analysis of etiologic factors in cerebral palsy with severe mental retardation. I. Analysis of gestational, parturitional and neonatal data. *European Journal of Pediatrics*, **123**, 67–81.

Editorial (1976). Worldwide decline in dizygotic twinning. *British Medical Journal*, **i**, 1553.

Editorial (1981). Bed rest in obstetrics, *Lancet*, **i**: 1137–1138.

Edmonds, H. W., and Hawkins, J. W. (1941). The relationship of twins, teretomas and ovarian dermoids. *Cancer Research*, **1**, 896–899.

Edmonds, L. D. and Layde, P. M. (1982). Conjoined twins in the United States 1970–1977. *Teratology*, **25**, 301–308.

Edwards, J. (1938). Season and rate of conception. *Nature* (Letter), 357.

Edwards, J. H. (1968). Multiple pregnancy. *Proceedings of the Royal Society of Medicine*, **61**, 227–229.

Edwards, J. H., Cameron, A. H. and Wingham, J. (1967). The Birmingham Twin Survey. Cited in Strong, S. J. and Corney, G. (1967). *The Placenta in Twin Pregnancy*, Pergamon Press, Oxford, p. 38.

Edwards, J. N., Dent, T. and Kahn, J. (1966). Monozygotic twins of different sex. *Journal of Medical Genetics*, **3**, 117–123.

Edwards, R. G. (1985). In vitro fertilisation and embryo replacement in in vitro fertilization and embryo transfer. *Annals of the New York Academy of Sciences*, **442**, 1–22.

Edwards, R. G. (1986). In vitro fertilization and twinning. Paper given at Fifth Congress of International Society for Twin Studies, Amsterdam (unpublished).

Edwards, R. G. and Steptoe, R. C. (1983). Current status of in vitro fertilisation and implantation of human embryos. *Lancet*, **ii**, 1265–1269.

Edwards, R. G., Fishel, S. B., Cohen, J., Fehilly, C. H., Purdy, J. M., Slater, J. M., Steptoe, R. C. and Webster, J. M. (1984). Factors influencing the success of in vitro fertilisation for alleviating human infertility. *Journal of In Vitro Fertilisation and Embryo Transfer*, 1, No. 1: 3–23.

Edwards, R. G., Mettler, L. and Walters, D. E. (1986). Identical twins and in vitro fertilization. *Journal of In Vitro Fertilisation and Embryo Transfer*, **3**, 114–117.

Ellis, R. F., Berger, G. S., Keith, L. and Depp, R. (1979). The Northwestern University Multihospital Twin Study. II Mortality of first versus second twin. *Acta Geneticae Medicae et Gemellologiae*, **28**, 347–352.

Elwood, J. H. and Nevin, N. C. (1973). Factors associated with anencephalus and spina bifida in Belfast. *British Journal of Preventive and Social Medicine*, **27**, 73–80.

Elwood, J. M. (1973). Changes in the twinning rate in Canada 1926–1970. *British Journal of Preventive Social Medicine*, **27**, 236–241.

Elwood, J. M. (1974). Clomiphene and anencephalic births. *Lancet* (letter), **i**, 31.

Elwood, J. M. (1978). Maternal and environmental factors affecting twin births in Canadian cities. *British Journal of Obstetrics and Gynaecology*, **85**, 351–358.

Elwood, J. M. (1985). Temporal trends in twinning. In: *Issues and Reviews in Teratology*, Kalter, H. (ed.), Plenum Press, New York, pp. 65–93.

Elwood, J. M. and McBride, M. L. (1979). Contrasting effects of maternal fertility and birth rank on the occurrence of NTDs. *Journal of Epidemiology and Community Health*, **33**, 78–83.

Elwood, J. M. and Elwood, J. H. (1980). *Epidemiology of Anencephalus and Spina Bifida*. Oxford University Press, Oxford.

Emanuel, I., Huang, S. W., Gutman, L. T., Yu, F. C. and Linn, C. C. (1972). The incidence of congenital malformations in a Chinese population: the Tapei collaborative study. *Teratology*, **5**, 159–169.

Emery, A. E. H. (1986). Identical twinning and oral contraception. *Biology and Society*, **3**(1), 23–27.

Enbom, J. A. (1985). Twin pregnancy with intrauterine death of one twin. *American Journal of Obstetrics and Gynecology*, **152**, 424–429.

Enders, T. and Stern, C. (1948). The frequencies of twins, relative to age of mothers in American populations. *Genetics*, **33**, 263–272.

Ericson, A., Kallen, B., Setterstrom, R., Eriksson, M. and Westerhol, P. (1984). Delivery outcome of women working in laboratories during pregnancy. *Archives of Environmental Health*, **39**, 5–10.

Eriksson, A. (1962). Variations in the human twining rate. *Acta Genetica et Statistica Medica*, **12**, 242–250.

Eriksson, A. W. (1973). Human twining in and around the Aland Islands. *Commentetiones Biologicae*, **64**, Helsingfors, Helsinki, 60.

Eriksson, A. W. and Fellman, J. (1967). Twinning in relation to the marital status of the mother. *Acta Genetica et Statistica Medica*, **17**, 385–398.

Eriksson, A. W. and Fellman, J. (1973). Differences in the twinning rates between Finns and Swedes. *American Journal of Human Genetics*, **25**, 141–151.

Eriksson, A. W., Kostense, P. J., Bressers, M., Tas, R. F. J. and Fellman, J. O. (1986). Twinning rates around years of privation. *Acta Geneticae Medicae et Gemellologiae*, **35**, Abstracts, p. 28–29.

Farrell, A. G. W. (1964). Twin pregnancy: a study of 1000 cases. *South African Journal of Obstetrics and Gynaecology*, **2**, 35–41.

Farroqui, M. D., Grossman, J. H. and Shauman, R. A. (1973). A review of twin pregnancies and perinatal mortality. *Obstetric and Gynaecological Survey*, **28**, 144–145.

Fedrick, J. (1976). Anencephalus in the Oxford record linkage study area. *Developmental Medicine and Child Neurology*, **18**, 643–656.

Fedrick, J. and Anderson, A. B. M. (1976). Factors associated with spontaneous preterm birth. *British Journal of Obstetrics and Gynaecology*, **83**, 342–350.

Fehrmann, H. (1980). Misdiagnosis of fetal heart rate during a twin labour. *British Journal of Obstetrics and Gynaecology*, **87**, 1174–1177.

Felszer, M. (1979). The incidence of twins in the Kingdom of Tonga and maternal and perinatal complications. *Fiji Medical Journal*, **7**, 156–162.

Ferguson, W. F. (1964). Perinatal mortality in multiple pregnancy. A review of perinatal deaths from 1609 multiple gestations. *Obstetrics and Gynecology*, **23**, 854.

Ferguson-Smith, M. A. (1966). X-Y chromosomal interchange in the aetiology of true hermaphroditism and of Xx Klinefelter's syndrome. *Lancet*, **ii**, 475–476.

Filkins, K., Russo, J., Brown, T., Schmerler, S. and Searle, B. (1984). Genetic amniocentesis in multiple gestations. *Prenatal Diagnosis*, **4**, 223–226.

Finberg, H. J. and Birnholz, J. C. (1979). Ultrasound observations in multiple gestation with first trimester bleeding: the blighted twin. *Radiology*, **132**, 137–142.

Fisher, R. A., Sheppard, D. M. and Lawler, S. D. (1982). Twin pregnancy with complete hydatidiform mole (46,XX) and fetus (46,YY): genetic origin proved by analysis of chromosome polymorphisms. *British Medical Journal*, **284**, 1218–1220.

Flannery, D. B. and Robinow, M. (1986). New hypotheses for twin studies of congenital anomalies. *Acta Geneticae Medicae et Gemellologiae*, **35**, Abstracts p. 44.

Fliegner, J. R. and Eggers, T. R. (1984). The relationship between gestational age and birthweight in twin pregnancy. *Australian and New Zealand Journal of Obstetrics and Gynecology*, **24**, 192–197.

Fontaine, G. and Vankemmel, P. (1978). Craniorachischisis in a double headed female fetus. *Teratology*, **18**, 289–290 (letter).

Foong, J. C. (1971). Further study of twinning in Singapore. *Journal of Singapore Paediatric Society*, **13**, 85–90.

Forbes, J. F. and Small, M. J. (1983). A comparative analysis of birthweight for gestational age standards. *British Journal of Obstetrics and Gynaecology*, **99**, 297–303.

Forrester, R. M., Lees, V. T. and Watson, G. H. (1966). Rubella syndrome: escape of a twin. *British Medical Journal*, **1**, 1403.

Fotheringham, J. (1974). Comparison of liver function in twins and singleton pregnancies. Medical student elective, Department of Obstetrics and Gynaecology, University of Aberdeen, supervised by Campbell, D. M.

Fraccaro, M. (1957). A contribution to the study of birthweight based on an Italian sample twin data. *Annals of Human Genetics*, **21**, 224–236.

Fraser, F. C. and Nora, J. J. (1975). *Genetics of Man*. Lee and Febiger, Philadelphia, pp. 177.

Fraser, F. C., Czeizel, A. and Hanson, C. (1982). Increased frequency of neural tube defects in siblings of children with other malformations. *Lancet*, **ii**, 144–145.

Fraumeni, J. F., Li, F. P. and Dalager, N. (1973). Teratomas in children: epidemiological features. *Journal of the National Cancer Institute*, **51**, 1425–1430.

Frezal, J., Kelley, J., Guillemot, M. L. and Lamy, M. (1964). Anencephaly in France. *American Journal of Human Genetics*, **16**, 336–350.

Frutiger, P. (1969). Zum Problem der Akardie. *Acta Anatomica*, **74**, 505–531.

Fujikura, T. and Froehlich, L. A. (1971). Twin placentation and zygosity. *Obstetrics and Gynecology*, **37**, 34–43.

Fujikura, T. and Froehlich, L. A. (1974). Mental and motor development in monozygotic co-twins with dissimilar birthweights. *Pediatrics*, **53**, 884–889.

Fullerton, W. T., Hytten, F. E., Klopper, A. and McKay, E. (1965). A case of quadruplet pregnancy. *Journal of Obstetrics and Gynaecology of the British Commonwealth*, **72**, 791–796.

Gaehtgens, G. (1936). Klinischer Beitrag zur Pathogenese des akuten Hydramnions. *Monatsschrift für Geburtschilfe und Gynakologie*, **103**, 40–48.

Galea, P., Scott, J. M. and Goel, K. M. (1982). Feto-fetal transfusion syndrome. *Archives of Disease in Childhood*, **57**, 781–794.

Gartler, S. M. and Riggs, A. D. (1983). Mammalian X-chromosome inactivation. *Annual Reviews in Genetics*, **17**, 155–190.

Gaspard, O. and Franchimont, P. (1974). HCS, hCG and hCG subunit serum levels during multiple pregnancies (1974). *Acta Geneticae Medicae et Gemellologiae*, **22**, 195–197.

Gedda, L. (1951). *Studio dei Gemelli*, Edizioni Orizzonte Medico, Rome.

Gedda, L. (1961). *Twins in History and Science*, Thomas, Springfield, Illinois.

Gedda, L., Sciacca, A., Branci, G., Villantico, S., Bonanni, G., Gueli, N. and Tatone, C. (1984). Situs viscerum specularis in monozygotic twins. *Acta Geneticae Medicae et Gemellologiae*, **33**, 81–85.

Gedda, L., Branci, G. and Furlan, C. (1986). Monthly frequency distribution of twin vs single births in Italian regions 1981–1982. *Acta Geneticae Medicae et Gemellologiae*, **35**, Abstracts, p. 27.

Geeves, R. C. (1928). An amorphous "Siamese " twin and its separation from a normal fetus. *Medical Journal of Australia*, **i**, 617–618.

Gemzell, C. and Roos, P. (1966). Pregnancies following treatment with human gonadotrophins with special reference to the problem of multiple births. *American Journal of Obstetrics and Gynecology*, **94**, 490–496.

Gericke, G. S. (1986). Genetic and teratological considerations in the analysis of concordant and discordant abnormalities in twins. *South African Medical Journal*, **69**, 111–114.

Gessner, I. H. (1966). Spectrum of congenital cardiac anomalies produced in chick embryos by mechanical interference with cardiogenesis. *Circulation Research*, **18**, 625–633.

Ghosh, S. and Ramanujacharyulu, T. K. T. S. (1979). Study of twin births in an urban community of Delhi. *Indian Journal of Medical Research*, **701**, 70–77.

Gigon, U., Moser, H. and Aufdermauer, P. (1981). Twin pregnancy with operative removal of one fetus with chromosomal mosaicism 46XX/45XO and term delivery of a healthy baby. *Zeitschrift für Geburtshilfe und Perinatologie*, **185**, 365–366.

Giles, P. (1908). Abandonment and exposure. In: *Encyclopaedia of Religion and Ethics*, Hastings, J. (ed.), Vol. 1, Clark, Edinburgh.

Giles, W. B., Trudinger, B. J. and Cook, C. M. (1985). Umbilical waveforms in twin pregnancy. *Acta Geneticae Medicae et Gemellologiae*, **34**, 233–237.

Gilgenkrantz, S., Marchal, C., Wendremaire, P. H. and Seger, M. (1981). Cytogenetic and antigenic studies in a pair of twins: a normal boy and a trisomic 21 girl with chimera. In: *Twin Research 3, Part A, Twin Biology and Multiple Pregnancy*, Gedda, L., Parisi, P. and Nance, W. E. (eds.), Alan R. Liss, New York, pp. 141–153.

Gillim, D. L. and Hendricks, C. H. (1953). Holoacardius: review of the literature and case report. *Obstetrics and Gynecology*, **2**, 647–653.

Giovannucci-Uzielli, M. L., Vecchi, C., Donzelli, G. P., Levi D'Ancona, V. and Lapi, E. (1981). The history of the Florentine sextuplets: obstetric and genetic considerations. In: *Twin Research 3, Part A, Twin Biology and Multiple Pregnancy*, Gedda, L., Parisi, P. and Nance, W. E. (eds.), Alan R. Liss, New York, pp. 217–220.

Golding, J. (1986a). Social class and twinning. *Acta Geneticae Medicae et Gemellologiae*, **35**, Abstracts, p. 29.

Golding, J. (1986b). Season of conception and risk of twinning. *Acta Geneticae Medicae et Gemellologiae*, **35**, Abstracts, p. 26.

Goswami, H. K. and Wagh, K. V. (1975). Twinning in India. *Acta Geneticae Medicae et Gemellologiae*, **24**, 347–350.

Grant, P. and Pearn, J. H. (1969). Foetus in foetu. *Medical Journal of Australia*, **1**, 1016–1019.

Graves, L. R., Adams, J. G. and Schreier, P. C. (1962). The fate of the second twin. *Obstetrics and Gynecology*, **19**, 246–250.

Grennert, L., Gennser, G., Persson, P., Kullander, S. and Thorell, J. (1976). Ultrasound and human-placental-lactogen screening for early detection of twin pregnancies. *Lancet*, **i**, 4–6.

Greulich, W. W. (1934). Heredity in human twinning. *American Journal of Physical Anthropology*, **19**, 391–431.

Groenewegen, K. and Van de Kaa, D. J. (1967). Resultaten van het demografisch enderzoek westellijk Nieun-Guinea. Deel 6: De progenituur van Papoes viouwen. Government Printing and Publishing Office, The Hague.

Gronow, M. J., Martin, M. J., McBain, J. C., Wein, P., Speirs, A. L. and Lapata, A. (1985). Aspects of multiple embryo transfer. *Annals of the New York Academy of Sciences*, **442**, 318–386.

Gross, R. E. and Clatworthy, H. W. (1951). Twin fetuses in fetu. *Journal of Pediatrics*, **38**, 502–508.

Gross, R. E., Clatworthy, H. W. and Meeker, I. A. (1951). Sacrococcygeal teratomas in infants and children: a report of 40 cases. *Surgery, Gynecology and Obstetrics*, **92**, 341–354.

Gruenwald, P. (1970). Environmental influences on twins apparent at birth. A preliminary study. *Biology of the Neonate*, **15**, 79–93.

Guerrero, R. (1970). Sex ratio: a statistical association with the type and time of insemination in the menstrual cycle. *International Journal of Fertility*, **15**, 221–225.

Guerrero, R. (1974). Association of the type and time of insemination within the menstrual cycle with the human sex ratio at birth. *New England Journal of Medicine*, **291**, 1056–1059.

Guerrero, R. and Rojas, O. I. (1975). Spontaneous abortion and aging of human ova and spermatozoa. *New England Journal of Medicine*, **293**, 573–575.

Guttmacher, A. F. (1937). An analysis of 521 cases of twin pregnancy. *American Journal of Obstetrics and Gynecology*, **34**, 76–84.

Guttmacher, A. F. (1939). An analysis of 573 cases of twin pregnancy. *American Journal of Obstetrics and Gynecology*, **38**, 277–288.

Guttmacher, A. F. and Kohl, S. G. (1958). The fetus of multiple gestations. *Obstetrics and Gynecology*, **12**, 528–541.

Guttmacher, A. F. and Nichols, B. L. (1967). Teratology of conjoined twins. *Birth Defects: Original Articles Series*, **3**(1), 3–7.

Guyton, A. C. (1981). Prepregnancy reproductive function of the female and the female hormones. In: *Textbook of Medical Physiology*, W. B. Saunders, Philadelphia, Eastbourne, Toronto, Fig. 81/7, p. 1016.

Hack, M., Brish, M., Serr, D. M., Insler, V. and Lunenfeld, B. (1970). Outcome of pregnancy after induced ovulation. *Journal of the American Medical Association*, **211**,(5), 791–797.

Hall, J. G., Reed, S. D., McGillivray, B. C., Herrman, J., Partington, M. W., Schinzel, A., Shapiro, J. and Weaver, D. D. (1983). Twinning in amyoplasia—a specific type of arthrogryposis with an apparent excess of discordantly affected identical twins. *American Journal of Medical Genetics*, **15**, 591–599.

Hall, M. H. (1970). Assessment of the effects of folic acid deficiency in pregnancy. MD Thesis, University of Aberdeen.

Hall, M. H. (1987). Personal communication.

Hall, M. H., Pirani, B. B. K. and Campbell, D. M. (1976). The cause of the fall in serum folate in normal pregnancy. *British Journal of Obstetrics and Gynaecology*, **83**, 132–136.

Hall, M. H., Campbell, D. M. and Davidson, R. J. L. (1979). Anaemia in twin pregnancy. *Acta Geneticae Medicae et Gemellologiae*, **28**, 279–282.

Hall, M. H., Chng, P. and MacGillivray, I. (1980). Is routine antenatal care worthwhile? *Lancet*, **ii**, 78–80.

Hall, M. H. and Carr-Hill, R. (1982). The weaker sex? Impact of sex ratio on onset and management of labour. *British Medical Journal*, **285**, 401–403.

Hall, M. H. and Carr-Hill, R. A. (1985). The significance of uncertain gestation for obstetric outcome. *British Journal of Obstetrics and Gynaecology*, **92**, 452–460.

Hall, M. H., Campbell, D. M., Fraser, C., Carr-Hill, R. and Samphier, M. (1985). Extent and antecedents of uncertain gestation. *British Journal of Obstetrics and Gynaecology*, **92**, 443–451.

Hammond, J. (1952). Fertility. In: *Marshall's Physiology of Reproduction*, 3rd edition, Parkes, A. J. (ed.), Vol. 2, Longmans, London.

Hamon, A. and Dinno, N. (1978). Dicephalus dipus tribrachius conjoined twins in a female infant. *Birth Defects: Original Articles Series*, **14**, 213–218.

Hanna, J. H. and Hill, J. M. (1984). Single intrauterine fetal demise in multiple gestation. *Obstetrics and Gynecology*, **63**, 126–130.

Hanson, J. W. (1975). Incidence of conjoined twinning. *Lancet*, **ii**, 1257 (letter).

Hardy, J., Drage, J. S. and Jackson, E. C. (1979). *The First Year of Life*, Johns Hopkins UP, Baltimore.

Hare, E. H., Moran, P. A. P. and MacFarlane, A. (1981). The changing seasonality of infant deaths in England and Wales 1972–1978 and its relation to seasonal temperature. *Journal of Epidemiology and Community Health*, **35**, 77–82.

Harlap, S. (1979). Gender of infants conceived on different days of the menstrual cycle. *New England Journal of Medicine*, **300**, 1445–1448.

Harlap, S., Shahar, S. and Baras, M. (1985). Overripe ova and twinning. *American Journal of Human Genetics*, **37**, 1206–1215.

Harper, P. S. (1981). *Practical Genetic Counselling*, John Wright, Bristol, 96–97

Harris, J. R. (1922). A recent twin murder in South Africa. *Folklore*, **33**, 214–223.

Harrison, K. A. (1969). Changes in blood volume produced by treatment of severe anaemia in pregnancy. *Clinical Science*, **36**, 197–207.

Harrison, K. A. and Rossiter, C. E. (1985). Child-bearing, health and social priorities: a survey of 22774 consecutive hospital births in Zaria, Northern Nigeria. 7. Multiple pregnancy. *British Journal of Obstetrics and Gynaecology*, **92**, (Suppl. 5), 49–60.

Harrison, K. A., Ekanem, A. D. and Chong, H. (1985). Child bearing, health and social priorities: a survey of 22774 consecutive hospital births in Zaria, Northern Nigeria. 10. Easily identifiable congenital malformations. *British Journal of Obstetrics and Gynaecology*, **92** (Suppl. 5), 81–85.

Harrison, K. B. and Warburton, D. (1986). Preferential X-chromosome activity in human female placental tissues. *Cytogenetics and Cell Genetics*, **41**, 163–168.

Hartikainen-Sorri, A. L. and Jouppila, P. (1984). Is routine hospitalization needed in antenatal care of twin pregnancy? *Journal of Perinatal Medicine*, **12**, 31–34.

Hartikainen-Sorri, A. L. (1985). Is routine hospitalization in twin pregnancy necessary? A follow-up study. *Acta Geneticae Medicae et Gemellologiae*, **34**, 189–192.

Harvey, M. A. S., Huntley, R. M. C. and Smith, D. W. (1977). Familial monozygotic twinning. *Journal of Pediatrics*, **90**, 246–248.

Hay, S. and Wehrung, D. A. (1970). Congenital malformations in twins. *American Journal of Human Genetics*, **22**, 662–678.

Hay, S. and Barbano, H. (1972). Independent effects of maternal age and birth order on the incidence of selected congenital malformations. *Teratology*, **6**, 271–280.

Heifetz, S. A. (1984). Single umbilical artery, a statistical analysis of 237 autopsy cases and review of the literature. *Perspective Pediatric Pathology*, **8**, 345–378.

Hellin, D. (1895). Die Ursache der Multiparitat der Unipaeren. *Tiere Uberhaupt und der Zwillingsschwangerschaft beim Menschen Insbesondere*, Seltz and Schaner, Munich.

Hellman, L. M., Kobayashi, M. and Cromb, E. (1973). Ultrasonic diagnosis of embryonic malformations. *American Journal of Obstetrics and Gynecology*, **115**, 615–623.

Hemon, D., Berger, C. and Lazar, P. (1979a). Analyse des variations géographiques de la fréquence des accouchements gemellaires en France. Une approche indirecte de l'étude des avortements spontanés. *Revue D'Épidémiologie et de Santé Publique*, **27**, 91–99.

Hemon, D., Berger, C. and Lazar, P. (1979b). The etiology of human dizygotic twinning with special reference to spontaneous abortions. *Acta Geneticae Medicae et Gemellologiae*, **28**, 253–258.

Hemon, D., Berger, C. and Lazar, P. (1981a). Twinning following oral contraceptive discontinuation. *International Journal of Epidemiology*, **10**(4), 319–328.

Hemon, D., Berger, C. and Lazar, P. (1981b). Some observations concerning the decline of dizygotic twinning rate in France between 1901 and 1968. *Twin Research 3, Part A, Twin Biology and Multiple Pregnancy*, Gedda, L., Parisi, P. and Nance, W. E. (eds.), Alan R. Liss, New York, pp. 49–56.

Hendricks, C. H. (1966). Twinning in relation to birthweight, mortality and congenital anomalies. *Obstetrics and Gynecology*, **27**, 47–53.

Henriksen, J. B., Flugsrud, L. B. and Orstavik, I. (1968). Cytomegali hos en nyfodt tvilling pavist ved isolation av cytomegalvirus. *Tidsskrift for den Norske Laegeforening*, **88**, 81.

Herlitz, G. (1941). Zur Kenntnis der anamischen und polyzytamischen Zustande bei Neugeborenen, sowie des Icterus gravis neonatorum. *Acta Paediatrica (Uppsala)*, **29**, 211–253.

Herrlin, K. M. and Hauge, M. (1967). The determination of triplet zygosity. *Acta Genetica et Statistica Medica*, **17**, 81–95.

Heuser, R. L. (1967). *Multiple births, United States 1964*, National Centre for Health Statistics, Series 21, No. 14, US Department of Health Education and Welfare, Washington DC.

Hickey, R. C. and Layton, J. M. (1954). Sacrococcygeal teratoma. Emphasis on the biological history and early therapy. *Cancer*, **7**, 1031–1043.

Hill, A. V. and Jeffreys, A. J. (1985). Use of minisatellite DNA probes for determination of twin zygosity at birth. *Lancet*, **ii**, 1394–1395.

Hirst, J. C. (1939). Maternal and fetal expectations with multiple pregnancy. *American Journal of Obstetrics and Gynecology*, **37**, 634–643.

Hoefnagel, D. and Benirschke, K. (1962). Twinning in Klinefelter's syndrome. *Lancet*, **ii**, 1282 (letter).

Holczberg, G., Biale, Y., Lewenthal, H. and Insler, V. (1982). Outcome of pregnancies in 31 triplet gestations. *Obstetrics and Gynecology*, **59**, 472–476.

Hollingsworth, M. J. and Duncan, C. (1966). The birthweight and survival of Ghanaian twins. *Annals of Human Genetics*, **30**, 13–24.

Holt, N. (1987). The role of X-inactivation in the genesis of monozygotic twinning. Bachelor of Medical Science Dissertation, University of Newcastle-upon-Tyne.

Hoogendoorn, D. (1973). Drop in the number of twins in the Netherlands. *Nederlands T. Geneesk*, **117**, 805–807.

Houlton, M. C., Marivate, M. and Philpott, R. H. (1982). Factors associated with pre-term labour and changes in the cervix before labour in twin pregnancy. *British Journal of Obstetrics and Gynaecology*, **89**(3), 190–194.

Hoyme, H. E., Higginbottom, M. C. and Jones, K. L. (1981). Vascular etiology of disruptive structural defects in monozygotic twins. *Pediatrics*, **67**, 288–291.

Hunter, A. G. W. and Cox, D. M. (1979). Counselling problems when twins are discovered at genetic amniocentesis. *Clinical Genetics*, **16**, 34–42.

Huxley, J. S. and DeBeer, G. R. (1934). *The Elements of Experimental Embryology*, University Press, Cambridge, pp. 154–163; 325–332.

Hytten, F. E. and Leitch, I. (1971). *The Physiology of Human Pregnancy*, 2nd edition, Blackwell Scientific Publications, Oxford.

Illsley, R. and Mitchell, R. G. (1984). The developing concept of low birthweight and the present state of knowledge. In: *Low birthweight: A Medical, Physiological and Social Study*, Illsley, R. and Mitchell, R. G. (eds.), Wiley, Chichester, pp. 5–32.

Illsley, R. and Samphier, M. (1985). Selective migration and the family cycle. Paper presented at British Association meeting in Glasgow (unpublished).

Imaizumi, Y. (1978)., Concordance and discordance of anencephaly in 109 twin pairs in Japan. *Japanese Journal of Human Genetics*, **23**, 389–393.

Imaizumi, Y. and Inouye, E. (1979). Analysis of multiple birth rates in Japan. I. Secular trend, maternal age effect, and geographical variation in twinning rates. *Acta Geneticae Medicae et Gemellologiae*, **28**, 107–124.

Imaizumi, Y., Asaka, A. and Inouye, E. (1980). Analysis of multiple birth rates in Japan. V. Seasonal and social class variations in twin births. *Japanese Journal of Human Genetics*, **25**, 299–307.

Imaizumi, Y. and Inouye, E. (1984). Multiple birth rates in Japan. Further analysis. *Acta Geneticae Medicae et Gemellologiae*, **33**, 107–114.

Imam, A. (1967). Cited by Nylander, PPS. *Acta Geneticae Medicae et Gemellologiae* (1970d), **19**, 458.

Imperato, P. J. (1971). Twins among the Bambara and Malinke of Mali. *Journal of Tropical Medicine and Hygiene*, **74**, 154–159.

Inouye, E. and Imaizumi, Y. (1981). Analysis of twinning rates in Japan. In: *Twin Research 3, Part A, Twin Biology and Multiple Pregnancy*, Gedda, L., Parisi, P. and Nance, W. E. (eds.), Alan R. Liss, New York, pp. 21–33.

International Clearinghouse for Birth Defects Monitoring Systems (1980). *Lancet*, **ii**, 1314.

Itzkowic, D. (1979). A survey of 59 triplet pregnancies. *British Journal of Obstetrics and Gynaecology*, **86**, 23–28.

James, W. B. and Lauersen, N. H. (1975). Hydatidiform mole with coexisting fetus. *American Journal of Obstetrics and Gynecology*, **122**, 267–272.

James, W. H. (1971). Excess of like sexed pairs of dizygotic twins. *Nature*, **232**, 277–278.

James, W. H. (1972). Secular changes in dizygotic twinning rates. *Journal of Biosocial Science*, **4**, 427–434.

James, W. H. (1974). Possible bias associated with the use of Weinberg's rule. *Journal of Reproductive Medicine*, **13**, 199.

James, W. H. (1976). Twinning and anencephaly. *Annals of Human biology*, **3**, 401–409.

James, W. H. (1977). Clomiphene, anencephaly and spina bifida. *Lancet*, **i**, 603 (letter).

James, W. H. (1978). A note on the epidemiology of acardiac monsters. *Teratology*, **16**, 211–216.

James, W. H. (1979). Is Weinberg's differential rule valid? *Acta Geneticae Medicae et Gemellologiae*, **28**, 69–71.

James, W. H. (1980a). Seasonality in twin and triplet births. *Annals of Human Biology*, **7**, 163–169.

James, W. H. (1980b). Sex ratio and placentation in twins. *Annals of Human Biology*, **7**, 273–276.

James, W. H. (1980c). Secular changes in twinning rates in England and Wales. *Annals of Human Biology*, **7**(5), 485–487.

James, W. H. (1980d). Gonadotrophin and the human secondary sex ratio. *British Medical Journal*, **281**, 711–712.

James, W. H. (1981). Differences between the events preceding spina bifida and anencephaly. *Journal of Medical Genetics*, **18**, 17–21.

James, W. H. (1982a). Second survey of secular trends in twinning rates. *Journal of Biosocial Science*, **14**, 481–497.

James, W. H. (1982b). The IQ advantages of the heavier twin. *British Journal of Psychology*, **73**, 513–517.

James, W. H. (1983). Twinning rates. *Lancet*, **i**, 934–935 (letter).

James, W. H. (1984). Coitus-induced ovulation and its implications for estimates of some reproductive parameters. *Acta Geneticae Medicae et Gemellologiae*, **33**, 547–555.

James, W. H. (1985). Dizygotic twinning, birthweight and latitude. *Annals of Human Biology*, **12**, 441–447.

James, W. H. (1986a). Hormonal control of sex ratio. *Journal of Theoretical Biology*, **118**, 427–441.

James, W. H. (1986b). Recent secular trends in dizygotic twinning rates in Europe. *Journal of Biosocial Science*, **18**, 497–504.

Jandial, V., Horne, C. H. W., Glover, R. G., Nisbet, A. D., Campbell, D. M. and MacGillivray, I. (1979). The value of measurement of pregnancy-specific proteins in twin pregnancies. *Acta Geneticae Medicae et Gemellologiae*, **28**, 319–325.

Janerich, D. T. (1975). Female excess in anencephaly and spina bifida: possible gestational influences. *American Journal of Epidemiology*, **99**, 1–6.

Jaschevatzky, O. E., Goldman, B., Kampf, D., Wexler, H. and Grunstein, S. (1980). Etiological aspects of double monsters. *European Journal of Obstetrics, Gynecology and Reproductive Biology*, **10**, 343–349.

Jassani, M. N., Merkatz, I. R., Brennan, J. N. and MacIntyre, M. N. (1980). Twin pregnancy with discordancy for Down's syndrome. *Obstetrics and Gynecology*, **55** (Suppl.), 455–465.

Jeanneret, O., and MacMahon, B. (1962). Secular changes in rates of multiple births in the United States. *American Journal of Human Genetics*, **14**, 410–425.

Jeanty, P., Roesch, F., Verhoogen, C. and Struyven, J. (1981). The vanishing twin. *Ultrasonics*, **2**, 25–31.

Jeffrey, R. L., Bowes, W. A. and Delaney, J. J. (1974). Role of bed rest in twin gestation. *Obstetrics and Gynecology*, **43**, 822–826.

Jeffreys, A. J., Wilson, V. and Thien, S. L. (1985). Individual-specific 'fingerprints' of human DNA. *Nature*, **316**, 76–79.

Johnson, S. F. and Driscoll, S. G. (1986). Twin placentation and its complications. *Seminars in Perinatology*, **10**, 9–13.

Jonas, E. G. (1963). The value of prenatal bed rest in multiple pregnancy. *Journal of Obstetrics and Gynaecology of the British Commonwealth*, **70**, 461–464.

Jones, K. L. and Benirschke, K. (1983). The developmental pathogenesis of structural defects: the contribution of monozygotic twins. *Seminars in Perinatology*, **7**, 239–243.

Jorgensen, G. (1970). Twin studies in congenital heart diseases. *Acta Geneticae Medicae et Gemellologiae*, **19**, 251–256.

Jung, J. H., Graham, J. M., Schultz, N. and Smith, D. W. (1984). Congenital hydranencephaly/porencephaly due to vascular disruption in monozygotic twins. *Pediatrics*, **73**, 467–469.

Junqueira, L. C. U. and de C. Pinto, V. A. (1951). Foetus in foetu acardico. Consideracoes em torno de um caso. *Review Paul. Medicine*, **38**, 118–122.

Junnarkar, A. R. and Nadkarni, M. G. (1979). Incidence of multiple births in an Indian rural community. *Journal of Epidemiology and Community Health*, **33**, 305–306.

Kaelber, C. T. and Pugh, T. F. (1969). Influence of intrauterine relations on the intelligence of twins. *New England Journal of Medicine*, **280**, 1030–1034.

Kajii, T., Ferrier, A., Niikawa, N., Takahara, H., Ohama, K. and Avirachen, S. (1980). Anatomic and chromosomal anomalies in 639 spontaneous abortuses. *Human Genetics*, **55**, 87–98.

Kallen, B. and Rybo, G. (1978). Conjoined twinning in Sweden. *Acta Obstetricia et Gynecologica Scandinavica*, **57**, 257–259.

Kallen, B. and Thorbert, G. (1985). Study of pregnancy outcome in a small area around a chemical factory and a chemical dump. *Environmental Research*, **37**, 313–319.

Kamimura, K. (1976). Epidemiology of twin births from a climatic point of view. *British Journal of Preventive and Social Medicine*, **30**: 175–176.

Kamin, L. J. (1978). Transfusion syndrome and the heritability of IQ. *Annals of Human Genetics*, **42**: 161–171.

Kandror, I. S. (1961). Physical development of newborn infants and children up to 3 years, born in the Arctic. *Pediatrics*, **40**: 41–46.

Kang, Y. S. and Cho, W. K. (1962). The sex ratio at birth and other attributes of the newborn from maternity hospitals in Korea. *Human Biology*, **34**: 38–48.

Kaplan, M. and Eidelman, A. E. (1983). Clustering of conjoined twins in Jerusalem, Israel: an epidemiologic survey. *American Journal of Obstetrics and Gynecology*, **143**: 636–637.

Kappel, B., Hansen, K. B., Moller, J. and Faaborg-Anderson, J. (1985). Bed rest in twin pregnancy. *Acta Geneticae Medicae et Gemellologiae*, **34**: 67–71.

Kappel, B., Sogaard, J., Nielsen, J. and Olsen, J. (1986). Seasonality in twin births in Denmark from 1936 to 1984. *Acta Geneticae Medicae et Gemellologiae*, **35**: Abstracts, p. 26.

Karn, M. (1952). Birthweight and length of gestation of twins, together with maternal age, parity and survival rate. *Annals of Eugenics*, **16**: 365–377.

Karn, M. (1953). Twin data: a further study of birthweight, gestation time, maternal age, order of birth and survival. *Annals of Eugenics*, **17**: 233–248.

Karp, L., Bryant, J. I., Tagatz, G., Giblett, E. and Fialkow, P. H. (1975). The occurrence of gonadal dysgenesis in association with monozygotic twinning. *Journal of Medical Genetics*, **12**: 70–78.

Kaufman, M. H. and O'Shea, K. S. (1978). Induction of monozygotic twinning in the mouse. *Nature*, **276**: 707–708.

Kellar, R., Matthews, G. D., MacKay, R., Brown, J. B. and Roy, E. J. (1959). Some clinical applications of oestrogen assay. *Journal of Obstetrics and Gynaecology of the British Commonwealth*, **66**: 804–814.

Kelsick, F. and Minkoff, J. (1982). Management of the breech second twin. *American Journal of Obstetrics and Gynecology*, **144**, 783–786.

Kemsley, W. F. F., Billewicz, W. Z. and Thomson, A. M. (1962). A new weight for height standard based on British anthropometric data. *British Journal of Preventive and Social Medicine*, **16**, 189–195.

Kendler, K. S. and Robinette, C. D. (1983). Month of birth by zygosity in the NAS-NRC twin registry. *Acta Geneticae Medicae et Gemellologiae*, **32**(2), 113–116.

Kenna, A. P., Smithells, R. W. and Fielding, D. W. (1975). Congenital heart disease in Liverpool 1960–1969. *Quarterly Journal of Medicine*, **44**, 17–44.

Kerenyi, T. D. and Chitkara, U. (1981). Selective birth in twin pregnancy with discordancy for Down's syndrome. *New England Journal of Medicine*, **304**, 1525–1527.

Kerin, J. F., Warnes, G. M., Quinn, P. H., Jeffrey, R., Kirby, C., Matthews, C. D.,

Seamark, R. F. and Cox, L. W. (1983). Incidence of multiple pregnancy after in vitro fertilisation and embryo transfer. *Lancet*, **ii**, 537–540.

Kerr, M. G. and Rashad, M. N. (1966). Autosomal trisomy in a discordant monozygotic twin. *Nature*, **212**, 726–727.

Khanna, K. K., Roy, P. B. and Bhatt, V. P. (1969). Female pseudohermaphroditism in conjoined twins. *Indian Journal of Medical Genetics*, **23**, 201–205.

Khoury, M. J. and Erickson, T. D. (1983). Maternal factors in dizygotic twinning: evidence from inter-racial crosses. *Annals of Human Biology*, **10**(5), 409–415.

Khunda, S. (1972). Locked twins. *Obstetrics and Gynecology*, **39**, 453–459.

Kidd, C. B., Innes, G. and Ross H. S. (1967). The prevalence of mental subnormality in two regions: some comparisons between North-East Scotland and Northern Ireland. *Ulster Medical Journal*, **36**, 139–144.

Kimball, A. P. and Rand, P. R. (1950). A manoeuvre for the simultaneous delivery of chin to chin locked twins. *American Journal of Obstetrics and Gynecology*, **59**, 1167–1168.

Kimmel, D. L., Moyer, E. K., Pearle, A. R., Winborne, L. W. and Gotwals, J. E. (1950). Cerebral tumour containing five human fetuses: case of fetus in fetu. *Anatomical Record*, **106**, 141–165.

Kindred, J. E. (1944). Twin pregnancies with one twin blighted. *American Journal of Obstetrics and Gynecology*, **48**, 642–684.

King, M. C., Friedman, G. D., Lattanzio, D., Rodgers, G., Lewis, A. M., Dupuy, M. E. and Williams, H. (1980). Diagnosis of twin zygosity by self-assessment and by genetic analysis. *Acta Geneticae Medicae et Gemellologiae*, **29**, 121–126.

Kirke, P. N. and Elwood, J. H. (1984). Anencephaly in the United Kingdom and Republic of Ireland. *British Medical Journal*, **289**, 1621 (letter).

Klebe, J. G. and Ingomar, C. J. (1972). The fetoplacental circulation during parturition illustrated by the interfetal transfusion syndrome. *Pediatrics*, **49**, 112–116.

Klein, J. (1964). Perinatal mortality in twin pregnancy. *Obstetrics and Gynecology*, **23**, 738–744.

Kloosterman, G. J. (1963). The "third circulation" in identical twins. *Nederlands Tijdschrift voor Verloskunde en Gynaecologie*, **63**, 395–412.

Klopper, A. (1976). Induction of ovulation. A review of current practice. *La Revue Française de'Endocrinologie Clinique, Nutrition et Metabolisme*, **17**, 531–539.

Knox, D. and Morley, D. (1960). Twinning in Yoruba women. *Journal of Obstetrics and Gynaecology of the British Empire*, **67**, 981–984.

Knox, E. G. (1970). Fetus-fetus interaction—a model aetiology for anencephalus. *Developmental Medicine and Child Neurology*, **12**, 167–177.

Kohorn, E. I. and Kaufman, M. (1974). Sonar in the first trimester of pregnancy. *Obstetrics and Gynecology*, **44**, 473–483.

Komaromy, B. and Lampé, L. (1977). The value of bed rest in twin pregnancies. *International Journal of Gynaecology and Obstetrics*, **15**, 262–266.

Kramer, A. A., Corey, L. and Nance, W. E. (1982). Rates of congenital heart disease and oral clefting in the offspring of Norwegian twins. March of Dimes *Birth Defects*, Conference Abstracts.

Kruger, J. and Propping, P. (1976). Twinning frequencies in Baden-Wurttemberg according to maternal age and parity from 1955 to 1972. *Acta Geneticae Medicae et Gemellologiae*, **25**, 36–40.

Kurachi, K., Aono, T., Minagawa, J. and Miyake, A. (1983). Congenital malformations of newborn infants after clomiphene-induced ovulation. *Fertility and Sterility*, **40**, 187–189.

Kurjak, A. and Latin, U. (1979). Ultrasound diagnosis of fetal abnormalities in multiple pregnancy. *Acta Obstetrica Gynecologica Scandinavica*, **58**, 153–161.

Kurtz, G. R., Davis, L. L. and Loftus, J. B. (1958). Factors influencing the survival of triplets. *Obstetrics and Gynecology*, **12**, 504–508.

Kyu, H., Thu, A. and Cook, P. J. L. (1981). Human genetics in Burma. *Human Heredity*, **31**, 291–295.

Lamy, M., DeGrouchy, J. and Schweisguth, O. (1957). Genetic and non-genetic factors in the aetiology of congenital heart disease: a study of 1188 cases. *American Journal of Human Genetics*, **9**, 17–41.

Lamy, M., Frezal, J., DeGrouchy, J. and Chryssostomidou, M. (1955). L'âge maternel et le rang de naissance dans un enchantillon de jumeaux. *Acta Genetica et Statistica Medica*, **5**, 403–419.

Landy, H. J., Keith, L. and Keith, D. (1982). The vanishing twin. *Acta Geneticae Medicae et Gemellologiae*, **31**, 179–194.

Lauritsen, J. G. (1976). Aetiology of spontaneous abortion. *Acta Obstetricia et Gynecologica Scandinavica*, Suppl. 52, 1–29.

Law, R. G. (1967). *Standards of obstetric care: the report of the North-West Metropolitan Regional Obstetric Survey*, E. & S. Livingstone, Edinburgh.

Layde, P. M., Erickson, J. O., Falek, A. and McCarthy, B. J. (1980). Congenital malformations in twins. *American Journal of Human Genetics*, **32**, 69–78.

Lazar, P. (1976). Effets des avortements spontanés sur le fréquence des naissances gémellaires. *Comptes Rendus Academic Sciences*, **282**, 243–246.

Lazar, P., Hemon, D. and Berger, C. (1978). Twinning rate and reproduction failures. In: *Twin Research: Biology and Epidemiology*, Nance, W. E., Allen, G. and Parisi, P. (eds.), Alan R. Liss, New York, pp. 125–132.

Leck, I. (1983). Spina bifida and anencephaly: fewer patients, more problems. *British Medical Journal*, **286**, 1679–1680.

Le Marec, B., Roussey, M., Oger, J. and Senecal, J. (1978). Excess twinning in the parents of spina bifida. In: *Twin Research: Biology and Epidemiology*, Nance, W. E., Allen, G. and Parisi, P. (eds.), Alan R. Liss, New York, pp. 121–123.

Lemire, R. J. and Beckwith, B. (1982). Pathogenesis of congenital tumours and malformations of the sacrococcygeal region. *Teratology*, **25**, 201–213.

Lemli, L. and Smith, D. W. (1963). The XO syndrome: a study of differential phenotype in 25 patients. *Journal of Pediatrics*, **63**, 577–588.

Lenstrup, C. (1984). Reactive value of antepartum non-stress test in multiple pregnancies. *Acta Obstetricia et Gynecologica Scandinavica*, **63**(7), 597–601.

Lenz, F. (1933). Zur frage der ursachen von zwillingsgeburten. *Archives für Rassen und Gesellschaftsbiologie*, **27**, 294–318.

Lenz, W. (1966). Malformations caused by drugs in pregnancy. *American Journal of Diseases of Children*, **112**, 99–106.

Leroy, B., Lefort, F. and Jeny, R. (1982). Uterine height and umbilical perimeter curves in twin pregnancies. *Acta Geneticae Medicae et Gemellologiae*, **31**, 195–198.

Levi, S. (1976). Ultrasonic assessment of the high rate of human multiple pregnancy in the first trimester. *Journal of Clinical Ultrasound*, **4**, 3–5.

Levi, S. and Reimers, M. (1978). Demonstration échographique de la fréquence relativement élevée des grossesses multiples humaines pendant la période embryonnaire In: *L'implantation de l'Oeuf*, DuMesnil due Buisson, S., Psychoyos, A. and Thomas, K. (eds.), Masson Editions, Paris, pp. 295–307.

Lewis, E. (1979). Mourning by the family after a stillbirth or neonatal death. *Archives of Disease in Childhood*, **54**, 303–306.

Lewis, E. (1983). Psychological consequences and strategies of management. In: *Advances in Perinatal Medicine*, 3rd edition, Mulinsky, A., Friedman, E. A. and Gluck, I. (eds.), Plenum Press, New York.

Lewis, E. and Page, A. (1978). Failure to mourn a stillbirth: an overlooked catastrophe. *British Journal of Medical Psychology*, **51**, 237–241.

Lewis, R. H. (1961). Foetus in foetu and the retroperitoneal teratoma. *Archives of Disease in Childhood*, **36**, 220–226.

Lilienfeld, A. M. and Pasamanick, B. (1955). A study of variations in the frequency of twin births by race and socio-economic status. *American Journal of Human Genetics*, **7**, 204–217.

Lil'in, E. T. and Gindilis, V. M. (1976). Genetiko-statisticheskii analiz mnogoplodia u cheloveka. *Genetika*, (English abstract), **12**, 118–127.

Lin, R. S. and Chen, K. P. (1968). A preliminary study in Taiwan. I. Epidemiological aspects. *Journal of Formosan Medical Association*, **67**, 329–342.

Lindley, M. and Migeon, B. R. (1979). Fetal mortality and sex ratio. *Science*, **206**, 1428.

Lindsten, J. (1963). *The Nature and Origin of Z-chromosome Aberrations in Turner's Syndrome*. Amquist and Wiksell, Stockholm.

Lipovetskaya, N. G. and Yampol'skaya, Y. A. (1975). Decrease in the birth rate of twins and multiple-pregnancy factors. *Genetika*, **11**, 150–157.

Lister, U. G. (1969). Cited by Nylander, P. P. S. (1970d). *Acta Geneticae Medicae et Gemellologiae*, **19**, 458.

Little, J. and Elwood, J. M. (1987). Problems in the assessment of seasonality in twinning rate with reference to twinning in North-East Scotland and Northern Ireland 1975–1979. In: *Seasonal Effects of Reproduction, Infection and Psychoses*, Miura, T. (ed.), SPB Academic Publishing, The Hague, Netherlands, pp. 61–72.

Little, J. and Nevin, N. C. (1988). Congenital anomalies in twins in Northern Ireland. I. Anomalies in general and specific anomalies other than neurbal tube defects and of the cardiovascular system 1974–1979. *Acta Geneticae Medicae et Gemellologiae* (in press).

Little, W. A. and Friedman, E. A. (1958). The twin delivery—factors influencing second twin survival. *Obstetrics and Gynecological Survey*, **13**, 611–623.

Livingston, J. E. and Poland, B. J. (1980). A study of spontaneously aborted twins. *Teratology*, **21**, 139–148.

Livingstone, W. P. (1918). *Mary Slessor of Calabar*, Hodder and Stoughton, London, New York, Toronto.

Lorber, J. (1984). The family history of "simple" congenital hydrocephalus: an epidemiological study based on 270 probands. *Zeitschrift für Kinderchirurgie und Grenzgebiete*, **39** (suppl. II), 94–95.

Lord, J. M. (1956). Intra-abdominal foetus-in-foetu. *Journal of Pathology and Bacteriology*, **72**, 627–641.

Loughnan, P. M., Gold, H. and Vance, J. C. (1973). Phenytoin teratogenicity in man. *Lancet*, **i**, 70–72.

Louw, J. H. and Barnard, C. N. (1955). Congenital intestinal atresia: observations on its origin. *Lancet*, **ii**, 1065–1067.

Louw, J. H., Cywes, S., Davies, M. R. Q. and Rode, H. (1981). Congenital jejuno-ileal atresia: observations on its pathogenesis and treatment. *Zeitschrift für Kinderchirurgie und Grenzgebiete*, **33**, 3–17.

Loucopoulos, A. and Jewelewicz, R. (1982). Management of multifetal pregnancies: sixteen years experience in the Sloane Hospital for Women. *American Journal of Obstetrics and Gynecology*, **143**, 902–905.

Lowry, J. F. (1979). Fetal mortality and sex ratio. *Science*, **206**, 1428.

Lykken, D. T. (1978). The diagnosis of zygosity in twins. *Behavior Genetics*, **8**(5), 437–473.

MacArthur, J. W. (1942). Relations of body size to litter size and to the incidence of paternal twins. *Journal of Heredity*, **33**, 87–91.

McArthur, N. R. (1952). A statistical study of human twinning. *Annals of Eugenics*, **16**, 338–350.

McBride, M. L. (1979). Sib risks of anencephaly and spina bifida in British Columbia. *American Journal of Medical Genetics*, **3**, 377–387.

McClure, H. I. (1937). Multiple pregnancy. *Ulster Medical Journal*, **6**, 284–292.

McCullough, J. M. and O'Rourke, D. H. (1986). Geographic distribution of consanguinity in Europe. *Annals of Human Biology*, **13**, 359–367.

McDonald, A. D. (1964). Mongolism in twins. *Journal of Medical Genetics*, **1**, 39–41.

MacDonald, R. R. (1962). Management of second twin. *British Medical Journal*, **1**, 518–522.

MacFarlane, A. and Scott, J. S. (1976). Pre-eclampsia/eclampsia in twin pregnancies. *Journal of Medical Genetics*, **13**, 208–211.

MacGillivray, I. (1958). Some observations on the incidence of pre-eclampsia. *Journal of Obstetrics and Gynaecology of the British Empire*, **65**, 536–539.

MacGillivray, I. (1975). Malformations and other abnormalities in twins. In: *Human Multiple Reproduction*, MacGillivray, I., Nylander, P. P. S. and Corney, G. (eds.), W. B. Saunders, London, pp. 165–175.

MacGillivray, I. (1980). Twins and other multiple deliveries. *Clinics in Obstetrics and Gynaecology*, **7**(3), 581–600.

MacGillivray, I. (1981). The probable explanation for the falling twinning rate in Scotland. In: *Twin Research 3, Part A, Twin Biology and Multiple Pregnancy*, Gedda, L., Parisi, P. and Nance, W. E. (eds.), Alan R. Liss, New York, pp. 15–19.

MacGillivray, I. (1983). *Pre-eclampsia. The Hypertensive Disease of Pregnancy*, W. B. Saunders, London, Philadelphia, Toronto, Chapters 1 and 2, pp. 1–22; Chapter 6, pp. 174–190.

MacGillivray, I. (1984)., Presidential address: The Aberdeen contribution to Twinning. *Acta Geneticae Medicae et Gemellologiae*, **33**(1), 5–11.

MacGillivray, I. (1986). Update on the value of bed rest in multiple pregnancy. Paper presented to Fifth Congress of International Society for Twin Studies, Amsterdam (unpublished).

MacGillivray, I., Campbell, D. M. and Duffus, G. M. (1971). Maternal metabolic response to twin pregnancy in primigravidae. *Journal of Obstetrics and Gynaecology of the British Commonwealth*, **78**, 530–534.

MacGillivray, I., Nylander, P. P. S. and Corney, G. (1975). *Human Multiple Reproduction*, W. B. Saunders, London.

MacGillivray, I. and Campbell, D. M. (1981). The outcome of twin pregnancies in Aberdeen. In: *Twin Research 3, Part A, Twin Biology and Multiple Pregnancy*, Gedda, L., Parisi, P. and Nance, W. E. (eds.), Alan R. Liss, New York, pp. 203–206.

MacGillivray, I., Campbell, D. M., Samphier, M. and Thompson, B. (1982). Preterm deliveries in twin pregnancies in Aberdeen. *Acta Geneticae Medicae et Gemellologiae*, **31**, 207–211.

McIntosh, R., Merritt, K. I., Richards, M. R., Samuels, M. H. and Bellows, M. T. (1954). Incidence of congenital malformations: a study of 5964 pregnancies. *Pediatrics*, **14**, 505–522.

McKeown, T. and Record, R. G. (1952). Observations on foetal growth in multiple pregnancy in man. *Journal of Endocrinology*, **8**, 386–401.

McKeown, T. and Record, R. G. (1953). The influence of placental size on foetal growth in man with special reference to multiple pregnancy. *Journal of Endocrinology*, **9**, 418–426.

McKeown, T. and Record, R. G. (1960). Malformations in a population observed for five years after birth. In: *CIBA Foundation Symposium on Congenital Malformations*, Wolstenholme, G. E. W. and O'Conner, C. M. (eds.), Churchill, London, pp. 2–21.

McMillen, M. M. (1979). Differential mortality by sex in fetal and neonatal deaths. *Science*, **204**, 89–91.

Macourt, D. C., Stewart, P. and Zaki, M. (1982). Multiple pregnancy and fetal abnormalities in association with oral contraceptive usage. *Australian and New Zealand Journal of Obstetrics and Gynecology*, **22**, 25–28.

Magnus, P. (1984). Distinguishing fetal and maternal genetic effects on variation in birthweight. *Acta Geneticae Medicae et Gemellologiae*, **33**, 481–486.

Majsky, A. and Kout, M. (1982). Another case of occurrence of two different fathers of twins by HLA typing. *Tissue Antigens*, **20**, 305.

Mannino, F. L., Jones, K. L. and Benirschke, K. (1977). Congenital skin defects and fetus papyraceus. *Journal of Pediatrics*, **91**, 559–564.

Marinho, A. O., Ilesanmi, A. O., Ladele, O. A., Asuni, O. H., Omigbodun, A. and Oyejide, C. O. (1986). A fall in the rate of multiple births in Ibadan and Igbo Ora, Nigeria. *Acta Geneticae Medicae et Gemellologiae*, **35**, 201–204.

Marivate, M., de Villiers, K. Q. and Fairbrother, P. (1977). Effect of prophylactic outpatient administration of fenoterol on the time and onset of spontaneous labour and fetal growth rate in twin pregnancy. *American Journal of Obstetrics and Gynecology*, **128**, 707–708.

Marsh, R. W. (1980). The significance for intelligence of differences in birthweight and health within monozygotic twin pairs. *British Journal of Psychology*, **71**, 63–67.

Martin, N. G., El Beaini, J. L., Olsen, M. C., Bhatnagar, A. S. and Macourt, D. (1984)., Gonadotrophin levels in mothers who had two sets of DZ twins. *Acta Geneticae Medicae et Gemellologiae*, **33**, 131–139.

Masson, G. M. (1973). Plasma estriol in normal and pre-eclamptic multiple pregnancies. *Obstetrics and Gynecology*, **42**, 568–573.

Medearis, A. L., Jonas, H. S., Stockbauer, J. W. and Danke, H. C. (1979). Perinatal deaths in twin pregnancy. A five year analysis of statistics in Missouri. *American Journal of Obstetrics and Gynecology*, **134**, 413–418.

Meir, P. R. and Saunders, B. (1982). Prenatal diagnosis and multiple gestation. *Birth Defects*, **18** (3pt a), 121–124.

Mellin, G. W. and Katzenstein, M. (1962). The saga of thalidomide: neuropathy to embryopathy, with case reports of congenital anomalies. *New England Journal of Medicine*, **267**, 1184–1193; 1238–1244.

Melnick, M. (1977). Brain damage in survivor after death of monozygotic co-twin. *Lancet*, **ii**, 12187.

Melnick, M. and Myrianthopoulos, N. C. (1979). The effects of chorion type on normal and abnormal developmental variation in monozygous twins. *American Journal of Medical Genetics*, **4**, 147–156.

Metneki, J. and Czeizel, A. (1983). Twinning rates. *Lancet*, **i**, 935 (letter).

Metneki, J., Czeizel, A. and Keller, I. (1983). Az ooszenott ikrek gyakorisaga, epidemiologiaja es koreredete. *Orvosi Hetilap*, **124**, 885–887.

Meyer, A. W. (1919). The occurrence of superfetation. *Journal of the American Medical Association*, **72**, 769–774.

Michels, V. V. and Riccardi, V. M. (1978). Twin recurrence and amniocentesis: male and MZ heritability factors. *Birth Defects: Original Articles Series*, **14**, 201–211.

Micklewitz, H., Kennedy, J., Kawada, C. and Kennison, R. (1981). Triplet pregnancies. *Journal of Reproductive Medicine*, **26**, 243–246.

Miettinen, M. (1954). On triplets and quadruplets in Finland. *Acta Paediatrica*, **43**, Suppl. 99, 9–103.

Milham, S. (1964). Pituitary gonadotrophin and dizygotic twinning. *Lancet*, **ii**, 566.

Milham, S. (1966). Symmetrical conjoined twins: an analysis of the birth records of 22 sets. *Journal of Pediatrics*, **69**, 643–647.

Milham, S. and Gittelsohn, A. M. (1965). Parental age and malformations. *Human Biology*, **37**, 13–22.

Millis, J. (1959). The frequency of twinning in poor Chinese in the Maternity Hospital, Singapore. *Annals of Human Genetics*, **23**, 171–174.

Mitchell, S. C., Korones, S. B. and Berendes, H. W. (1971a). Congenital heart disease in 56,109 births: incidence and natural history. *Circulation*, **43**, 323–332.

Mitchell, S. C., Sellmann, A. H., Westphal, M. C. and Park, J. (1971b). Etiologic correlates in a study of congenital heart disease in 56,109 births. *American Cardiology*, **28**, 653–657.

Mittler, P. (1971). *The Study of Twins*, Penguin Books, Hardmondsworth.

Miura, T., Nakamura, I., Shimura, M., Nonaka, K. and Amau, Y. (1984). Twinning rate by month of mother's birth in Japan. *Acta Geneticae Medicae et Gemellologiae*, **33**, 123–130.

Modan, B., Kallner, H., Modan, M. and Nemser, L. (1968). Differential twinning in Israeli major ethnic groups. *American Journal of Epidemiology*, **88**, 189–194.

Moir, J. C. (1964). *Operative Obstetrics*, Baillière Tindall and Cox, London, p. 225.

Moore, C. M., McAdams, A. J. and Sutherland, J. (1969). Intrauterine disseminated intravascular coagulation: a syndrome of multiple pregnancy with a dead twin fetus. *Journal of Pediatrics*, **74**, 523–528.

Mori, K. (1975). Genetic aspects of congenital heart disease. *Journal of Tokyo Womens Medical College*, **45**, 118–135.

Mortimer, B. and Kirschbaum, J. D. (1942). Human double monsters (so called Siamese twins): anatomic presentation. *American Journal of Diseases of Children*, **64**, 697–704.

Morton, N. E. and Schull, W. J. (1953). *Studies on Consanguinity and Heritability*, Hiroshima: Atomic Bomb Casualty Commission, National Research Council.

Morton, N. E., Chung, C. S. and Mi, M. P. (1967). Genetics of inter-racial crosses in Hawaii. *Monographs in Human Genetics*, **3**, Karger, Basel.

Mosteller, M., Townsend, J. I., Corey, L. A. and Nance, W. E. (1981). Twinning rates in Virginia: secular trends and the effects of maternal age and parity. In: *Twin Research 3, Part A, Twin Biology and Multiple Pregnancy*, Gedda, L., Parisi, P. and Nance, W. E. (eds.), Alan R. Liss, New York, pp. 57–59.

Mudaliar, A. L. (1930). Double monsters: a study of their circulatory system and some other anatomical abnormalities and the complications in labour. *Journal of Obstetrics and Gynaecology of the British Empire*, **37**, 753–768.

Mueller-Heubach, E., Hechman, L. and Tyndall, C. (1985). Factors affecting the management of twin delivery. *Archives of Gynaecology*, 237 Suppl., Abstracts XIth World Congress of Gynaecology and Obstetrics, Berlin West, Springer-Verlag, Berlin, p.169.

Mulcahy, M. T., Roberman, B. and Reid, S. E. (1984). Chorion biopsy, cytogenetic diagnosis and selective termination in a twin pregnancy at risk of haemophilia. *Lancet*, **ii**, 866–867.

Muller, P., Calvert, J. and Rihm, G. (1970). Mosaique 45, XO/46, XX/47, XXX chez deux jumelles monozygotes: concordances et discordances cliniques et biologiques. *Annals of Endocrinology (Paris)*, **31**, 1143–1152.

Mulligan, T. O. (1970). Cited by Nylander, P. P. S. (1971c). *Annals of Human Genetics*, **34**, 410.

Munnell, E. W. and Taylor, H. C. (1946). Complications and fetal mortality in 136 cases of multiple pregnancy. *American Journal of Obstetrics and Gynecology*, **52**, 588–597.

Munsinger, H. (1977). The identical twin transfusion syndrome: a source of error in estimating IQ resemblances and heritability. *Annals of Human Genetics*, **40**, 307–321.

Myrianthopoulos, M. C. (1970). An epidemiologic survey of twins in a large prospectively studied population. *American Journal of Human Genetics*, **22**, 611–629.

Myrianthopoulos, M. C. (1975). Congenital malformations in twins: epidemiologic survey. *Birth Defects: Original Articles Series*, **XI**(8): 1–39.

Myrianthopoulos, M. C. (1978). Congenital malformations. The contribution of twin studies. *Birth Defects: Original Article Series*, **14**, 151–159.

Myrianthopoulos, M. C., and Chung, C. S. (1974). Congenital malformations in singletons: epidemiologic survey. *Birth Defects: Original Articles Series*, **X**(11), 1–58.

Naeye, R. L. (1963). Human intrauterine parabiotic syndrome and its complications. *New England Journal of Medicine*, **268**, 804–809.

Naeye, R. L. (1965). Organ abnormalities in a human parabiotic syndrome. *American Journal of Pathology*, **46**, 829–842.

Nance, W. E. (1981). Malformations unique to the twinning process. In: *Twin Research 3, Part A, Twin Biology and Multiple Pregnancy*, Gedda, L., Parisi, P. and Nance, W. E. (eds.), Alan R. Liss, New York, pp. 123–133.

Nance, W. E. and Uchida, I. (1964). Turner's syndrome, twinning and an unusual variant of glucose-6-phosphate dehydrogenase. *American Journal of Human Genetics*, **16**, 380–392.

Nance, W. E. and Corey, L. A. (1976). Genetic models for the analysis of data from the families of identical twins. *Genetics*, **83**, 811–826.

Napolitani, F. D. and Schreiber, I. (1960). The acardiac monster: a review of the world literature and presentation of two cases. *American Journal of Obstetrics and Gynecology*, **80**, 582–589.

Neel, J. V. (1958). A study of major congenital defects in Japanese infants. *American Journal of Human Genetics*, **10**, 398–445.

Neilson, J. P., Crowther, C., Verkuyl, D. A. A. and Bannerman, C. (1986). Cervical assessment in the management of twin pregnancy. *Acta Geneticae Medicae et Gemellologiae*, **35**, Abstracts, p. 68.

Nejedly, C. (1951). Su di un caso di gravidanza gemellare monocoriale biamniotica con un fetu papiraceo. *Minerva Ginecol*, **3**, 20–22.

Nelson, T. R. (1955). A clinical study of pre-eclampsia. *Journal of Obstetrics and Gynaecology of the British Empire*, **62**, 48–66.

Neto, R. M., Castilla, E. E. and Paz, J. E. (1981). Hypospadias: an epidemiological study in Latin America. *American Journal of Medical Genetics*, **10**, 5–19.

Nevin, N. C., McDonald, J. R. and Walby, A. L. (1978). A comparison of neural tube defects identified by two independent routine recording systems for congenital malformations in Northern Ireland. *International Journal of Epidemiology*, **7**, 319–327.

New Zealand Yearbook (1982). Department of Statistics, Wellington.

Newman, H. H. and Patterson, J. T. (1909). A case of normal identical quadruplets in the 9-banded armadillo and its bearing on the problems of identical twins and of sex determination. *Biological Bulletin*, **17**, 181–187.

Nichols, B. L., Blattner, R. J. and Rudolph, A. J. (1967). General clinical management of thoracopagus twins. *Birth Defects: Original Articles Series*, **III**(1), 38–51.

Nielsen, J. (1966). Diabetes mellitus in parents of patients with Klinefelter's syndrome. *Lancet*, **i**, 1376 (letter).

Nielsen, J. (1970). Twins in sibships with Klinefelter's syndrome and the YYY syndrome. *Acta Geneticae Medicae et Gemellologiae*, **19**, 399–404.

Nielsen, J. and Dahl, G. (1976). Twins in the sibships and parental sibships of women with Turner's syndrome. *Clinical Genetics*, **10**, 93–96.

Nissen, E. D. (1958). Twins: collision, impaction, compaction and interlocking. *Obstetrics and Gynecology*, **11**, 514–526.

Noonan, J. A. (1963). Cardiovascular anomalies in twins (abstract). *Proceedings of the Society of Pediatric Research*, 54.

Noonan, J. A. (1978). Twins, conjoined twins, and cardiac defects. *American Journal of Diseases of Children*, **132**, 17–18.

Nora, J. J., Gilliland, J. C., Sommerville, R. J. and McNamara, D. G. (1967). Congenital heart disease in twins. *New England Journal of Medicine*, **277**, 568–571.

Nylander, P. P. S. (1967). Twinning in West Africa. *World Medical Journal*, **14**, 178–180.

Nylander, P. P. S. (1969). The frequency of twinning in a rural community in Western Nigeria. *Annals of Human Genetics*, **33**, 41–44.

Nylander, P. P. S. (1970a). The determination of zygosity—a study of 608 pairs of twins born in Aberdeen. *Journal of Obstetrics and Gynaecology of the British Commonwealth*, **77**(6), 505–510.

Nylander, P. P. S. (1970b). The inheritance of dizygotic twinning. A study of 18,737 maternities in Ibadan, Western Nigeria. *Acta Geneticae Medicae et Gemellologiae*, **19**, 36–39.

Nylander, P. P. S. (1970c). Placental forms and zygosity determination of twins in Ibadan, Western Nigeria. *Acta Geneticae Medicae et Gemellologiae*, **19**, 49–54.

Nylander, P. P. S. (1970d). Twinning in Nigeria. *Acta Geneticae Medicae et Gemellologiae*, **19**, 457–464.

Nylander, P. P. S. (1971a). Biosocial aspects of multiple births. *Journal of Biosocial Science*, Suppl. 3, 29–38.

Nylander, P. P. S. (1971b). Ethnic differences in twinning rates in Nigeria. *Journal of Biosocial Science*, **3**, 151–157.

Nylander, P. P. S. (1971c). The incidence of triplets and higher multiple births in some rural and urban populations in Western Nigeria. *Annals of Human Genetics*, **34**, 409–415.

Nylander, P. P. S. (1973). Serum levels of gonadotrophins in relation to multiple pregnancy in Nigeria. *Journal of Obstetrics and Gynaecology*, **80**, 651–653.

Nylander, P. P. S. (1975a). The causation of twinning. In: *Human Multiple Reproduction*, MacGillivray, I., Nylander, P. P. S. and Corney, G. (eds.), W. B. Saunders, London, pp. 77–86.

Nylander, P. P. S. (1975b). Frequency of multiple births. In: *Human Multiple Reproduction*, MacGillivray, I., Nylander, P. P. S. and Corney, G. (eds.), W. B. Saunders, London, pp. 87–97.

Nylander, P. P. S. (1975c). Factors which influence twinning rates. In: *Human Multiple Reproduction*, MacGillivray, I., Nylander, P. P. S. and Corney, G. (eds.). W. B. Saunders, London, pp. 98–106.

Nylander, P. P. S. (1978). Causes of high twinning frequencies in Nigeria. In: *Twin Research: Biology and Epidemiology*, Nance, W. E., Allen, G. and Parisi, P. (eds.). Allan R. Liss, New York, pp. 35–43.

Nylander, P. P. S. (1979a). The twinning incidence in Nigeria. *Acta Geneticae Medicae et Gemellologiae*, **28**, 261–263.

Nylander, P. P. S. (1979b). Perinatal mortality in twins. *Acta Geneticae Medicae et Gemellologiae*, **28**, 363–368.

Nylander, P. P. S. (1981). The factors that influence twinning rates. *Acta Geneticae Medicae et Gemellologiae*, **30**, 189–202.

Nylander, P. P. S. (1983). The phenomenon of twinning. In: *Obstetrical Epidemiology*, Barron, S. L. and Thomson, A. M. (eds.), Academic Press, London, pp. 143–165.

Nylander, P. P. S. and Osunkoya, B. O. (1970). Unusual monochorionic placentation with heterosexual twins. *Obstetrics and Gynecology*, **36**, 621–625.

Nylander, P. P. S. and Corney, G. (1971). Placentation and zygosity of triplets and higher multiple births in Ibadan, Nigeria. *Annals of Human Genetics*, **34**, 417–426.

Nylander, P. P. S. and MacGillivray, I. (1975). Complications of twin pregnancy. In: *Human Multiple Reproduction*, MacGillivray, I., Nylander, P. P. S. and Corney, G. (eds.), W. B. Saunders, London, pp. 137–146.

Nylander, P. P. S. and Corney, G. (1977). Placentation and zygosity of twins in Northern Nigeria. *Annals of Human Genetics*, **40**, 323–329.

O'Connor, M. C., Murphy, H. and Dalrymple, I. J. (1979). Double blind trial of ritodrine and placebo in twin pregnancy. *British Journal of Obstetrics and Gynaecology*, **86**, 706–709.

O'Connor, M. C., Arias, E., Royston, J. P. and Dalrymple, I. J. (1981). The merits of special antenatal care for twin pregnancies. *British Journal of Obstetrics and Gynaecology*, **88**, 222–230.

Ohama, K., Ueda, K., Okamoto, E. and Kujiwara, A. (1985). Two cases of dizygotic twins with androgenetic mole and normal conceptus. *Hiroshima Journal of Medical Sciences*, **34**, 371–375.

Olivier, G., Sophonn, S. and Van Hong, N. (1965). Fréquence de la gémellite en Indochine. *Bulletin Académique Nationale Médecine*, **149**, 589–691.

Olofsson, P. and Rydhstrom, H. (1985). Twin delivery: how should the second twin be delivered? *American Journal of Obstetrics and Gynecology*, **153**, 479–481.

Onyskowova, Z., Dolezal, A. and Jedlicka, V. (1971). The frequency and the character of malformations in multiple birth: a preliminary report. *Teratology*, **4**, 496–497.

Ornoy, A., Navot, D., Menashi, M., Laufer, N. and Chemke, J. (1980). Asymmetry and discordance for congenital anomalies in conjoined twins: a report of six cases. *Teratology*, **22**, 145–154.

Osborne, R. H. and De George, F. V. (1957). Selective survival in dyzygotic twins in relation to the ABO blood groups. *American Journal of Human Genetics*, **9**, 321–330.

Owen, J. B. (1976). *Sheep Production*, Baillière Tindall, London.

Paintin, D. B. (1962). The epidemiology of antepartum haemorrhage. A study of all births in a community. *Journal of Obstetrics and Gynaecology of the British Commonwealth*, **69**, 614–624.

Papiernik, E., Gerard, L., Hult, A. M. and Schneider, L. (1976). Hypothesis of an ovular regulation of pregnancy weight gain. *Acta Geneticae Medicae et Gemellologiae*, **25**, 328–330.

Paredes, A., Turner, H. H., and Zanartu, J. (1962). Psychologic study of identical twins with ovarian dysgenesis. *Journal of Nervous and Mental Disorders*, **143**, 28–33.

Parisi, P. (1986). Incidence of twinning: variability and interpretations. *Acta Medicae Geneticae et Gemellologiae*, **35**, Abstracts, p. 28.

Parisi, P. and Caperna, G. (1981). The changing incidence of twinning: one century of Italian statistics. In: *Twin Research 3, Part A, Twin Biology and Multiple Pregnancy*, Gedda, L., Parisi, P. and Nance, W. E. (eds.), Alan R. Liss, New York, pp. 35–48.

Parisi, P., Gatti, M., Prinzi, G. and Caperna, G. (1983). Familial incidence of twinning. *Nature*, **304**, 626–628.

Parsons, P. A. (1964). Birthweight and survival of unlike-sexed twins. *Annals of Human Genetics*, **28**: 1–10.

Patel, N., Bowie, W., Campbell, D. M., Howat, R., Melrose, E., Redford, D., McIlwaine, G. and Smalls, M. (1984). *Scottish Twin Study 1983 Report*, Social Paediatric and Obstetric Research Unit, University of Glasgow and Greater Glasgow Health Board.

Patten, P. T. (1970). Perinatal mortality by birth order in multiple pregnancy. *Australian and New Zealand Journal of Obstetrics and Gynecology*, **10**, 22–29.

Peal, W. J. (1965). East African sources of steroidal components of potential value as hormone precursors. *Proceedings of East African Academy*, **III**, 9–13.

Pedersen, I. K., Philip, J., Sele, V. and Starup, J. (1980). Monozygotic twins with dissimilar phenotypes and chromosome complements. *Acta Obstetricia et Gynecologica Scandinavica*, **59**(5): 459–462.

Pedreira, C. M., Peixoto, U. S. and Rocha, L. M. G. I. (1959). Estude de gemelaridade na populacao de Salvador-Bahlia. *Anais da I Reuniao Brasileira de Genetica Humana*, 137–140.

Penrose, L. S. (1937). Congenital syphilis in monovular twin. *Lancet*, **i**, 322.

Persson, P. H. and Grennert, L. (1979). Diagnosis and treatment of twin pregnancy. *Acta Geneticae Medicae et Gemellologiae*, **28**, 311–317.

Pescia, G., Ferrier, P. E. and Wyss-Hutin, D. (1975). 45 X Turner's syndrome in monozygotic twin sisters. *Journal of Medical Genetics*, **12**, 390.

Petres, R. E. and Redwine, F. O. (1981). Selective birth in twin pregnancy. *New England Journal of Medicine*, **305**, 1218–1219 (letter).

Philip (1981). Cited by Rodeck, C. H. and Wass, D. (1981). *Prenatal diagnosis*, **1**, 43.

Philippe, P. (1981). Features of pedigree transmission of twin births at Isle-aux-Coudres (Quebec). *Human Heredity*, **31**, 116–118.

Phillpott, R. H. (1980). Obstructed labour. *Clinics in Obstetrics and Gynaecology*, **7**(3), 601–619.

Pickering, R. M. (1987). Maternal characteristics and the distribution of birthweight standardized for gestational age. *Journal of Biosocial Science*, **19**, 17–26.

Ping, Y. W. and Chin, C. L. (1967). Incidence of twin births among the Chinese in Taiwan. *American Jouranl of Obstetrics and Gynecology*, **98**, 881–884.

Pollard, G. N. (1969). Multiple births in Australia 1944–1963. *Journal of Biosocial Science*, **1**, 389–404.

Pollard, R. (1985). Twinning Rates in Fiji. *Annals of Human Genetics*, **49**, 65–73.

Porter, I. H. and Hook, E. B. (1980). *Human Embryonic and Fetal Death*, Academic Press, New York.

Portes, L. and Granjon, A. (1946). Les Présentations au cours des accoucaments gémellaires. *Gynecologie et Obstetrique*, **45**, 1459.

Potter, A. M. and Taitz, L. S. (1972). Turner's syndrome in one of monozygotic twins with mosaicism. *Acta Paediatrica Scandinavica*, **61**, 473–476.

Potter, E. L. (1962). *Pathology of the Fetus and the Newborn*, Year Book Publishers, Chicago, p. 155.

Potter, E. L. (1963). Twin zygosity and placental form in relation to the outcome of the pregnancy. *American Journal of Obstetrics and Gynecology*, **87**, 566–577.

Potter, E. L. and Fuller, H. (1949). Multiple pregnancies at the Chicago Lying-in Hospital 1941–1947. *American Journal of Obstetrics and Gynecology*, **58**, 139–146.

Potter, E. L. and Craig, J. M. (1976). *Pathology of the Fetus and the Infant* 3rd edition, Yearbook Medical Publishers, Chicago, pp. 220–221.

Powell-Phillips, W. D., Wittmann, A. and Davison, B. M. (1979). Fetal monitoring of a triplet pregnancy. *British Journal of Obstetrics and Gynaecology*, **86**, 666–667.

Powers, W. F. and Miller, T. C. (1979). Bed rest in twin pregnancy: identification of a critical period and its cost implications. *American Journal of Obstetrics and Gynecology*, **134**(1), 23–30.

Prescott, P. (1980). Sensitivity of a double-blind trial of ritodrine and placebo in twin pregnancy. *British Journal of Obstetrics and Gynaecology*, **87**, 393–395.

Pritchard, C. W. and Thompson, B. (1982). Starting a family in Scotland. *Journal of Biosocial Science*, **14**, 127–139.

Propping, P. and Kruger, J. (1976). Uber die Haufigkiet von Zwillingsgeburten. *Deutsche Medizinische Wochenschrift*, **101**: 506–512.

Puissant, F. and Leroy, F. (1982). A reappraisal of perinatal factors in twins. *Acta Geneticae Medicae et Gemellologiae*, **31**, 213–219.

Quigley, M. and Wolf, D. P. (1984). Human in vitro fertilization and embryo transfer at the University of Texas, Houston. *Journal of In Vitro Fertilization and Embryo Transfer*, **1**(1), 29–33.

Race, R. R. and Sanger, R. (1975). *Blood Groups in Man*, 6th edition, Blackwell Scientific Publications, Oxford.

Rachtootin, P. and Olsen, J. (1980). Secular changes in the twinning rate in Denmark. *Scandinavian Journal of Social Medicine*, **8**, 89–94.

Ramos, A. (1961). Introducao a anthropologia Brasileira. *Colecao Estudos Brasileros, Rio de Janeiro*, **1**, 422.

Ramzin, M. S., Stucki, D., Napflin, S., Allemann, F. and Gamper, S. (1982). Early prenatal loss in twin pregnancies. Paper given at Workshop on Multiple Pregnancies, International Society for Twin Studies, Paris (unpublished).

Rao, P. S. S., Inbaraj, S. G. and Muthurathnam, S. (1983). Twinning rates in Tamilnadu. *Journal of Epidemiology and Community Health*, **37**, 117–120.

Rausen, A. R., Seki, M. and Strauss, L. (1965). Twin transfusion syndrome. A review of 19 cases studied at one institution. *Journal of Pediatrics*, **66**, 613–628.

Record, R. G. (1952). Relative frequencies and sex distribution of human multiple births. *British Journal of Social Medicine*, **6**, 192–196.

Record, A. G., Armstrong, E. and Lancashire, R. J. (1978). A study of the fertility of mothers of twins. *Journal of Epidemiology and Community Health*, **32**, 183–189.

Redwine, F. O. and Hays, P. M. (1986). Selective birth. *Seminars in Perinatology*, **10**, 73–81.

Redwine, F. O. and Petres, F. E. (1984). Selective birth in a case of twins discordant for Tay Sachs disease. *Acta Geneticae Medicae et Gemellologiae*, **33**, 35–38.

Reed, T., Uchida, J. A., Norton, J. A. and Christian, J. C. (1978). Comparisons of dermatoglyphic patterns in monochorionic and dichorionic monozygotic twins. *American Journal of Human Genetics*, **30**, 383–391.

Registrar General (1958). *Statistical Review of England and Wales for the year 1956. Part III Commentary*, HMSO, London.

Registrar General for Scotland Annual Report (1983). No. 129, HMSO, Edinburgh.

Rehan,, N. and Tafida, D. S. (1980). Multiple births in Hausa women. *British Journal of Obstetrics and Gynaecology*, **87**: 997–1004.

Reisman, L. E. and Pathak, (1966). Bilateral renal cortical necrosis in the newborn. *American Journal of Diseases of Children*, **111**, 541–543.

Reveley, A. M., Gurling, H. M. D. and Murray, R. M. (1981). Mortality and psychosis in twins. In: *Twin Research, 3, Part B, Intelligence, Personality and Development*, Gedda, L., Parisi, P. and Nance, W. E. (eds.), Alan R. Liss, New York, pp. 175–178.

Riccardi, V. M. and Bergmann, C. A. (1977). Anencephaly with incomplete twinning (Diprosopus). *Teratology*, **16**, 137–140.

Richards, M. R., Merritt, K. K., Samuels, M. H. and Langmann, A. G. (1955). Congenital malformations of the cardiovascular system in a series of 6053 infants. *Pediatrics*, **12**, 12–32.

Richter, J., Miura, T., Nakamura, I. and Nonaka, K. (1984). Twinning rates and seasonal changes in Gorlitz, Germany from 1611 to 1860. *Acta Geneticae Medicae et Gemellologiae*, **33**, 121–124.

Roberts, A. M. (1972). Gravitational separation of X and Y spermatozoa. *Nature*, **238**, 223–225.

Roberts, C. J. and Lloyd, S. (1973). Observations on the epidemiology of simple hypospadias. *British Medical Journal*, **i**, 768–770.

Roberts, C. J. and Lowe, C. R. (1975). Where have all the conceptions gone? *Lancet*, **i**, 498–499.

Robertson, E. G. and Neer, K. J. (1983). Placental injection studies in twin gestation. *American Journal of Obstetrics and Gynecology*, **147**, 170–174.

Robertson, J. G. (1964). Twin pregnancy. Influence of early admission on fetal survival. *Obstetrics and Gynecology*, **23**, 854–860.

Robinson, H. P. and Caines, J. S. (1977). Sonar evidence of early pregnancy failure in patients with twin conceptions. *British Journal of Obstetrics and Gynaecology*, **84**, 22–25.

Robson, E. B. (1955). Birthweight in cousins. *Annals of Human Genetics*, **19**, 262–268.

Rodeck, C. H. (1984). Fetoscopy in the management of twin pregnancies discordant for a severe abnormality. *Acta Geneticae Medicae et Gemellologiae*, **33**, 57–60.

Rodeck, C. H. and Wass, D. (1981). Sampling pure fetal blood in twin pregnancies by fetoscopy using a single uterine puncture. *Prenatal Diagnosis*, **1**, 43–49.

Rogers, J. G., Voullaire, L. and Gold, H. (1982). Monozygotic twins discordant for trisomy 21. *American Journal of Medical Genetics*, **11**, 143–146.

Rogers, S. C. (1969). Epidemiology of stillbirths from congenital abnormalities in England and Wales 1961–1966. *Developmental Medicine and Child Neurology*, **11**, 617–629.

Rogers, S. C. (1976). Anencephalus, spina bifida, twins and teratoma. *British Journal of Preventive and Social Medicine*, **30**, 26–28.

Rola-Janicki, A. R. (1974). Multiple births in Poland in 1949–1971. *Acta Geneticae Medicae et Gemellologiae*, **22**, 202–209.

Romans-Clarkson, S. E., Clarkson, J. E., Dittmer, I. D., Flett, R., Linsell, C., Mullen, P. E. and Mullin, B. (1986). Impact of a handicapped child on mental health of patients. *British Medical Journal*, **293**, 1395–1397.

Ron-El, R., Caspi, E., Schreyer, P., Weinberg, Z., Arieli, S. and Goldberg, M. D. (1981). Triplet and quadruplet pregnancies. *Obstetrics and Gynecology*, **57**, 458–463.

Roos, F. J., Roter, A. M. and Molina, F. A. (1957). A case of triplets including anomolous twins and a fetus compressus. *American Journal of Obstetrics and Gynecology*, **73**, 1342–1345.

Rosenquist, G. C. (1963). Parabiotic syndrome. *New England Journal of Medicine*, **269**, 161–162.

Ross, L. J. (1959). Congenital cardiovascular anomalies in twins. *Circulation*, **20**, 327–342.

Ross, R. C. and Phillpott, N. W. (1953). Five year survey of multiple pregnancies. *Canadian Medical Association Journal*, **49**, 247–249.

Rothman, K. J. (1977). Fetal loss, twinning and birthweight after oral contraceptive use. *New England Journal of Medicine*, **297**, 468–471.

Rovinsky, J. J. and Jaffin, H. (1965). Blood and plasma volume in multiple pregnancy. *American Journal of Obstetrics and Gynecology*, **93**, 1–13.

Rovinsky, J. J. and Jaffin, H. (1966). Cardiovascular haemodynamics in pregnancy. *American Journal of Obstetrics and Gynecology*, **95**, 781–794.

Rudolph, A. J., Michaels, J. P. and Nichols, B. L. (1967). Obstetric management of conjoined twins. *Birth Defects: Original Articles Series*, **III**(1), 28–57.

Russell, J. K. (1952). Maternal and fetal hazards associated with twin pregnancies. *Journal of Obstetrics and Gynaecology of the British Empire*, **59**, 209–213.

Ryden, A. L. (1934). Kasuisticher Beitrag zur Kenntnis der Geburt von Toracopagen. *Zentralblatt für Gynaekologie*, **58**, 972–975.

Rydhstrom, H. and Ohrlander, S. (1985). Twin deliveries in Sweden 1973–1981. The value of an increasing caesarean section rate. *Archives of Gynecology*, **237**, 168. XIth World Congress of Gynecology and Obstetrics, Berlin West, Seps 15–20, 1985 Abstracts. Springer-Verlag, Berlin.

Saier, F., Burden, D. and Cavanagh, D. (1975). Fetus papyraceus: an unusual case with congenital anomaly of the surviving fetus. *Obstetrics and Gynecology*, **45**, 217–220.

Samphier, M. (1982). Birthweight in twins by maternal and fetal factors. Paper given at Workshop on Multiple Pregnancies, International Society for Twin Studies, Paris (unpublished).

Samphier, M. and Thompson, B. (1981). The Aberdeen Maternity and Neonatal Databank. In: *Prospective Longitudinal Research*, Mednick, S. A. and Baert, A. E. (eds.), Oxford University Press, London, pp. 61–65.

Samueloff, A., Evron, S. and Sadovsky, E. (1983). Fetal movements in multiple pregnancy. *American Journal of Obstetrics and Gynecology*, **146**, 789–792.

Sande, H. A. and Eyjolfsson, D. (1985). Hydatidiform mole with a coexistent fetus. *Acta Obstetricia et Gynecologica Scandinavica*, **64**, 353–355.

Satge, P., Correa, P., Charreau, M., Quenum, C. and Sanokho, A. (1966). A propos de deux cas de maladies des inclusions cytomegaliques et en particulier d'une forme subaique encéphalique et anicterique chez un nouveau-ne Africain jumeau dizygote. *Bulletin de la Société Médicale d'Afrique Noire de Lange Française*, **11**, 41–53.

Saunders, M. C., Dick, J. S., Brown, I. Mc. L., McPherson, K. and Chalmers, I. (1985). The effects of hospital admission for bed rest on the duration of twin pregnancy. *Lancet*, **ii**, 793–795.

Say, B., Gungor, E. and Durmus, Z. (1967). Twin births in Turkey. *Lancet*, **i**, 52 (letter).

Scarr, S. (1969). Effects of birthweight on later intelligence. *Social Biology*, **16**, 249–256.

Schenker, J. G., Jarkoni, S. and Granat, M. (1981). Multiple pregnancies following induction of ovulation. *Fertility and Sterility*, **35**, 105–123.

Schinzel, A. A. G. L., Smith, D. W. and Miller, J. R. (1979). Monozygotic twinning and structural defects. *Journal of Pediatrics*, **95**, 921–930.

Schmidt, H. D., Rosing, F. W. and Schmidt, D. E. (1983). Causes of an extremely high local twinning rate. *Annals of Human Biology*, **10**(4), 371–380.

Schmidt, M. and Salzano, F. M. (1980). Dissimilar effects of thalidomide in dizygotic twins. *Acta Geneticae Medicae et Gemellologiae*, **29**, 295–297

Schneider, L., Bessis, R., Hajeri, H. and Papiernik, E. (1978). On twin care: early detection of twin pregnancies with the use of charts of normal uterine height and waist measurements. In: *Twin Research: Clinical Studies*, Nance, W. E., Allen, G. and Parisi, P. (eds.). Allan R. Liss, New York. pp. 143–146.

Schneider, L., Bessis, R. and Simonnet, T. (1979). The frequency of ovular resorption during the first trimester of twin pregnancy. *Acta Geneticae Medicae et Gemellologiae*, **28**, 271–272.

Schneider, K. T. M., Vetter, K., Huch, R. and Huch, A. (1985). Acute polyhydramnios complicating twin pregnancies. *Acta Geneticae Medicae et Gemellologiae*, **34**, 179–184.

Scialli, A. R. (1986). The reproductive toxicity of ovulation induction. *Fertility and Sterility*, **45**, 315–323.

Scott, J. M. and Ferguson-Smith, M. A. (1973). Heterokaryotypic monozygotic twins and the acardiac monster. *Journal of Obstetrics and Gynaecology of the British Commonwealth*, **80**, 52–59.

Scragg, R. F. R. and Walsh, R. J. (1970). A high incidence of multiple births in one area of New Britain. *Human Biology*, **42**, 442–449.

Scrimgeour, J. B. and Baker, T. G. (1974). A possible case of superfetation in man. *Journal of Reproduction and Fertility*, **36**, 69–73.

Segreti, W. O., Winter, P. M. and Nance, W. E. (1978). Familial studies of monozygotic twinning. In: *Twin Research: Biology and Epidemiology*, Nance, W. E., Allen, G. and Parisi, P. (eds.). Allan R. Liss, New York, pp. 55–60.

Selvin, S. and Janerich, D. T. (1972). Seasonal variation in twin births. *Nature*, **237**, 289–290.

Severn, C. B. and Holyoke, E. A. (1973). Human acardiac anomalies. *American Journal of Obstetrics and Gynecology*, **116**, 358–365.

Shah, S. B. and Patel, D. N. (1984). Twinning and structural defects. *Indian Pediatrics*, **21**, 475–478.

Shahar, S. and Morton, N. E. (1986). Origin of teratomas and twins. *Human Genetics*, **74**, 215–218.

Shapiro, L. R., Zemek, L. and Shulman, M. J. (1978). Familial monozygotic twinning: an autosomal dominant form of monozygotic twinning with variable penetrance. In: *Twin Research: Biology and Epidemiology*, Nance, W. E., Allen, G. and Parisi, P. (eds.), Alan R. Liss, New York, pp. 61–63.

Shearer, W. T., Schreiner, R. L., Marshall, R. E. and Barton, L. L. (1972). Cytomegalovirus infection in a newborn dizygous twin. *Journal of Pediatrics*, **81**, 1161–1165.

Sheets, J. W. (1986). Depopulation and twin births in the Hebrides. *Biology and Society*, **3**, 118–124.

Sherman, G. H. and Lowe, E. W. (1970). Do twins carry a high risk for mother and baby? *Journal of the National Medical Association (New York)*, **62**, 217–220.

Shiota, K. (1984). Spontaneous abortion: a screening device for abnormal conceptuses. In: *Advances in Reproductive Health Care*, Hafez, E. S. E. (ed.), MTP Press, Lancaster, pp. 173–181.

Shipley, P. W., Wray, J. R., Hechter, H. H., Arellano, M. G. and Borhani, N. O. (1967). Frequency of twinning in California—its relationship to maternal age, parity and race. *American Journal of Epidemiology*, **85**, 147–156.

Siemens, H. W. (1926). Ueber den Einfluss der Ernährung auf die Fruchtbarkeit, insbesondere auf die Zwillingsfruchtbarkeit beim Menschen. *Archives Rassen Biologie*, **18**, 426–431.

Sinha, D. P., Nandakumar, V. C., Brough, A. K. and Beebeejaum, M. S. (1979). Relative cervical incompetence in twin pregnancy. Assessment and efficacy of cervical suture. *Acta Geneticae Medicae et Gemellologiae*, **28**, 327–331.

Skelly, H., Marivate, M., Norman, R., Kenoyer, G. and Martin, R. (1982). Consumptive coagulopathy following fetal death in a triplet pregnancy. *American Journal of Obstetrics and Gynecology*, **142**, 595–596.

Skjaerris, J. and Aberg, A. (1982). Prevention of prematurity in twin pregnancy by orally administered Terbutaline. *Acta Obstetricia et Gynecologica Scandinavica*, Suppl. 108, 39–40.

Smith, A. (1966). Observations on the determinants of human multiple birth. In: *Report of Registrar General for Scotland 1964*, HMSO, Edinburgh, p. 70.

Smith, J. J. and Benjamin, F. (1968). Posthaemorrhagic anaemia and shock in the newborn at birth. *Obstetrics and Gynecology*, **23**, 511–521.

Smithells, R. W. and Franklin, D. (1964). Anencephaly in Liverpool. *Developmental Medicine and Child Neurology*, **6**, 231–240.

Solowy, M. K. and Shepard, F. M. (1971). Ancenphaly in Central Virginia. *Clinical Pediatrics*, **10**, 43–45.

Soltan, H. C. (1968). Genetic characteristics of families of XO and XXY patients, including evidence of source of X chromosome in 7 aneuploid patients. *Journal of Medical Genetics*, **5**, 173–180.

Soma, H., Masaomi, T., Kyokawa, T., Tsuneo, A. and Tokoro, K. (1975). Serum gonadotrophin levels in Japanese women. *Obstetrics and Gynecology*, **46**, 311–312.

Spiers, P. S. (1973). Multiple ovulation and risk of anencephaly and spina bifida. *Lancet*, **ii**, 1149 (letter).

SPSS X (1983). *Users Guide.*, SPSS Inc., McGraw-Hill Book Co.

Spurway, J. H. (1962). Fate and management of the second twin. *American Journal of Obstetrics and Gynecology*, **83**, 1377–1388.

Stein, Z., Susser, M., Warburton, D., Wittes, J. and Kline, J. (1975). Spontaneous abortion as a screening device: the effect of fetal survival on the incidence of birth defects. *American Journal of Epidemiology*, **102**, 275–290.

Stein, Z., Stein, W. and Susser, M. (1986). Attention of trisomies as a maternal screening device: an explanation of the association of trisomy 21 with maternal age. *Lancet*, **i**, 944–947.

Stevenson, A. C., Johnston, H. A., Stewart, M. I. P. and Golding, D. R. (1966). Congenital malformations. A report of a study of a series of consecutive births in 24 centres. *Bulletin of the World Health Organization*, **34** (Suppl.), 1–127.

Stevenson, A. C., Davison, B. C. C., Say, B., Ustaoglu, S., Leyci, D., Abul-Emen, M. and Toppozada, H. L. (1971). Contribution of fetal/maternal incompatibility to aetiology of pre-eclampstic toxaemia. *Lancet*, **ii**, 1286–1289.

Stevenson, A. C., Say, B., Ustaoglu, S. and Durmus, Z. (1976). Aspects of pre-eclamptic toxaemia of pregnancy, consanguinity and twinning in Ankara. *Journal of Medical Genetics*, **13**, 1–8.

Stockard, C. R. (1921). Developmental rate and structural expression. I. An experimental study of twins, double monsters and single deformities and the interaction among embryonic organs during their origin and development. *American Journal of Anatomy*, **28**, 115–277.

Strong, S. J. and Corney, G. (1967). *The Placenta in Twin Pregnancy*, Pergamon Press, Oxford.

Studdeford, W. E. (1936). Is superfetation possible in the human being? *American Journal of Obstetrics and Gynecology*, **31**, 845–855.

Sutherland, A. I. (1980). Genetic and non-genetic aspects of reproductive performance in man and the rabbit. Ph.d. Thesis (unpublished), University of Edinburgh.

Sutherland, A., Cooper, W., Howie, W., Liston, W. A. and MacGillivray, I. (1981). Incidence of severe pre-eclampsia amongst mothers and mothers-in-law of preeclamptics and controls. *British Journal of Obstetrics and Gynaecology*, **88**, 785–791.

Suzuki, I. M., Matsundsu, A., Wakita, K., Niskjuma, M. and Odsanai, K. (1980). Hydatidiform mole with a surviving co-existing fetus. *Obstetrics and Gynecology*, **56**, 384–388.

Swapp, G. H. and Gomez, E. (1975). Personal communication. Insulin clearance in twin pregnancy.

Syrop, C. H. and Varner, M. W. (1985). Triplet gestation: maternal and neonatal implications. *Acta Geneticae Medicae et Gemellologiae*, **34**, 81–88.

Szendi, B. (1939). Double monsters in light of recent biological experiments and investigations regarding heredity. Contribution to problem of determination of sex. *Journal of Obstetrics and Gynaecology of the British Empire*, **46**, 836–847.

Szymonowicz, W., Preston, H. and Yu, V. Y. H. (1986). The surviving monozygotic twin. *Archives of Disease in Childhood*, **61**, 454–458.

Tada, S., Yasukochi, H., Ohtaki, C., Fukuta, A. and Takanashi, R. (1974). Fetus in fetu. *British Journal of Radiology*, **47**, 146–148.

TambyRaja, R. L., Atputharajah, V. and Slamon, Y. (1978). Prevention of prematurity in twins. *Australian and New Zealand Journal of Obstetrics and Gynecology*, **18**, 179–183.

TambyRaja, R. L. and Ratnam, S. S. (1981). Plasma steroid changes in twin pregnancy. In: *Twin Research, 3, Part A, Twin Biology and Multiple Pregnancy*, Gedda, L., Parisi, P. and Nance, W. E. (eds.), Alan R. Liss, New York, pp. 189–195.

Tan, K. L., Goon, S. M., Salmon, Y. and Wee, J. H. (1971). Conjoined twins. *Acta Obstetricia et Gynecologica Scandinavica*, **50**, 373–380.

Tan, K. L., Tan, R., Tan, S. H. and Tan, A. M. (1979). The twin transfusion syndrome: clinical observations on 35 affected pairs. *Clinical Pediatrics*, **18**, 111–114.

Tanimura, T. and Tanaka, O. (1977). Twin embryos in Japan. *Japanese Journal of Human Genetics*, **22**, 227–228.

Tanner, J. M. (1978). *Fetus into Man*. Open Books Publishing, London.

Taylor, E. S. (1976). Editorial. *Obstetric and Gynaecological Survey*, **31**, 535.

Tchouriloff, M. (1877). *Bulletin de la Societé d'Anthropologie de Paris*, **12**, 440–446.

Templeton, A. and Kelman, G. (1974). Personal communication (Tidal volume in twin pregnancy).

Thom, H., Buckland, C. M., Campbell, A. G. M., Thompson, B. and Farr, V. (1984). Maternal serum alpha-feto-protein in monozygotic and dizygotic twin pregnancy. *Prenatal Diagnosis*, **4**(5), 341–346.

Thompson, B., Sauvé, B., MacGillivray, I. and Campbell, D. M. (1981). Reproductive performance in twin sisters. In: *Twin Reserach 3, Part A, Twin Biology and Multiple Pregnancy*, Gedda, L., Parisi, P. and Nance, W. E. (eds.), Alan R. Liss, New York, pp. 169–173.

Thompson, B., Campbell, D. M. and MacGillivray, I. (1982). Twinning and oral contraception in North-East Scotland. paper given at Workshop on Multiple Pregnancies, International Society for Twin Studies, Malmo, Sweden (unpublished).

Thompson, B., Pritchard, C. and Corney, G. (1983). Perinatal mortality in twins by zygosity and placentation. paper given at Fourth Congress of International Socity for Twin Studies, London (unpublished).

Thompson, B., Fraser, C., Hewitt, A. and Skipper, D. (1988). *Having a First Baby*

Experiences in 1951 and 1985 Compared: Two Social, Obstetric and Dietary Studies of Married Primigravidae in Aberdeen. Aberdeen University Press (in press).

Thomson, A. M., Billewicz, W. Z. and Hytten, F. E. (1968). The assessment of fetal growth. *Journal of Obstetrics and Gynaecology of the British Commonwealth*, **75**, 903–916.

Tietze, C. (1983). *Induced Abortion: a World Review*, 5th edition, The Population Council, New York.

Timonen, S. and Carpen, E. (1968). Multiple pregnancies and photoperiodicity. *Annales Chirurgiae et Gynaecologiae, Fenniae*, **57**, 135–138.

Tippett, P. (1983). Blood group chimaeras: a review, *Vox Sanguinis, Basel*, **44**, 333–359.

Tresmontant, R., Heluin, G. and Papiernik, E. (1983). Cost of care and prevention of preterm births in twin pregnancies. *Acta Geneticae Medicae et Gemellologiae*, **32**, 99–103.

Uchida, I. A. and Rowe, R. D. (1957). Discordant heart anomalies in twins. *American Journal of Human Genetics*, **9**, 133–140.

Uchida, I. A., de Sa, D. J. and Whelan, D. T. (1983a). 45x/46xx mosaicism in discordant monozygotic twins. *Pediatrics*, **71**, 413–417.

Uchida, I. A., Freeman, V. C., Gedeon, M. and Goldmaker, J. (1983b). Twinning rate in spontaneous abortion. *American Journal of Human Genetics*, **35**, 987–993.

United Nations Department of Economic and Social Affairs. (1975). *Demographic Yearbook*, United Nations, New York.

United Nations Department of Economic and Social Affairs (1981). *Demographic Yearbook*, United Nations, New York.

Vallois, H. V. (1949). La répartition des groupes sanguins en France: l'ouest armorico-vendeen. *Archiv der Julius Klaus-Stiftung für Vererbungsforschung Sozialanthropologie und Rassenhygiene*, **24**, 508–516.

Vallotton, M. B. and Forbes, A. P. (1967). Autoimmunity in gonadal dysgenesis and Klinefelter's syndrome. *Lancet*, **i**, 648–651.

Van Allen, M. I., Smith, D. W. and Shepard, T. H. (1983). Twin reversed arterial perfusion (TRAP) sequence: a study of 14 twin pregnancies with acardius. *Seminars in Perinatology*, **7**, 285–293.

Van der Molen, H. J. (1963). Determination of plasma progesterone during pregnancy. *Clinica Chimica Acta*, **8**, 943–953.

Van der Pol, J. G., Bleker, O. P. and Treffers, P. E. (1982). Clinical bed rest in twin pregnancy. *European Journal of Obstetrics, Gynecology and Reproductive Biology*, **14**, 75–80.

Van Staey, M., De Bie, S., Matton, M. and Th. De. Roose, J. (1984). Familial congenital esophageal atresia. Personal case report and review of the literature. *Human Genetics*, **66**, 260–266.

Varma, T. R. (1979). Ultrasound evidence of early pregnancy failure in patients with multiple conceptions. *British Journal of Obstetrics and Gynaecology*, **86**, 290–292.

Vessey, M., Doll, R., Peto, R., Johnson, B. and Wiggins, P. (1976). A longterm follow up study of women using different methods of contraception – an interim report. *Journal of Biosocial Science*, **8**, 373–427.

Vestergaard, P. (1972). Triplets pregnancy with a normal foetus and a dicephalus dibrachius sirenomelus. *Acta Obstetricia et Gynecologica Scandinavica*, **51**, 93–94.

Viljoen, D. L., Nelson, M. M. and Beighton, P. (1983). The epidemiology of conjoined twinning in Southern Africa. *Clinical Genetics*, **24**, 15–21.

Vogel, F. and Motulsky, A. G. (1979). *Human Genetics: Problems and Approaches*, Springer Verlag, New York.

Vowles, M., Pethybridge, R. J. and Brimblecombe, F. S. W. (1975). Congenital malformations in Devon, their incidence, age and primary source of detection. In: *Bridging in Health*, McLachlan, G. (ed.), Nuffield Provincial Hospitals Trust, London, pp. 201–215.

Waardenburg, P. J. (1926). Quoted in Gedda, L. (1961). *Twins in History and Science*, Charles C. Thomas, Illinois.

Waboso, M. F. (1966). The causes of perinatal mortality at the Maternity Hospital, Calabar eastern group of provinces with some suggestions for preventive measures. *Journal of Nigerian Medical Association*, **3**, 368.

Wallace, L. R. (1951). Flushing of ewes. *New Zealand Journal of Agriculture*, **83**, 377–380.

Walter, S. D. and Elwood, J. M. (1975). A test for seasonality of events with a variable population at risk. *British Journal of Preventive and Social Medicine*, **29**, 18–21.

Ware, H. D. (1971). The second twin. *American Journal of Obstetrics and Gynecology*, **110**, 855–873.

Waterhouse, J. A. H. (1950). Twinning in twin pedigrees. *British Journal of Social Medicine*, **4**, 197–216.

Weatherall, J. A. C., Vlietnick, R. E. and Van den Berghe, H. (1979). EEC concerted action project—European congenital anomalies and twins (EURO-CAT). *Acta Geneticae Medicae et Gemellologiae*, **28**, 377–379.

Webster, F. and Elwood, J. M. (1985). A study of the influence of ovulation stimulants and oral contraception on twin births in England. *Acta Geneticae Medicae et Gemellologiae*, **34**, 105–108.

Weekes, A. R. L., Menzies, D. N. and de Boer, C. H. (1977). The relative efficacy of bed rest, cervical suture and no treatment in the management of twin pregnancy. *British Journal of Obstetrics and Gynaecology*, **84**, 161–164.

Wehefrith, E. (1925). Uber die Vererbung der Zwillingsschwangerschaft. *Zeitschrift für Konstitutionslehre*, **11**(2), 554–575.

Weinberg, W. (1902). Beitrage zur Physiologie und Pathologie der Mehrlingsgeburten beim Menschen. *Pflugers Archiv für die gesamte Physiologie des Menschen und der Tiere*, **88**, 346–430.

Weinberg, W. (1909). Die Analage zur Mehrlingsgeburt beim Menschen und ihre Vererbung. *Archive für Rassen und Gesselschaftsbiologie*, **6**, 322–339, 470–482, 609–630.

Wharton, B., Edwards, J. H. and Cameron, A. H. (1968). Monoamniotic twins. *Journal of Obstetrics and Gynaecology of the British Commonwealth*, **75**, 158–163.

White, C. and Wyshak, G. (1964). Inheritance in human dizygotic twinning. *New England Journal of Medicine*, **271**, 1003–1012.

Willerman, L. and Churchill, J. A. (1967). Intelligence and birthweight in identical twins. *Child Development*, **38**, 623–629.

Williamson, E. M. (1965). Incidence and family aggregation of major congenital malformations of the central nervous system. *Journal of Medical Genetics*, **2**, 161–172.

Willis, R. A. (1962). *The Borderland of Embryology and Pathology*, 2nd edition, Butterworth, London.

Wilson, R. S. (1979). Twin growth initial deficit, recovery and trends in concordance from birth to nine years. *Annals of Human Biology*, **6**, 205–220.

Wilson, R. S. (1983). The Louisville twin study: developmental syndromes in behaviour. *Child Development*, **54**, 298–316.

Windham, G. C., Bjerkedal, T. and Sever, L. E. (1982). The association of twinning and neural tube defects: studies in Los Angeles, California and Norway. *Acta Geneticae Medicae et Gemellologiae*, **31**, 165–172.

Windham, G. C. and Sever, L. E. (1982). Neural tube defects among twin births. *American Journal of Human Genetics*, **34**, 988–998.

Windham, G. C. and Bjerkedal, T. (1984). Malformations in twins and their siblings, Norway 1967–1979. *Acta Geneticae Medicae et Gemellologiae*, **33**, 87–95.

Witschi, E. (1952). Over-ripeness of the egg as a cause of twinning and teratogenesis: a review. *Cancer Research*, **12**, 763–786.

Wittmann, B. K., Baldwin, V. J. and Nichol, B. (1981). Antenatal diagnosis of twin transfusion syndrome by ultrasound. *Obstetrics and Gynecology*, **58**, 123–127.

Wood, C. and Pinkerton, J. H. M. (1966). Uterine activity following the birth of the first twin. *Australian and New Zealand Journal of Obstetrics and Gynecology*, **6**, 95–99.

Woodward, J. (1986). The bereaved twin. *Acta Geneticae Medicae et Gemellologiae*, **35**, Abstracts, p. 14.

Wyshak, G. (1975). Twinning rates among women at the end of their reproductive span and their relation to age at menopause. *American Journal of Epidemiology*, **102**, 170–178.

Wyshak, G. (1978a). Statistical findings on the effects of fertility drugs on plural births. In: *Twin Research: Biology and Epidemiology*, Nance, W. E., Allen, G. and Parisi, P. (eds.) Alan R. Liss, New York, pp. 17–33.

Wyshak, G. (1978b). Menopause in mothers of multiple births and mothers of singletons only. *Social Biology*, **25**, 52–61.

Wyshak, G. (1981). Reproduction and menstrual characteristics of mothers of multiple births and mothers of singletons only: a discriminant analysis. In: *Twin Research 3, Part A, Twin Biology and Multiple Pregnancy*, Gedda, L. Parisi, P. and Nance, W. E. (eds.), Alan R. Liss, New York, pp. 95–105.

Wyshak, G. (1985). Pregnancy loss in mothers of multiple births and in mothers of singletons only. *Annals of Human Biology*, **12**, 85–89.

Wyshak, G. and White, C. (1963). Birth hazard of the second twin. *Journal of the American Medical Association*, **186**, 869–970.

Wyshak, G. and White, C. (1965). Genealogical study of human twinning. *American Journal of Public Health*, **55**, 1586–1593.

Wyshak, G. and White, C. (1969). Fertility of twins and parents of twins. *Human Biology*, **41**, 66–82.

Yee, B., Tu, B. and Platt, L. D. (1982). Coexisting hydatidiform mole with a live fetus presenting as a placenta praevia on ultrasound. *American Journal of Obstetrics and Gynecology*, **144**, 726–728.

Yen, S. and MacMahon, B. (1968). Genetics of anencephaly and spina bifida? *Lancet*, **ii**, 623–662.

Yen, S. S. C., Yen, S. S., Vela, P. and Rankin, J. (1970). Hormonal relationship during the menstrual cycle. *Journal of the American Medical Association*, **211**, 1513–1517.

Yoshida, K. and Soma, H. (1984). A study of twin placentation in Tokyo. *Acta Geneticae Medicae et Gemellologiae*, **33**, 115–120.

Yoshioka, J., Kadomoto, Y., Mino, M., Morikawa, Y., Kasubuchi, Y. and Kusunoki, T. (1979). Multicystic encephalomalacia in liveborn twin with a stillborn macerated co-twin. *Journal of Pediatrics*, **95**, 798–800.

Zahalkova, M. (1974). Multiple births in Southern Moravia. *Acta Geneticae Medicae et Gemellogiae*, Suppl. 22, 210–213.

Zahalkova, M. (1979). Clustering of twin births in space and time. *Acta Geneticae Medicae et gemellologiae*, **28**, 259–260.

Zahalkova, M. and Zudova, Z. (1984). Spontaneous abortions and twinning. *Acta Geneticae Medicae et Gemellologiae*, **33**, 25–26.

Zake, E. Z. (1984). Case reports of 16 sets of conjoined twins from a Uganda hospital. *Acta Geneticae Medicae et Gemellologiae*, **33**, 75–80.

Zimmerman, A. A. (1967). Embryologic and anatomic considerations of conjoined twins. *Birth Defects: Original Articles Series*, **II**(1), 18–27.

Index